Endovascular Techniques in the Management of Cerebrovascular Disease

Edited by

Thomas J Masaryk MD
Director, Section of Neuroradiology
The Imaging Institute;
Center for Cerebrovascular Disease
The Neurological Institute
The Cleveland Clinic
Cleveland, OH
USA

Peter A Rasmussen MD
Director, Department of Neurological Surgery
Center for Cerebrovascular Disease
The Neurological Institute
The Cleveland Clinic
Cleveland, OH
USA

Henry Woo MD
Director, Department of Neurological Surgery
Cerebrovascular Center
Stony Brook University Medical Center
Stony Brook, NY
USA

David Fiorella MD PHD
Section of Neuroradiology
The Imaging Institute
The Center for Cerebrovascular Disease
The Neurological Institute
The Cleveland Clinic
Cleveland, OH
USA

informa
healthcare

© 2008 Informa UK Ltd

First published in the United Kingdom in 2008 by Informa Healthcare, Telephone House, 69–77 Paul Street, London EC2A 4LQ. Informa Healthcare is a trading division of Informa UK Ltd. Registered Office: 37/41 Mortimer Street, London W1T 3JH. Registered in England and Wales number 1072954.

Tel: +44 (0)20 7017 5000
Fax: +44 (0)20 7017 6699
Website: www.informahealthcare.com

Although every effort has been made to ensure that all owners of copyright material have been acknowledged in this publication, we would be glad to acknowledge in subsequent reprints or editions any omissions brought to our attention.

A CIP record for this book is available from the British Library.

Library of Congress Cataloging-in-Publication Data

Data available on application

ISBN-10: 1 84184 607 4
ISBN-13: 978 1 84184 607 1

Distributed in North and South America by
Taylor & Francis
6000 Broken Sound Parkway, NW, (Suite 300)
Boca Raton, FL 33487, USA

Within Continental USA
Tel: 1 (800) 272 7737; Fax: 1 (800) 374 3401
Outside Continental USA
Tel: (561) 994 0555; Fax: (561) 361 6018
Email: orders@crcpress.com

Book orders in the rest of the world
Paul Abrahams
Tel: +44 207 017 4036
Email: bookorders@informa.com

Composition by Exeter Premedia Services Pvt Ltd, Chennai, India
Printed and bound in India by Replika Press Pvt Ltd

Contents

Contributors

Bryson Borg MD
Department of Neuroradiology
Keesler Air Force Base
Biloxi, MS
USA

David Fiorella MD PHD
Section of Neuroradiology
The Imaging Institute
Center for Cerebrovascular Disease
The Neurological Institute
The Cleveland Clinic
Cleveland, OH
USA

Vivek A Gonugunta MD FRCS
Endovascular Surgical Neuroradiology
Center for Cerebrovascular Disease
The Neurological Institute
The Cleveland Clinic
Cleveland, OH
USA

Irene Katzan MD
Department of Neurology
Center for Cerebrovascular Disease
The Neurological Institute
The Cleveland Clinic
Cleveland, OH
USA

Michael E Kelly MD FRCSC
Endovascular Surgical Neuroradiology
Center for Cerebrovascular Disease
The Neurological Institute
The Cleveland Clinic
Cleveland, OH
USA

Thomas J Masaryk MD
Section of Neuroradiology
The Imaging Institute
Center for Cerebrovascular Disease
The Neurological Institute
The Cleveland Clinic
Cleveland, OH
USA

Shaye Moskowitz MD PhD
Endovascular Surgical Neuroradiology
Center for Cerebrovascular Disease
The Neurological Institute
The Cleveland Clinic
Cleveland OH
USA

Peter A Rasmussen MD
Department of Neurological Surgery
Center for Cerebrovascular Disease
The Neurological Institute
The Cleveland Clinic
Cleveland, OH
USA

Raymond D Turner IV MD
Endovascular Surgical Neuroradiology
Center for Cerebrovascular Disease
The Neurological Institute
The Cleveland Clinic
Cleveland, OH
USA

Henry Woo MD
Department of Neurological Surgery
Cerebrovascular Center
Stony Brook University Medical Center
Stony Brook, NY
USA

Preface

In his biography of Cleveland native Harvey Cushing, John Fulton describes the fortuitous series of circumstances that conspired to create the specialty of neurological surgery. The compulsive and competitive Dr Cushing trained as a surgeon under the precise tutelage of William Hallsted. On the recommendation of his friend and mentor, William Osler, Cushing spent the year following completion of his surgical residency traveling Europe. It was then, under the guidance of Professor Theodor Kocher in the laboratory of Professor Hugo Kronecker in Berne, Switzerland, that Cushing described the relationship between intracranial pressure and systemic blood pressure regulated by the vasomotor center in the medulla that would ultimately be known as the 'Cushing reflex'. Prior to this time, vital signs (and in particular blood pressure) were not routinely charted during surgical procedures. Cushing continued his experiments as he toured Europe, performing studies in dogs in Professor Angelo Mosso's laboratory in Turin, Italy. While in Italy, Cushing was serendipitously introduced to Scipione Riva-Rocci's elegantly simple sphygmomanometer, which he promptly recognized as a significant addition to the operating room. Upon his return home the combination of his compulsive personality, watchful (albeit indirect) management of systemic and intracranial pressure, and career-long obsession with hemostasis (Cushing developed the silver hemoclip, and, with physicist W Bovie, introduced electrocoagulation) precipitated the beginning of neurosurgical practice.

In 1979, I came to Cushing's home town as a medical student at the suggestion of my father. A local medical imaging company, Technicare, had just installed their first commercial digital subtraction angiography system at the Cleveland Clinic. Drs Paul Duscheneau, Mickey Weinstein, and Michael Modic were furiously imaging patients with the new device and publishing papers. The link between imaging and computers was strikingly powerful. . . my father had me hooked. I was extraordinarily fortunate to continue to benefit from this confluence of technology with the help of Dr Ralph Alfidi and my colleagues Jeff Ross, Paul Ruggieri, and Mike Modic, and perhaps more importantly the indulgence of my wife, Midge, and our four daughters.

Ingenious innovators such as Serbinenko, Engleson, Guglielmi and others have helped transform imaging from diagnostic adjunct to sophisticated guidance for definitive treatments (in a fashion analogous to the evolution of neurosurgical management hemostasis and intracranial pressure). Therapeutic devices will continue to develop in parallel with advances in image guided techniques. Presently, many of these are complimentary to conventional, open, neurosurgical procedures. As some techniques replace surgery, it seems unrealistic for radiologists to presume that surgeons will either watch idly or that, as imagers, they can remain uninvolved in pre- and post-procedure care and follow-up. In this respect I have been blessed to work as a true team with Peter, Henry, and David as well as the dedicated nurses and technologists in the angiography suite and the operating room at the Cleveland Clinic. Each contributes a unique and valuable skill set based on their training background; everyone recognizes that as a whole, the team functions better because of it . . . and (I truly believe) patients do better. In 2003 the group established the second formally credentialed fellowship in Endovascular Surgical Neuroradiology. In our own way, we each felt that a new specialty had arrived.

To each and every one, our sincerest thanks.

Thomas J Masaryk
2008

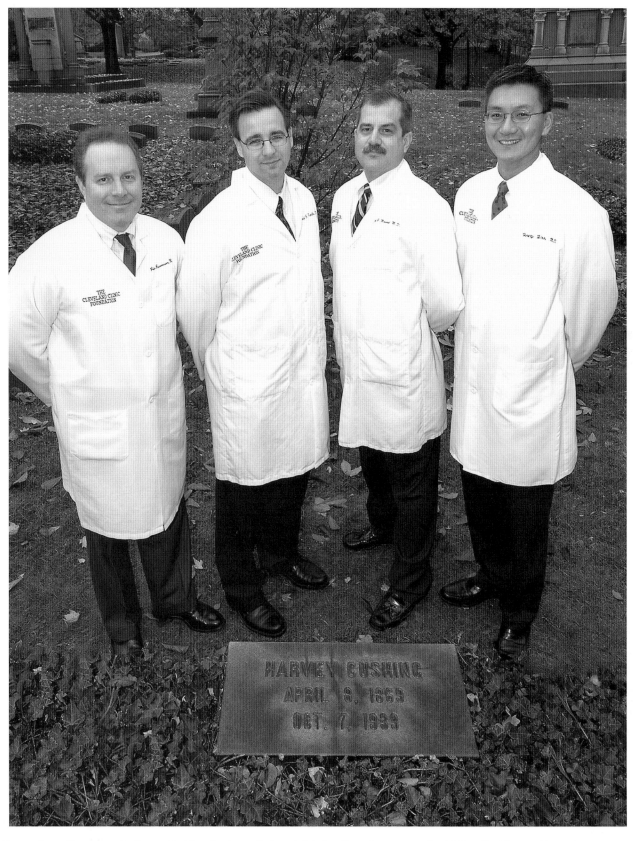

Team photo. Front row: Dr Harvey Cushing. Back row (left to right): Drs Peter Rasmussen, David Fiorella, Thomas Masaryk, Henry Woo.

1

Imaging: informed decision-making

Bryson Borg, David Fiorella and Thomas J Masaryk

Neurosurgery and neuroradiology have historically been complementary specialties: neurosurgery demands logical decision making and accurate therapeutic planning while diagnostic neuroradiology supplies ever more clinical data points through the evolution and application of digital imaging technologies. Endovascular surgical neuroradiology (also known as endovascular neurosurgery) combines the clinical needs of the former with the technical sophistication of the latter in a single specialty. The importance of mastery of the imaging concepts as a prerequisite to expeditious, yet thoughtful, decision making and safe clinical practice cannot be underestimated.

This is perhaps best exemplified in the setting of acute stroke, where the operative word is indeed 'expeditious'. Intravenous thrombolysis using simple, single-slice CT scanning became the only approved therapy in the USA for acute ischemic stroke within the first 3 hours of onset on the basis of the National Institute of Neurological Disorders and Stroke rt-PA Stroke Study Group (the NINDS rt-PA Trial).[1] Similar trials performed in Europe demonstrated no benefit to thrombolytic therapy.[2–4] A major difference in the trials was the time window for treatment: 3 hours in the North American study, 6 hours in Europe. Indeed, review of the US data demonstrates significantly better outcomes the sooner patients are treated (Figure 1.1).[5]

Hence the first caveat of acute stroke imaging: patients should be emergently transported to a facility with *immediate imaging* capability and a mechanism in place for rapid, *accurate interpretation.* Pre-emptive warning should be provided to the radiology department to facilitate imaging as rapidly as possible, regardless of the modality employed. National guidelines developed by the NINDS and adopted by the American Heart Association (AHA) suggest that acute stroke patients should be imaged within 20 minutes of initial arrival in the emergency department. The importance of efficient, detailed, and accurate communication among the transport team, clinical services, and radiology personnel cannot be overemphasized. (Indeed, the medical–legal implications are so great that the American College of Radiology has explicit recommendations regarding the documentation of the imaging and interpretation process and the communication to the requesting service.)[6] Familiarity with frequently used clinical scoring scales (Glasgow Coma Scale, National Institutes of Health Stroke Scale, Hunt–Hess Grade) by the imaging service and conversely the imaging signposts (hyperdense middle cerebral artery, decreased attenuation in greater than one-third of the vascular territory, Fisher Score) by the clinical services greatly facilitate the decision-making process.

CT scanning

Shortly following Roentgen's discovery of the X-ray at the end of the 19th century, Johan Rand, a Czech mathematician, began publishing his treatises on line integrals. Allan Cormack postulated, and documented, that the attenuation of X-rays through an object could be represented by such mathematical modeling.[7,8] With the subsequent development and refinement of the analog-to-digital converter and the application of evolving computer technology, Godfrey Hounsfield produced the first transaxial tomographic maps of X-ray attenuation utilizing filtered back-projection reconstruction in the early 1970s.[9] In 1979 Hounsfield and Cormack were awarded the Nobel Prize in Medicine.

While the basic principles of CT have remained the same, the engineering refinements have been impressive. Specifically, the X-ray source and opposing detector continue to be mechanically rotated about the patient but with broader coverage by the beam and detector at ever faster speeds of rotation. Eventually, data acquisition became so fast that the patient could be simply 'pulled through' the scanner during rotation and completely isotropic three-dimensional data sets could be acquired utilizing special 'spiral reconstruction' methods.[10] Recent innovations using this technology have included small portable scanners designed for neurologic intensive care units, which move to the bedside, and multi-row spiral scanners (Figure 1.2a).[11,12] Another exciting innovation is the high-end, vascular scanner with two X-ray sources and two sets of multi-row detectors. Such scanners may not only permit faster scanning, but also dual energy ('subtracted') angiographic studies (Figure 1.2b).[13]

CT scanning of the brain for cerebrovascular disease

There are advantages and disadvantages to the use of CT scanning in cerebrovascular disease. Advantages include:

- ready accessibility
- rapid acquisition
- high sensitivity to acute blood
- high-quality vascular imaging of occlusions, stenoses, and aneurysms is obtainable with contemporary scanners
- three-dimensional stereotactic targeting
- targeted relative perfusion maps.

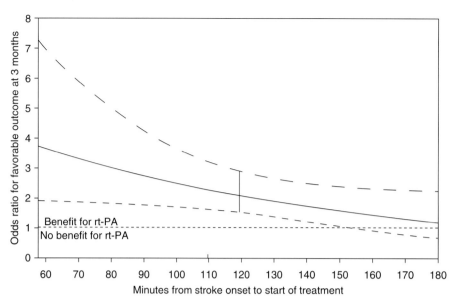

Figure 1.1
Graph derived from NINDS data demonstrating odds ratio of favorable stroke outcome versus time to treatment. The data indicates that there may be marginal benefit to patients after 3 hours (not otherwise pre-selected, by imaging). Reprinted with permission from Neurology 2000; 55:1649–55.

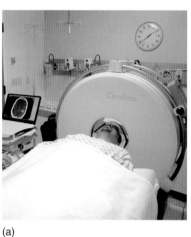

(a)

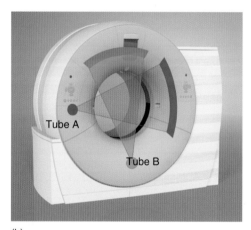

(b)

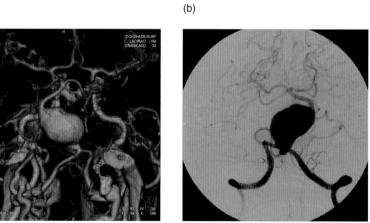

(c)

(d)

Figure 1.2
(a) Portable, ICU CT brain scanner. Geometry of gantry and use of spiral technology eliminates need for special shielding, power source and movable gantry table. Scans are reconstructed on a laptop computer. (Courtesy of Neurologica)
(b) Schematic representation of dual X-ray source/dual detector CT scan which may permit not only rapid acquisitions, but also dual energy subtraction angiography. (c) Dual energy CTA of a giant proximal basilar aneurysm. (Courtesy of Siemens Medical Systems)
(d) Corresponding conventional digital subtraction angiogram.

Disadvantages include:

- less sensitivity to hyperacute infarction than diffusion-weighted MRI
- limited coverage for perfusion maps
- qualitative, not quantitative nature of perfusion imaging (unless performed with xenon)
- ionizing radiation, particularly to the lens
- artifact, particularly in the posterior fossa.

Conventional CT scanning of the brain

CT for acute stroke is commonly performed using 5–8 mm contiguous transverse sections obtained without intravenous contrast administration. Primary goals of the initial head CT head are:

- to exclude intracranial hemorrhage (Figure 1.3);
- to identify early signs of ischemic stroke (see below); and

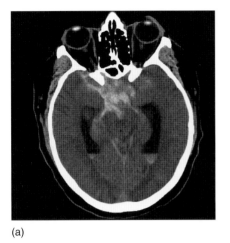
(a)

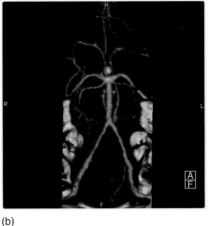
(b)

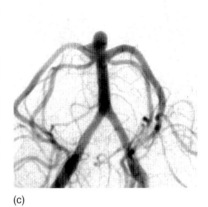
(c)

Figure 1.3
(a) CT scan of the brain demonstrating diffuse subarachnoid blood within the basal cisterns. (b) Simultaneously performed CT angiogram demonstrates a basilar summit aneurysm. (c) Confirmatory catheter angiography.

Table 1.1 Fisher Grading System

Fisher Group	Blood on CT	Number of patients	Vasospasm		
			Angiographic		Clinical vasospasm (DIND)
			Slight	Severe	
1	No subarachnoid blood detected	11	2	2	0
2	Diffuse or vertical layers <1 mm thick	7	3	0	0
3	Localized clot and/or vertical layer ≥ 1mm	24	1	23	23
4	Intracerebral or intraventricular clot with diffuse or no subarachnoid hemorrhage	5	2	0	0

Fisher CM, Kistler JP, Davis JM. Relation of cerebral vasospasm of subarachnoid hemorrhage visualized by CT scanning. Neurosurgery 1980; 6: 1–9. Reprinted with permission.

- to exclude neoplastic, inflammatory, or other processes that can mimic stroke clinically.

CT has an extraordinarily high sensitivity for detecting acute intracranial hemorrhage. The importance of appreciating early signs of stroke is exemplified by missed cases in ECASS trial, resulting in poorer outcomes after thrombolytic therapy.[14–17] The conspicuity of infarcts on unenhanced CT images can be increased by the use of variable window width and center level settings at a workstation (in contrast to standard fixed windows on the printed films) in order to accentuate the gray matter–white matter contrast,[18] as well as by contrast enhancement.[19]

Findings of acute ischemia within hours of onset, if present, are usually very subtle. Early CT findings of cerebral ischemia (which may or may not be visible) include:[20]

- hypoattenuation of gray matter structures
- mass effect
- hyperdense arteries.

Hypoattenuation of gray matter structures

There may be blurring of the gray matter–white matter junction, owing to cytotoxic edema, which can be seen as early as 2 hours after onset.[21] A specific example of the phenomenon is the so-called insular ribbon sign[22] (Figure 1.4), in which the temporal lobe insula (which is composed of gray matter) becomes isodense to adjoining white matter. This sign of early middle cerebral artery (MCA) occlusion can be explained by its water-shed position far from the collateral supply of both the anterior and posterior cerebral arteries, which leads to early irreversible damage.[22]

Another example is 'obscuration of the lentiform nucleus sign' or decreased attenuation of the basal ganglia gray matter, which becomes isodense to adjacent white matter structures such as the internal capsule and the external capsule (see Figure 1.4).[21] This region is supplied by lenticulostriate branches of the MCA that are end vessels and therefore prone to early irreversible damage after proximal MCA occlusion.[23] A key parameter to document in the report is the geographic extent to which these changes are present. Specifically, retrospective review of the ECASS results suggest that when these subtle CT changes of completed strokes involve more than one-third of the suspected involved vascular territory, outcomes with thrombolytics are generally poor.[14]

Mass effect

Examples of early mass effect include asymmetry or narrowing of the Sylvian fissure (in MCA infarcts) or subtle effacement of cortical sulci (Figure 1.5).[20]

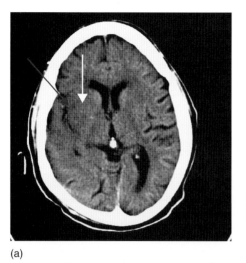

(a)

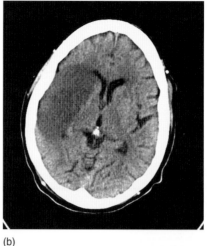

(b)

Figure 1.4
CT signs of early infection.
(a) Decreased attenuation coefficient involving the insula (red arrow), indicates early MCA ischemia. Obscured lentiform nucleus (white arrow) reflecting ischemia in the distribution of the M1 segment/lenticulostriate artery branches. (b) Follow-up scan demonstrating completed MCA infarct with local mass effect.

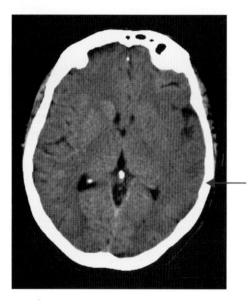

Figure 1.5
Early left MCA infarct demonstrating loss of grey-white contrast on the left with subtle mass effect resulting in effacement of the local sulci (red arrow).

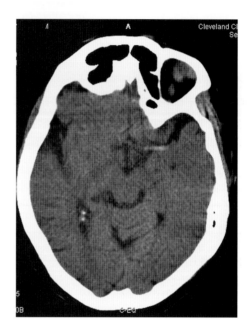

Figure 1.6
Hyperdense middle cerebral artery reflecting embolic thrombus on the left (arrow).

Hyperdense arteries

A typical example is the 'hyperdense MCA sign' (HMCAS), which represents fresh thrombus in an occluded MCA. The MCA appears hyperdense relative to the contralateral MCA with unenhanced CT (Figure 1.6).[24,25] Unlike the other early signs, this sign indicates occlusion of the MCA, not infarction within the MCA territory, and it can be seen within minutes of the acute event. The specificity of this sign has been reported as 100%, but sensitivity is only about 30%.[25] The hyperdense dot signs refer to thrombus in other smaller branches.[26] There are potential pitfalls related to the HMCAS, including the fact that a patent vessel with atherosclerotic changes can appear hyperdense, and that a hyperdense appearance can be due to presence of contrast in the circulation, (e.g. as may happen when a patient undergoes an emergent CT scan of the head after cardiac catheterization).

Although not routinely used in clinical practice, ischemic MCA stroke scans can be interpreted in a standardized fashion and scored according to a qualitative scale, the Alberta Stroke Program Early CT Score (ASPECTS), which reduces the observer variability reported in many clinical trials (Figure 1.7).[19,27,28]

The sensitivity of detecting acute hemorrhage is excellent with CT scanning, exceeding 90%,[29] although the specificity of increased attenuation continues to concern many.[30] The increased attenuation coefficient of blood is primarily related to the attenuation coefficient of hemoglobin (contracted thrombus is 80–85 hounsfield units (HU)), which may degrade with time from ictus onset or even severe anemia to lessen the sensitivity of CT.[31] Fisher et al. developed a grading scale that is often used in clinical practice; it has some predictive value in assessing the risk of developing vasospasm secondary to SAH (Table 1.1).[32]

CT angiography

As alluded to above, the dissemination of faster spiral CT scan technology and the increased public awareness of acute stroke therapies has prompted the increasing adoption of advanced imaging techniques (CT angiography and relative perfusion mapping) in the setting of emergent cerebrovascular

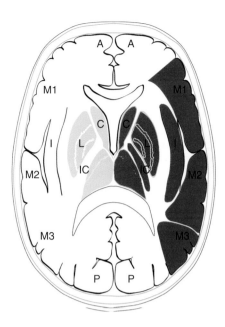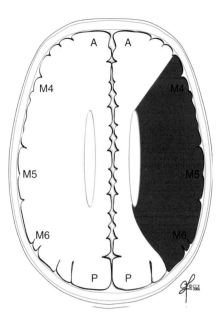

Figure 1.7
ASPECTS (Alberta Stroke Program Early CT Score) diagram demonstrating 10 compartments of the middle cerebral territory, each compartment scoring one point on a cumulative scale. Score of 10 is normal. ASPECTS score > 7 consistent with significant injury. Adapted with permission from Stroke 2004; 35: e103–5.

accidents (CVAs). (Minor drawbacks to this approach are the need for large-bore intravenous access, the need for iodinated contrast and concern over contrast reactions, and additional radiation exposure.)[33]

Despite these concerns, the introduction of helical or spiral CT scanning, coupled with multi-row detectors, has greatly rejuvenated the role of CT in modern cerebrovascular imaging.[34] The relatively high-kilovoltage, thinly collimated X-rays used in contemporary CT scanners result in linear attenuation, due to tissue density, thereby providing excellent contrast resolution. The enormous increase in gantry rotation speed, coupled with improved heat tolerance of the X-ray tube, provides improved temporal resolution such that dynamic, thin-section, volumetric spiral CT examination can be performed as an 'arterial snap-shot' approaches the anatomic information provided by catheter angiography.[35]

Data acquisition

The important first step with any dynamic contrast study is to determine the exact time to start scanning after intravenous contrast administration in order to capture the bolus while it resides only within the vessels of interest. Two methods are used:

- bolus tracking, in which the software measures the attenuation values for a region of interest (e.g. the common carotid artery), and spiral scanning is automatically started as soon as a certain threshold is exceeded;[36] and
- test bolus administration, in which bolus transit time to the carotid arteries is estimated by injecting a small test volume of contrast with axial 'same-level' scans performed in the lower neck; scanning with the examination bolus is then initiated with an appropriate time delay.[37]

Post-processing

Before starting the post-processing, it is frequently helpful to review the source data and axial images for calcifications, high-grade

stenoses or occlusion. Subsequently a variety of post-processing computer algorithms can be applied to create two- and three-dimensional angiographic displays:

- multi-planar reformation (MPR), which essentially involves sagittal, axial, and coronal anatomic reconstructions (Figure 1.8); curved multi-planar reformation (cMPR) can be manually applied along the vessel course to provide excellent linear demonstration of the vessel lumen;
- maximum intensity projection (MIP), which is most commonly used three-dimensional technique for vascular imaging, in which a single layer of brightest voxels along a line of site (or projection) at a specified angle (orthogonal or oblique) is displayed (see Figure 1.8); a major drawback is that there is no depth information (i.e. it displays only the density of objects, not spatial information), and evaluation of the vascular lumen in regions of dense calcifications may be impossible with conventional MIP techniques;
- shaded surface display (SSD), in which the first layer of voxels within defined density thresholds is used for display, leading to the visualization of the surface of all structures that fulfill the threshold conditions. Depth information is preserved but the attenuation information is scaled proportionately. While very helpful in evaluation for intracranial aneurysms, SSD is less useful for the evaluation for stenoses, particularly those that are calcified;
- volume rendering (VR), in which all the information in the volume data set is used to select groups of voxels within a defined threshold density, after which a color and shading or opacity are assigned (e.g. low opacity for semitransparent structures); VR maintains both depth and density information, and it is perhaps the best three-dimensional technique for intra- and extracranial vessels (see Figures 1.2, 1.8).

Image interpretation and analysis

The overall accuracy of CT angiography for detecting thromboses and stenoses of large intracranial and extracranial arteries is approximately 95–99%.[38–41] It is comparable to catheter angiography in distinguishing between total and near-total occlusions.[42]

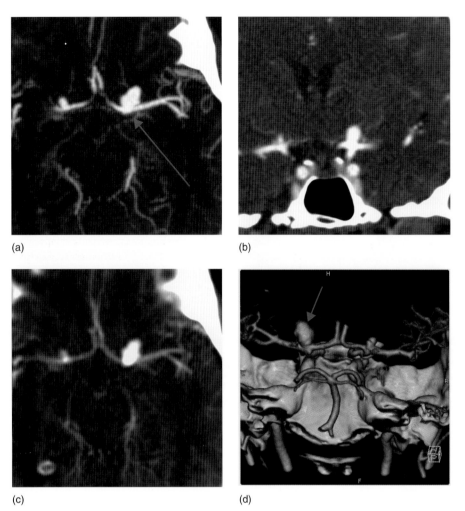

(a)

(b)

(c)

(d)

Figure 1.8
Aneurysm reconstruction.
(a) Multiplanar reconstruction of CT angiogram demonstrating left carotid terminus aneurysm.
(b) Maximum intensity projection (MIP), coronal and (c) axial of carotid terminus aneurysm.
(d) Volume rendered 3D CT angiogram, viewed from behind.

The following approach is very helpful in interpreting extra and intracranial CT angiography:

1. All three-dimensional methods are subject to some loss of information, and therefore source data images are inspected first for quality of the study, calcifications, stenoses, and occlusions.
2. MIP images inspected in multi-planar format are examined for vascular detail. Thin MIPs (10–20 mm) are preferred for intracranial circulation.
3. Finally, if there is arterial wall calcification, curved MIP and VR are examined to evaluate vascular lumen and plaque dimensions.

Perfusion Imaging

Perfusion of normal brain tissue is maintained within a narrow range by auto-regulation of the cerebral vasculature. Cerebral blood volume (CBV) is normally 4–5 mL per 100 g. Normal blood flow in human gray matter is about 50–60 mL per 100 g per minute.[43] Decreasing cerebral blood flow to < 35 mL per 100 g per minute (50–60% of normal) leads to the cessation of protein synthesis, although tissue can survive with no further additional insult to cerebral blood flow (CBF). With CBF reduced to < 20 mL per 100 g per minute (30–40% of normal) there is loss of neural function, and the tissue is at risk. (At these levels

Table 1.2 Cerebral blood flow (CBF) and oxygen utilization

Effects of variations in CBF	
CBF (ml per 100 g tissue per minute)	*Condition*
45–65	Normal brain at rest
75–80	Gray matter
20–30	White matter
25	EEG becomes flatline
15	Physiologic paralysis
12	Brain stem auditory evoked response changes
10	Alterations in cell membrane transport (cell death; cerebrovascular accident)

CBF = CPP/CVR = MAP − ICP/CVR
CBF, cerebral blood flow; CPP, cerebral perfusion pressure;
CVR, cerebrovascular resistance; ICP, intracranial pressure;
MAP, mean arterial pressure.

the patient will be neurologically impaired, but may recover.) Finally, when CBF falls to < 10 mL per 100 g for minute (< 20% of normal) there is irreversible cell death (Table 1.2).

The evolution of cerebral hemodynamic compromise can be described in stages.[44] In stage 1, the cerebral vasculature attempts to maintain normal CBF by vasodilating (CBV increased). As hemodynamic compromise progresses to stage 2, CBF diminishes as autoregulatory vasodilatation is superseded. The brain continues to remain viable by increasing the fraction of oxygen extracted from the circulation – so called misery perfusion. If hemodynamic compromise continues, the final stage is cell death and infarction.

The imaging techniques utilized to evaluate cerebral perfusion can categorized as follows:

- indicator dilution methods involving injection of a tracer detected over time;
- techniques that identify the degree of pre-existing auto-regulatory reserve and vasoreactivity by imaging before and after a vasodilatory stimulus (e.g. Diamox SPECT); and
- techniques that measure oxygen extraction fraction (O15–PET).

Perfusion techniques may also be categorized as those that use diffusible tracers or those that rely on non-diffusable contrast agents.[45] This is an important distinction in that the mathematical models used to quantify the data are unique to each.

CT perfusion

One of the early attempts at CTP imaging relied on stable xenon gas, which had the characteristics of being biologically inert, having a k-edge similar to that of iodinated contrast, being soluble in both water and lipid, and being freely diffusible across the blood–brain barrier. With this technique the measurement of CBF is a determination both of the amount of contrast agent in the feeding arteries as well as the amount that has passed into the brain parenchyma. Quantification of CBF requires knowledge of the arterial concentration (arterial input function, or AIF) and the tissue concentrations, or the partition coefficient between these two compartments. Following a baseline non-contrast scan, serial CT scans at preset locations are acquired during

xenon inhalation at a concentration of approximately 28% over 4.3 minutes. The initial scans can be used as masks to produce subtracted images, which can be used to calculate tracer accumulation over time. Xenon concentrations can be measured in the expiratory ventilation circuit to calculate the AIF. The Kety–Schmidt equation is then solved voxel by voxel via iterative calculation to produce quantitative CBF maps. Despite the singular advantage of quantitative blood flow, this technique has historically been arduous and is practiced at only a limited number of centers.

Non-diffusable tracer techniques have become more popular with the advent of temporally faster spiral scanners. The central volume principle states that CBF = CBV divided by mean transit time (MTT) from the time of arterial input to venous drainage. Calculation of MTT and CBF requires knowledge of the AIF, which, in the context of an intact blood–brain barrier, can be approximated by mathematical deconvolution. Contemporary CTP as well as MR perfusion measures brain perfusion by analyzing this dynamic enhancement of cerebral vasculature and parenchyma after a single intravenous bolus injection of contrast material.

Data acquisition

CTP has been performed with single-slice scanners but the examination is limited to 1 cm thickness.[46] With multi-slice CT, a 2–3 cm-thick section can be examined. The anatomic region that clinical symptoms indicate is most likely affected by ischemia must be selected *a priori* for the examination (e.g. basal ganglia in most cases of MCA disease). A bolus of contrast material is injected at a high rate (usually 8 ml/s) using a power injector, and tissue attenuation is monitored as the contrast first reaches and then perfuses the brain with one image per second acquired during wash-in and wash-out. For each voxel from these scans, a time-attenuation plot is generated that corresponds to the relative wash-in–wash-out of contrast (Figure 1.9). From these plots parameters such as time-to-peak can be measured or calculated (ascending slope of the curve is the CBF, while the area under the time-attenuation curve is the CBV) for each voxel in the image.

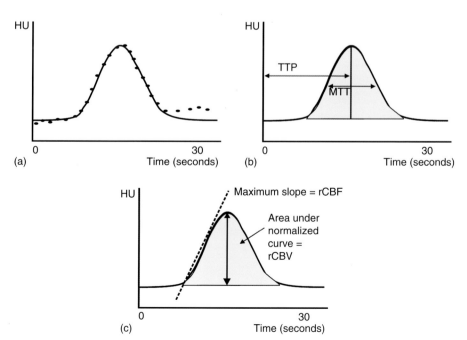

Figure 1.9
CT perfusion imaging based on time density curve created voxel by voxel during bolus administration of iodinated contrast. (a) Time attenuation plot. (b) Mean transit time calculated as the FWHM of the curve while time to peak (TTP) is calculated from the start to peak attenuation. (c) Relative cerebral blood volume (rCBV) is calculated as the area under the curve while relative cerebral blood flow (rCBF) is the upslope. HU, hounsfield units.

A simplified CTP technique called perfused blood volume (PBV) is used by some institutions to triage patients for thrombolysis. With this technique, data acquired for CT angiography are used at the same time to assess perfusion of the whole brain CBV but, unlike the quantitative dynamic perfusion technique described above, PBV images do not provide information about CBF or mean transit time, which may be important parameters for assessing 'tissue at risk'.[37,47,48]

Post-processing

Semiautomatic post-processing is used to create scaled, color maps of TTP or MTT, CBF, and CBV in less than 1 minute (see Figure 1.9).[49] Two mathematical approaches are used to calculate these parameters:[50]

1. The maximum slope model requires a rapid, tight bolus to calculate the slope of the time-attenuation curve, which is used to approximate CBF. CBV is calculated from an enhancement ratio relative to the superior sagittal sinus. It is relatively insensitive to motion.
2. Deconvolution analysis models calculate regional MTT by deconvolving the time-attenuation curve.[51] This method requires an arterial input function to deconvolve the curve, and it utilizes the central volume principle to calculate $CBF = CBV/MTT$.[52–54] This method theoretically provides absolute values for CBF and CBV. Nevertheless, there are variables (choice of input function, recirculation correction), which may limit the accuracy of these values.[55]

For practical purposes, 'r' is added before CBF and CBV indicating relative rather than absolute values of CBV and CBF because both techniques used for measurement of these parameters are limited in giving absolute values for a variety of reasons. Fiorella et al. recently demonstrated the variability in post-processing dynamic CTP data, suggesting that the current techniques are not sufficient to allow the use of quantitative values in clinical practice.[56]

Image interpretation and analysis

CTP has much higher sensitivity than unenhanced CT for detecting early ischemia.[57] During interpretation of CTP studies, color-coded parameter maps (Figure 1.10) are first visually assessed by comparing the cerebral hemispheres, with a sensitivity of over 90% in larger ischemic lesions.[57,58] When unilateral or regional ischemic lesions are suspected, corresponding regions of interest in the two hemispheres can be drawn for comparison, yielding a percentage of reduction of both CBF and CBV for the affected hemisphere versus the normal side. As discussed above, TTP and MTT are very sensitive indicators of hemodynamic disturbances, while CBF and CBV may help to predict the outcome of an ischemic lesion.

In cases where there is arterial stenosis or occlusion with good cerebrovascular compensation or good collateral circulation, there may be prolonged TTP, normal CBF and normal or increased CBV. In patients with oligemic tissue, TTP may be prolonged, CBF reduced (but still > 60%) and CBV reduced (but still > 80%). In areas where tissue is at risk, TTP will be prolonged, CBF reduced (but still > 30%), and CBV reduced (but still > 60%). And in areas of completed infarction there will be marked prolongation or non-measurable TTP, CBF (reduced to < 30%) and CBV (reduced to < 40%). These parameter guidelines are based on comparison studies between CT and diffusion weighted MRI attempting to differentiate between reversible 'penumbra' and irreversible infarction.[57,59]

As noted previously, an additional, simplified CTP technique (PBV) is used by some institutions to triage patients for thrombolysis. In this technique, data acquired for CT angiography are also used to approximate only the CBV for assessing areas of severe oligemia.[38,47,48]

Magnetic resonance imaging

Edward M Purcell and Felix Bloch were independently awarded the 1952 Nobel Prize in Physics for thier development of new methods for nuclear magnetic precession (i.e. nuclear magnetic resonance, or NMR). Purcell first observed NMR signaling in 1945 while working at the Massachusetts Institute of Technology Radiation Laboratory. Along with similar research by Nicolaas Bloembergen and Robert Pound, this work was later expanded to a comprehensive theory of nuclear magnetic relaxation; while his contributions with Herman Carr on improved spin-echo techniques laid the groundwork for future techniques in MRI.[60] Although Damadian patented the design and use of NMR for detecting cancer in 1974, he did not describe a method for generating pictures. The use of magnetic field gradients to localize and map the signals described by Purcell to a digital image matrix is

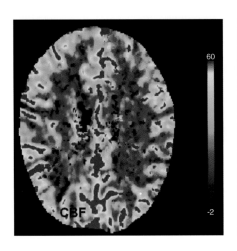
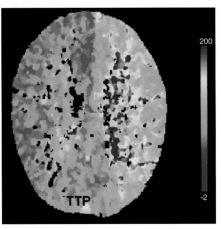

Figure 1.10
Clinical study demonstrating vascular occlusion with delayed time to peak (TTP) on the right image. In the left image MCA territory with more subtle diminished relative cerebral blood flow (CBF) (left image).

credited to Paul Lauterbur and Sir Peter Mansfield, who were themselves awarded the 2003 Nobel Prize in Physiology and Medicine for their ingenuity.[61] While the technique is exceptionally valuable in many cases of cerebrovascular disease, one must be aware of magnetic interactions between therapeutic implants and the main or gradient fields. Although beyond the scope of this text, an extensive review of this subject can be found in the work of Shellock.[62]

Magnetic resonance imaging for the evaluation of cerebrovascular disease

There are advantages and disadvantages to the use of MRI in cerebrovascular disease. Advantages include:

- extraordinary sensitivity of diffusion-weighted imaging to acute cerebral hemispheric ischemia
- contrast sensitivity to parenchymal blood breakdown products
- non-ionizing radiation
- vascular imaging without or with exogenous contrast
- selective vascular imaging of arteries or veins
- perfusion scanning of the entire brain
- three-dimensional stereotactic targeting.

Disadvantages include:

- hostile environment for acutely ill patients, (inherently takes more time)
- contraindicated in some patients with implants, whether risking actual harm to the patient (e.g. those with cerebral aneurysm clips, pacemakers, DBS electrodes) or merely degrading the image due to artifact (e.g. carotid stent, platinum coil)
- limited by patient motion/ artifact
- Gd-DTPA not FDA approved as a susceptibility contrast agent for perfusion imaging

Magnetic resonance imaging of the brain

Clinical MRI is predicated upon the relaxation properties of excited hydrogen nuclei in water. When the object to be imaged is placed in a powerful, uniform magnetic field, the spinning protons align either parallel to or against the main magnetic field. The difference in the number of parallel and anti-parallel nuclei is only about one in a million. However, the vast quantity of nuclei produce a detectable change in field – a radio signal. (The magnetic dipole moment of the nuclei precess about the axis of the main field; the frequency with which the dipole moments precess is called the Larmor frequency, governed by the Larmor equation. At conventional field strengths used in clinical practice the frequency approaches that of citizen band radio.) The tissue is then briefly exposed to stimulating pulses of synchronous (i.e. resonant) electromagnetic energy (i.e. a radiofrequency (RF) pulse) in a plane perpendicular to the magnetic field, causing some of the magnetically aligned hydrogen nuclei to assume a temporary non-aligned higher energy state. (The frequency of the pulses is also governed by the Larmor equation.) Upon termination of the stimulating pulse, the protons 'relax' by emitting a radio signal as they again align parallel to the magnetic field. In order to localize the signal from tissue in three-dimensional space within the magnet, three orthogonal magnetic gradients are applied. The first is the slice selection, which is applied during the RF pulse. Next comes the phase encoding gradient, and then finally the frequency encoding gradient, during the signal sampling period. In order to create the image, spatial information must be recorded along with the received tissue-relaxation RF signal. For this reason, the linearly variable magnetic fields, or gradients, are applied in addition to the strong static, or baseline, main field to allow encoding of the position of the nuclei. When received, the signals are recorded in a temporary memory termed k-space; this is the spatial frequency weighting in two or three dimensions of a real space object as sampled by MRI. The RF information is subsequently inverse-Fourier transformed by a computer into real space to obtain the desired image.

While CT provides good spatial resolution, MRI provides far better contrast resolution (the ability to distinguish subtle differences between two tissues). The basis of this ability is the complex library of RF pulse sequences, which is optimized to provide image contrast based on subtle chemical sensitivities of MRI. For example, injured tissue tends to develop edema, which makes a T2-weighted sequence that is sensitive for detection of pathology, and it is generally able to distinguish pathologic tissue from normal tissue. A notable eccentricity of conventional MRI is the changing, evolutionary pattern of fresh blood on different pulse sequences, caused by the changes in oxidative state of iron (hemoglobin): oxy-, deoxy-, met-hemoglobin, and finally ferritin or hemosiderin. Such changes occur over a period of days to months, producing paramagnetic effects (bright) on T1-weighted scans and susceptibility effects (dark) on gradient echo studies (Table 1.3).

Table 1.3 MR signal changes in hemorrhage at high field (1.0–3.0T) relative to cortex

Heme moiety	Time of appearance	T_1	T_2
Oxyhemoglobin	Immediately – first several hours	Unchanged or decreased	Increased
Deoxyhemoglobin	Hours—several days	Unchanged or decreased	Decreased
Intracellular methemoglobin	First several days	Increased	Increased
Extracellular methemoglobin	Several days – months	Increased	Increased
Ferritin/hemosiderin	Several days – indefinitely	Unchanged or decreased	Decreased

Adapted from Gomori et al.[64]

The term 'conventional MRI' typically denotes those imaging techniques that do not require special, high-speed gradient systems (i.e. spin echo and gradient echo) from those that do (e.g. echo planar diffusion and perfusion imaging). Conventional MRI continues to have a role in the patient who presents with stroke symptoms because it can reliably rule in or rule out non-ischemic processes, and because it is better able to discriminate between acute, subacute, and chronic infarcts (Figure 1.11). It can also differentiate venous from arterial ischemic infarcts by demonstrating vasogenic edema and hemorrhage (a common finding even in early venous infarcts) (Figure 1.12), and it can detect incidental arterial stenosis or occlusions by showing diminished or absent normal flow voids on spin echo images. It can also detect carotid or vertebral dissections using fat-suppressed pulse sequence.[65]

Diffusion imaging of the brain

Diffusion-weighted imaging (DWI) is a high-speed imaging technique with remarkable sensitivity and specificity to acute infarction compared to CT and conventional MRI. DWI can depict infarcted tissue in the cerebral hemispheres as early as minutes after the occlusion of the feeding vessel.[66,67] In DWI, the sensitivity is derived from additional pulsed gradients that are applied before and after the signal-producing RF pulse. These gradients sensitize the sequence to random molecular (Brownian) motion or 'diffusion' of water protons. (This motion may be restricted or limited by cell membranes, e.g. intracellular water of ischemic edema, versus free water in the extracellular space.) The gradients are applied in three different directions (anterior–posterior, superior–inferior, and side-to-side) during three different image acquisitions. Because of the directionality of the brain's fiber tracts, this helps to counteract the problems caused by anisotropy (direction-dependant movement). Ultimately, these image data sets can be combined to produce a so-called a trace image, which is typically used for interpretation/ diagnostic screening.

This diffusion sensitivity is quantified by a term, the b-value of a pulse sequence (determined primarily by the magnitude and duration of motion sensitizing gradients). The higher the b-value, the greater the sensitivity to restricted diffusion (i.e. ischemic edema). Any process causing restriction of diffusion appears brighter on DWI, and vice versa. Calculated images can also be

created from these data sets that display the correlation coefficient of diffusion as a gray scale image. Images are acquired at multiple b-values in order to calculate apparent diffusion co-efficients (ADC) and generate ADC map images. Any process causing restricted diffusion appears darker on ADC map images, and vice versa.

Acute ischemic lesions are characterized by high signal intensity on DWI and low ADC values. The signal intensity of acute stroke on DWI increases during the first week after symptom onset and decreases thereafter, but it may retain a significant amount of brightness for longer periods.[66] The signal on DWI often remains hyperintense for weeks,[68] while ADC values gradually increase over 7–10 days (seen as lesions getting brighter on ADC map images).[69] Lesion size on DWI is a good predictor of minimal completed infarct volume.[70]

Several patterns of ischemic lesions can be differentiated on DWI in patients with underlying anterior circulation ischemic disease:[71,72]

- typical large confluent 'cortical territorial infarct' (Figure 1.13a) (e.g. MCA or anterior cerebral artery occlusion in absence of adequate collateral circulation);
- 'subcortical infarcts' due to deep perforator occlusions (e.g. proximal M1 occlusion in the presence of good collateral vessels);
- 'typical territorial infarct with fragmentation' (e.g. spontaneous or induced thrombolysis of a large vascular territory with dissemination of emboli in the same territory (Figure 1.13b));
- 'shower of infarcts' (e.g. fragmented embolus of cardiac or cervical carotid origin to multiple vascular territories (Figure 1.13c)); and
- 'Border zone infarcts', which may be cortical (superficial) or subcortical watershed infarcts (Figure 1.13d).

Microembolism during endarterectomy and carotid stenting has been shown by intraoperative Doppler sonography,[73] while DWI can show evidence of infarcts caused by these microemboli.[74–77] The incidence of intraprocedure microembolism is related to multiple risk factors, including symptomatic status of the patient and plaque morphology. Fortunately, most of the resulting micro-infarcts are clinically silent.[78] However, this opens a new avenue of stroke prediction based on clinically silent micro-infarcts seen on DWI.[79]

Posterior circulation acute infarcts (Figure 1.14) have basically the same imaging features (i.e. they are brighter on DWI and

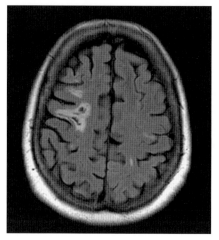

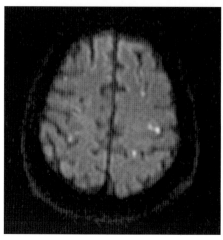

(a)   (b)

Figure 1.11

(a) T2 weighted FLAIR examination demonstrating focal defect in the right frontal lobe with diffuse, punctate changes in both hemispheres. (b) Diffusion weighted imaging demonstrates the largest defect on the right to be chronic while the bi-hemispheric defects are acute focal areas of infarction.

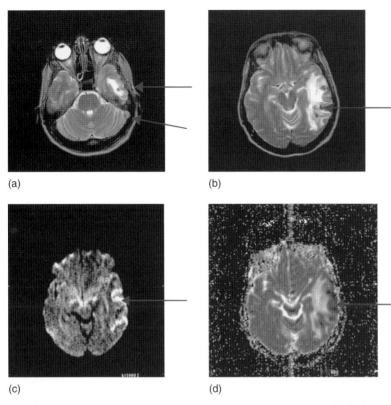

(a)   (b)

(c)   (d)

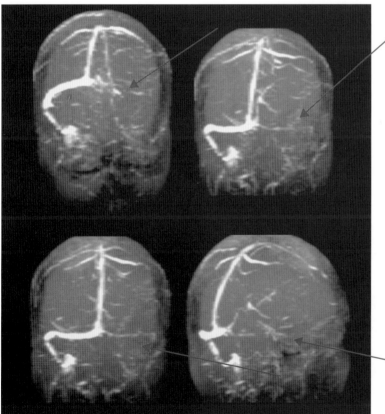

(e)

Figure 1.12
Vernous infarction (a) T2 weighted scan demonstrating heterogeneous defect in the left inferior temporal lobe of mixed increased and decreased signal (open arrow). Notice lack of "flow void" in the left sigmoid sinus. (b) Higher slice demonstrating finger-like projection of subcortical high signal consistent with vasogenic edema with areas of low signal in the adjacent cortex (arrow) suspicious for susceptibility artifact of blood breakdown products. (c,d) Diffusion tensor image and ADC map confirm ischemia only in the cortex (bright on diffusion, low on ADC) with "T2 shine-through" (bright on diffusion, bright on ADC) secondary to vasogenic edema. (e) MR venogram confirming transverse-sigmoid sinus thrombosis resulting in a hemorrhagic temporal lobe infarction and venous hypertension.

darker on ADC maps). However, DWI has relatively lower sensitivity to brainstem and cerebellar infarcts for a variety of reasons:

- image degradation occurs close to the skull base by susceptibility artifact (because of bones, the paranasal sinus, and dental amalgam) in the presence of strong diffusion gradients;
- lesions are usually smaller, and therefore they may not show up on DWI or may not be appreciated by some readers; and
- the different degree of packing of infratentorial fiber tracts and gray matter relative to the hemispheres.[80,81]

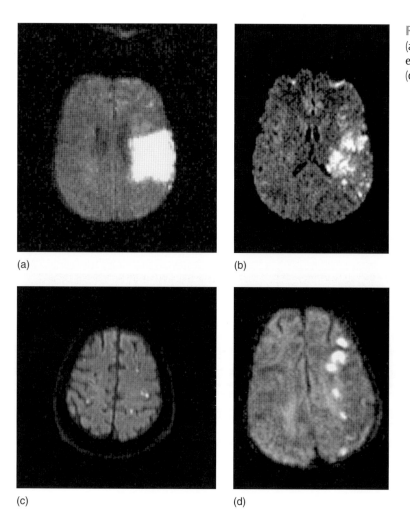

Figure 1.13
(a) MRD cortical infarct, (b) MRD fragmented embolus–MCA infarct, (c) MRD embolic shower, (d) watershed infarction MRD.

Venous infarcts can be bright on DWI but because there is often a combination of cytotoxic and vasogenic edema, the signal is more heterogenous and the evolutionary pattern is different (see Figure 1.12).[82–84]

It is important to remember that other pathologic entities (notably abscess or neoplasm) may also be increased in signal on DWI (Figure 1.15). In the case of an abscess, this distinction can be particularly difficult, although with other pathologic processes the DWI may be less hyperintense, a function of so-called T2 shine-through.[86] Additionally, because DWI is inherently a very highly T2-weighted sequence, lesions with vasogenic edema appear brighter on DWI, not because of restricted diffusion but because of its T2 characteristic; hence the shine-through effect. This is the major advantage of the ADC map: these mimics of stroke do not have low signal on the ADC map as an infarct would.

Hence, this pitfall can be avoided by examining the ADC map (Figure 1.16). However, a potential pitfall in this approach has been termed 'pseudo-normalization' of the infarct on the ADC map (usually on day 5), which is due to a balancing effect between cytotoxic and vasogenic edema at about this time.[66,87] Fortunately, the diagnosis has usually been established by this point in the clinical time course, and patients are seldom imaged as remotely as that from the onset of ictus.

Magnetic resonance angiography

MRA has proven to be a useful, non-invasive tool for evaluation of the intra-and extracranial vasculature since its first clinical application over 10 years ago.[88] It is an established clinical tool in extracranial carotid disease, with sensitivity and specificity of around 90%.[89,90] While technical details of MRA techniques are beyond the scope of this chapter, the three major techniques currently used for MRA are summarized below.[91,92] The goal of each method is to distinguish between flowing blood and surrounding stationary soft tissues.

Time-of-flight (saturation) method

The time-of-flight (TOF) method is commonly used and has a very high sensitivity to flow. There are two- and three-dimensional TOF techniques. The accuracy of the TOF method, particularly as a non-invasive complement to carotid duplex scanning, is well established.[93] The basic mechanism is suppression of the stationary background tissues by repeated RF pulses while a good signal is acquired from fresh flowing, fully magnetized blood entering the image slice or volume ('flow related enhancement').

Phase contrast (subtraction) method

The phase contrast method is a more time-consuming technique, and it is not commonly used in routine neurovascular evaluation. It is based on the phase shifts between stationary tissues and flowing blood, and it can provide both qualitative information and quantitative (direction and velocity) information about blood

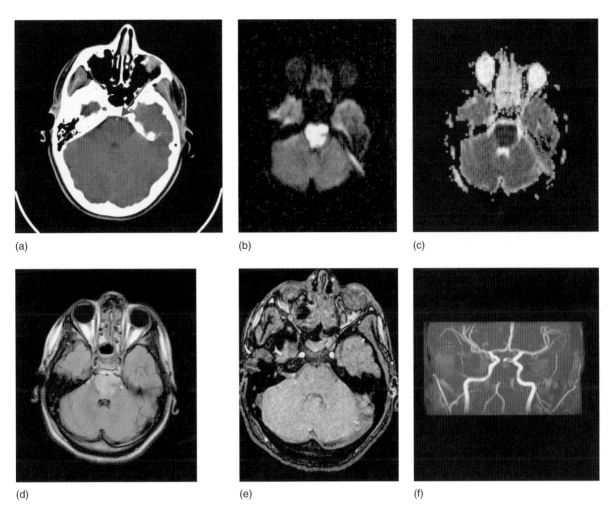

(a)   (b)   (c)

(d)   (e)   (f)

Figure 1.14

(a) Hyperdense basilar artery on CT, suspicious for thrombotic embolus. (b) Delayed diffusion scan demonstrates clear-cut infarction, confirmed with ADC map (c). (d) FLAIR T2 weighted scan shows infarct. Confirmed basilar occlusion on native (e) and MIP (f) MR angiogram.

flow in the vessels. Technically this method is very analogous to DWI, but the imaging gradients are scaled to detect macroscopic, faster arterial or venous flow, rather than the microscopic molecular, Brownian motion of DWI.

Contrast MRA (luminal opacification) method

Analogous to CT angiography (Figure 1.17), contrast MCA enables vessels take visualized by virtue of enhancement of the lumen with MRI contrast agents during the arterial phase of an intravenously administered bolus of a paramagnetic contrast agent. Likewise, this is a dynamic technique, and therefore the timing of the start of acquisition is critical; the two methods used for this purpose are essentially the same as discussed above under CTA (timing bolus and bolus tracking). Contrast MRA is increasingly being used for examining the extracranial vasculature,[89] and it is considered an adequate diagnostic test before surgery.[94,95] Additionaly, intracranial studies performed with exceedingly short echo times (to minimize susceptibility artifact from coils) may be used in lieu of conventional angiography to follow aneurysms after treatment for coil compaction.[96–98]

For three-dimensional post-processing, only multi-planar reformation and maximum intensity projection (MIP) methods (as discussed above under CTA) are routinely used for MRI studies. For practical purposes, the following points are important to remember during image analysis and interpretation:

- always thoroughly inspect the source data images to avoid misinterpretations related to post-processing errors and artifacts;[99,100]
- diminished signal or flow defect should not be attributed solely to stenosis or occlusion unless other technical causes are excluded (e.g. the presence of a metallic stent, signal loss due to vascular looping or tortuosity, flow saturation or intravoxel dephasing;[99,100] note that maximum intensity projection images (a post-processing method) are prone to overestimate stenosis);[89,100]
- the question of occlusion versus near occlusion and tandem or diffuse stenosis is best solved by contrast MRA (if not primarily performed) or by correlation with ultrasound.

As one can appreciate, it is critical to understand the technical aspects and flow dynamics in order to grade stenosis accurately as well as to lower the observer variability.[101]

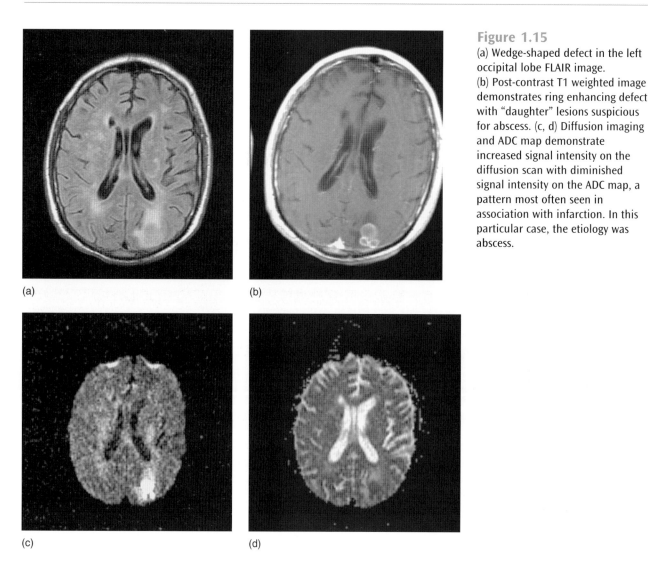

(a)   (b)

(c)   (d)

Figure 1.15
(a) Wedge-shaped defect in the left occipital lobe FLAIR image.
(b) Post-contrast T1 weighted image demonstrates ring enhancing defect with "daughter" lesions suspicious for abscess. (c, d) Diffusion imaging and ADC map demonstrate increased signal intensity on the diffusion scan with diminished signal intensity on the ADC map, a pattern most often seen in association with infarction. In this particular case, the etiology was abscess.

Magnetic resonance perfusion imaging

MR perfusion imaging can be performed by several techniques: arterial spin labeling and the more common, dynamic method of bolus infusion of susceptibility contrast. Like CT perfusion, a bolus of contrast material is rapidly infused intravenously and a hemodynamic map is generated that is based on the degree of susceptibility produced by the contrast material.[102] In clinical practice this represents an 'off-label' use of Gd-DTPA in which the agent is used not to increase signal (its normal use as a paramagnetic contrast) but to decrease signal on the basis of its susceptibility effect on T2-weighted sequences used for perfusion imaging (Figure 1.18). This hemodynamic map makes possible the calculation of the same parameters as discussed above under CTP (although the time-intensity curve is inverted); MTT, TTP, CBV, and CBF maps are then generated for interpretation.

The significance of MR perfusion imaging in the setting of stroke (often in combination with DWI) is basically threefold:

- identify tissue at risk;
- to predict the final infarct volume[103,104] and hence the clinical outcome; and

- to detect cerebral hemodynamic impairment,[105] (e.g. in the right cerebral hemisphere when the right internal carotid artery is occluded).

The key points of MR perfusion imaging in acute stroke studies can be summarized as follows:[70,106–109]

- infarct size on initial CBV map is the best predictor of final infarct volume, compared to other parameters;
- CBF and MTT map defects (meaning decreased flow and increased mean transit time) generally have poor correlation with final infarct volume;
- CBF and MTT map defects indicate hemodynamic impairment and are better predictors of lesion growth (probably as a result of threshold effects);
- TTP, if increased (>6 seconds) indicates hemodynamic impairment, – increased TTP is the most commonly seen perfusion abnormality in early stroke but, like MTT and CBF, it overestimates the final infarct volume.[110]

MR and CT perfusion studies, in conjunction with parenchymal scanning and angiographic techniques, already appear to be having an impact in patient selection for treatment of acute cerebrovascular disease, extending the time window for treatment in those patients with the necessary vascular reserve to sustain viable brain tissue beyond 3 hours.[111,112]

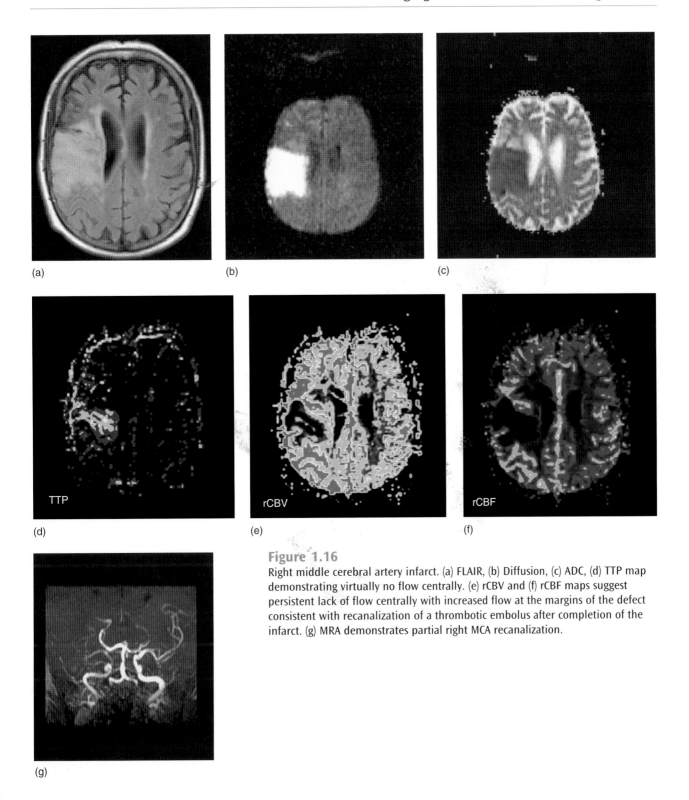

(a)   (b)   (c)

(d) TTP   (e) rCBV   (f) rCBF

(g)

Figure 1.16

Right middle cerebral artery infarct. (a) FLAIR, (b) Diffusion, (c) ADC, (d) TTP map demonstrating virtually no flow centrally. (e) rCBV and (f) rCBF maps suggest persistent lack of flow centrally with increased flow at the margins of the defect consistent with recanalization of a thrombotic embolus after completion of the infarct. (g) MRA demonstrates partial right MCA recanalization.

Nuclear medicine

In the 1950s and early 1960s, Hal Anger developed a device to detect iatrogenically administered, gamma-emitting, radioisotopes within the body for diagnostic and therapeutic purposes. His work serves as the basis for most contemporary nuclear imaging. The Anger camera consists of a series of lead collimators, placed between the detector surface and the patient; these collimators serve to minimize scatter. The detector is a scintillation crystal, which produces light flashes when an impinging gamma-ray reaches and interacts with the crystal. The scintillations are detected by an array of photomultiplier tubes optically coupled to the crystal. The photomulipliers produce an output signal in the form of an electrical current, which is proportional to the energy of the incident-stimulating gamma-ray. The electrical signal may be amplified, sorted by a pulse height analyzer, and then registered as a 'count'. Depending on the position of the event, the phototubes are variably activated. Hence, the entire system response yields positional information, although the spatial resolution is less than that of CT or MRI.

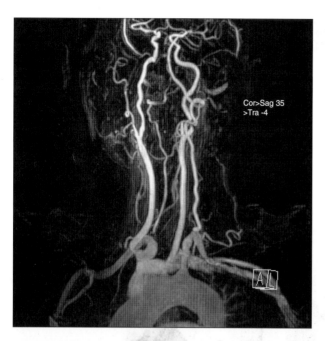

Figure 1.17
Gadolinium enhanced MR angiography of the aortic arch and cervical vessels.

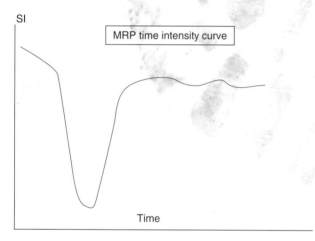

Figure 1.18
Time intensity curve of MR perfusion study (MRP) utilizing gadolinium-DTPA, in this instance a susceptibility contrast agent, which produces a transient decrease in signal intensity with time.

Single photon emission computed tomography imaging for cerebrovascular disease

Advantages of single photon (computed) tomography (SPECT or SPET) include:

- its ready accessibility; and
- its ability to test cerebrovascular reserve.

Its disadvantages include the fact that it:

- is time-consuming;
- provides limited spatial resolution; and
- is non-quantitative.

SPECT is a nuclear imaging technique much like CT, except that rather than producing cross-sectional images from external X-rays passing through the body, gamma-emitting radiopharmaceuticals (single photon emitters or positron emitters) are detected in multiple views by rotating a single (or, preferably, multiple) Anger camera(s) about the area of interest. Scintillation crystals for SPECT imaging are typically composed of sodium iodide with trace amounts of thallium. Using back projection techniques, cross-sectional images are then computed with the axial field of view determined by the axial field of view of the gamma-camera. Data reconstruction must account for emitted rays and also those attenuated within the patient (i.e. photons emanating from deep inside the patient are considerably attenuated by surrounding tissues). Whereas in CT, attenuation is a key component of the imaging process, in SPECT attenuation degrades the image and this must be corrected or accounted for.

A radioisotope such as technetium-99 m is attached to a delivery compound that passes through the blood–brain barrier and is avidly taken up by the brain parenchyma, with uptake proportional to cerebral blood flow.[113] Two common delivery compounds are hexamethylpropyleneamine oxime (HMPAO) and ethyl cysteinate dimer (ECD). Scans may be performed before and after administration of a cerebral vasodilator (e.g. Diamox) to provide a qualitative assessment of the level of vasomotor reserve (Figure 1.19).[45]

Positron emission tomography imaging for cerebrovascular disease

The main advantage of positron emission tomography (PET) is that it provides quantitative physiologic data.
Its disadvantages include:

- expense;
- low spatial and contrast resolution;
- its technically demanding nature; and
- the fact that it cannot be performed emergently.

PET is a tomographic nuclear imaging procedure first described in the early 1970s by Hoffman and Phelps. It uses radiopharmaceutical-labeled positron emitters (i.e. electron annihilation reaction induced gamma-rays). Positron emitters are attractive on the basis of their active participation in physiologic pathways, but they have the drawback of exceedingly short half-lives (e.g. O-15 has a half life of approximately 2 minutes), which necessitates a cyclotron for on-site production.

The PET principle is as follows. A low dose of labelled positron emitter such as C-11, N-13, O-15 or F-18 is injected into the patient, who is scanned by the tomographic system. Scanning consists of either a dynamic series of images or a static image obtained after an interval during which the radiopharmaceutical enters the biochemical process of interest. The scanner detects the spatial and temporal distribution of the radiolabel by detecting gamma-rays during the so-called emission scan. The gamma-rays emitted occur by positive beta-decay, the annihilation reaction between the positron and a shell electron of a neighbouring atom, which produces two 511 keV gamma-rays, that travel in diametrically opposite directions (owing to the conservation of energy and momentum laws). The two gamma-rays are detected by a

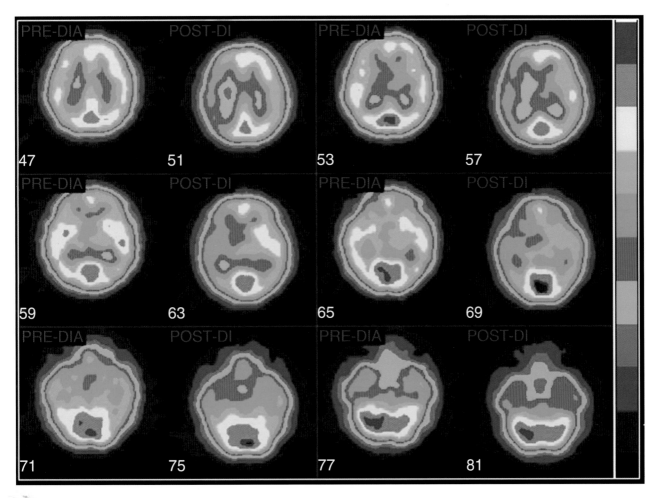

Figure 1.19
Acetazolamide SPECT study of right MCA ischemia. Notice the defect worsens on the "Post" scans indicative of a lack of additional vascular reserve in the right MCA territory with acetazolamide stimulated vasodilatation.

coincidence counting detection system, and, after proper filtering, the collected raw data sinograms are reconstructed into a cross-sectional image. Because the 'coincidence event' must have occurred along a straight line connecting two detectors, and because the probability of absorption of the two gamma-rays is independent of the position of the event along that imaginary line, PET is an inherently quantitative imaging method allowing the measurement of regional concentrations of the radiopharmaceutical injected after proper calibration. To achieve quantitative detection, several problems have to be overcome, including Compton scattering, random coincidences, and tissue absorption. It is worth noting that, owing to the high energy gamma-rays emitted by beta-decay, these systems require special detectors (e.g. bismuth germanate, BGO).

Dynamic data acquisition is performed when the data are to be quantified. In this technique, scans are acquired over times as short as 30 seconds. The most important technique for analysis of dynamic data is input deconvolution. Using this mathematical technique, quantitative tissue perfusion can be performed.

The major problems with three-dimensional data acquisition are the large number of random coincidences counted and the data acquisition and reconstruction time. Presently oxygen extraction fraction (OEF) as determined by PET is being used to define patients who may be amenable to extracerebral–intracerebral bypass.[114–117]

Ultrasound

Cardiovascular and cerebral ultrasonography was first performed in the early 1950s at Lund University by cardiologist Inge Edler and physicist Carl Hertz. Hertz was familiar with using ultrasonic reflectoscopes for non-destructive materials testing, and together they developed the idea of using this method in medicine. In December 1953, the method was used to generate an 'echo-encephalogram', and Edler and Hertz published their ideas in 1954.[118]

The Doppler effect was first described by the Austrian mathematician and physicist, Johann Christian Doppler (1803–1853) in 1842. Although it was first described in reference to light emitted by stars, the Doppler effect is applicable to any kind of wave, whether electromagnetic or mechanical, and thus also to ultrasound. Shortly thereafter, in 1880, the brothers Jacques and Pierre Curie demonstrated the 'piezoelectric effect'. Piezoelectric crystal are capable of generating high frequency pressure waves in a predetermined direction, as well as detecting their echo from reflected objects (stationary or moving).

It wasn't until 1959 that DL Franklin et al. produced a piezoelectric flowmeter that could be mounted directly on blood vessels, in which short ultrasound pulses were transmitted through the vessel lumen between two piezoelectric crystals, and the difference in transit time between upstream and downstream ultrasound pulses was used for measurement of instantaneous flow velocity.[119] Subsequently, Doppler frequency shift was used for the detection of blood velocity patterns transcutaneously, first desribed by S Satomura in 1959.[120]

Today's ultrasound instruments represent serial refinements of these early observations, primarily through evolution of Doppler spectral analysis (again with the aid of the analog-to-digital converter and improved computer technology allowing real-time Fourier transformation). Although coupled with increasingly sophisticated imaging (e.g. color flow, power Doppler), the primary diagnostic metric continues to be velocity measurements (as a reflection of underlying vascular pathology), the imaging component primarily being used as a means to ensure the accuracy and reproducibility. Indeed, 'reproducibility' is the operative word relative to cerebrovascular ultrasound.

Doppler ultrasound for cerebrovascular disease

Advantages of Doppler ultrasound include:

- its ready accessibility and the fact that it can be performed at the bedside; and
- the fact that it can test for flow-limiting stenoses as well as emboli.

Its disadvantages include the facts that it is:

- operator-dependent;
- potentially time-consuming;
- able to give only poor spatial resolution of distal vasculature; and
- non-quantitative.

Transcranial Doppler was initially described by Aaslid et al. in the 1980s utilizing a 2 MHz transducer.[121] Subsequently it has gained popularity as means to follow patients (serially and reproducibly) who have suspected vasospasm following subarachnoid

hemorrhage (at the bedside); document and follow focal, atherosclerotic intracranial stenoses pre- and post-treatment; detect microemboli; and also confirm clinical suspicions of brain death (Figure 1.20) (Table 1.4).[73,122–125] More recently, transcranial and intravascular ultrasound probes have been used as an adjunct to thrombolytic therapy for acute stroke.[126,127]

Doppler ultrasound is likewise popular and readily available for extracranial disease. And, like transcranial studies, these examinations are not only subject to the vagaries of individual operators, but the velocity measurements may also be significantly affected by hardware and signal processing. Thus these studies require diligent attention to technique with a systematic quality-assurance progam in order to serve as reliable (reproducible) indicators of extent of stenosis. This was perhaps best demonstrated during the ACAS trial in which all screening ultrasound laboratoriess were vetted before patients were recruited; substantial variability was found in velocity measurements, based on hardware manufacturer.[128]

Cerebral angiography

In the same year that Cushing recorded his seminal observations regarding intracranial pressure, Roentgen was awarded the Nobel Prize for his discovery of X-rays. Already in use in medicine, Haschek and Lindenthal were creating radiographs of blood vessels by performing experiments in cadavers using radio opaque solutions.[129] However, it wasn't until the late 1920s that the first attempt to create cerebral angiograms in humans were made by Egaz Moniz, using crude halide solutions; many of the first patients did not survive.[130,131] (Moniz, a neurologist, also received a Nobel Prize for his work on frontal leukotomy in 1949.)

In the first half of the 20th century, fluoroscopic imaging was dreadfully dim. It was not until the introduction of the image intensifier and television systems in the 1950s that image quality improved to the extent that intravascular maneuvers could be performed with any degree of safety. The formulation of more physiologic (and safe) iodinated contrast agents, the development of rapid film changers, and the introduction of new techniques

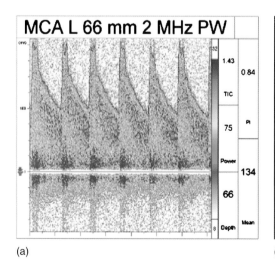

(a)

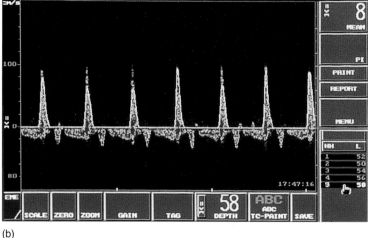

(b)

Figure 1.20

TransCranial Doppler (TCD) of (a) dramatic left MCA vasospasm velocity profiles over time. Notation on the right indicates the depth of insonation (66 mm) as well as mean velocity (134 cm/sec). (b) Relatively blunted and "bi-phasic" velocity profiles reflective of extraordinarily high intracranial pressure and consistent with brain death.

Table 1.4 Interpretation of transcranial Doppler for vasospasm

Mean MCA velocity	MCA:ICA ratio*	Interpretation
< 120 cm per second	< 3	Normal
120–200 cm per second	3–6	Mild vasospasm
> 200 cm per second	> 6	Severe vasospasm

*The Lindegaard ratio.
MCA, middle cerebral artery; ICA, internal cerebral artery.

for vascular access at approximately the same time (1952) led to the rise of cerebral angiography as a legitimate diagnostic tool,[132] and by extension neuroradiology as a subspecialty.

Film screen angiography, while having excellent spatial resolution, was low in contrast and had the distinct disadvantage that each image was serially developed in a chemical film processor. But, as with the imaging modalities described above, the introduction of the analog-to-digital converter and of real-time, computerized signal processing led to the digitization of angiography and the potential for dynamic, real-time, high-contrast subtracted angiograms (Figure 1.21a,b).[13,133–135] While image quality initially did not compete with the film screen, the near real-time feedback of any maneuver performed under fluoroscopy immediately transformed the angiography system from a diagnostic device to a therapeutic tool.

The digitization of cerebral angiography took place in the mid- and late 1970s. Simultaneously with these developments, physicians began to perform bolder and more ambitious percutaneously paced, catheter-directed treatments. In 1974 Serbinenko described the use of balloon-tipped catheters and detachable balloons for the treatment of cerebral aneurysms.[136] In 1978, Andres Gruntzig captivated the imagination of an even broader audience with the first reports of coronary balloon angioplasty.[136,137] The inevitable introduction of real-time digital roadmapping for complex catheterizations solidified the role of the angiography system as more than a 'camera'. In the interval since the late 1970s the technological evolution in endovascular surgical neuroradiology have been primarily catheter- and implantable device-related.

Nevertheless, transaxial rotation of the C-arm with the image intensifier (through an arc of 270°) detecting exposures from the X-ray source at three frames per second can produce projections that may be reconstructed in a fashion comparable to CT. Unfortunately the contrast resolution of image intensifiers is limited such that the vasculature can only be visualized with intra-arterial injections. Nevertheless, three-dimensional surface-rendered and multi-planar reconstructions of lesions such as aneurysms and vascular malformations with this technique can be extraordinarily helpful in the planning and execution of endovascular treatment (Figure 1.21c–e).[138–140]

Digital catheter angiography for cerebrovascular disease

Advantages of digital catheter angiography are that it can provide:

- the highest resolution and contrast images of cerebral vascular anatomy (the 'gold standard');

- dynamic images showing arterial, capillary, and venous phases;
- three-dimensional stereotactic imaging; and
- parenchymal imaging.

Its disadvantages include

- its invasive nature and associated risks;
- the use of ionizing radiation; and
- the expense.

Digital angiography systems potentially stand at the threshold of another round of innovation with the introduction of digital, flat-panel detectors and the gradual passing of older image intensifier systems. X-ray detectors based on flat-panel arrays derived from a hydrogenated amorphous silicone (a-Si:H) have become increasingly available in recent years. These detectors are available in two basic types: direct X-ray detectors and indirect X-ray detectors.[141] In direct X-ray detectors the flat-panel array is coupled to a photo-conductor, which detects the X-rays and produces an electrical charge that is then stored in the pixel storage capacitance until read out. In indirect detectors, the flat–panel array is coated with a phosphor material, which converts the detected X-rays to visible photons; these are then detected using a photoelectric converter in the pixel structure and stored in the pixel until read out (Figure 1.22a,b).

Evaluation of existing flat-panel X-ray detector technology shows that all current panels are based on thin film transistor (TFT) arrays. The TFT array consists of photo-diodes that collect light from a phosphor (selenium, cesium, or gadolinium); the photo-diodes cover the TFT array and convert incident x-rays to photons. Detector signal processing electronics convert the analog photo-diode signal to a true digital signal. TFT technology requires all connections between photo-diode to run horizontally, occupying potential active area. The TFT technology in medical applications limits active photo-diode area to about 50%, meaning that 50% of photons produced miss an active area and are discarded or contribute to noise by scattering into the adjacent detector areas.

Complementary metal oxide silicone (CMOS) is an alternate technology for producing flat-panel X-ray detectors.[142] CMOS allows much higher density circuits to be fabricated. CMOS is a three-dimensional process that allows active fill areas to approach 100%. CMOS flat panels have nearly double the efficiency of their TFT counterparts. The ability to incorporate the electronics on the same substrate as the detector array also allow significant reduction in heat. This technology also potentially allows more compact plates, greatly increased manufacturing yield by reducing physical connections, and improved system reliability and reduced service cost. Nevertheless, it remains to be seen whether this type of technology can be adapted for medical applications, and in particular angiographic systems, in an economic fashion.

One significant difference in the use of direct digital detectors versus image intensifiers in angiography systems is the much higher contrast sensitivity of the FD detectors as well as the lack of distortion (e.g. pin-cushion artifact) normally associated with image intensifiers.[143,144] Three-dimensional rotational acquisitions and reconstructions much more closely approximate conventional CT.[144–146] This may have significant implications in the detection of complications such as vascular perforation and hemorrhage (Figure 1.22c,d).[147] Additionally, when used with image fusion software and stereotactic techniques, such systems are likely to broaden the range of therapeutic maneuvers that are

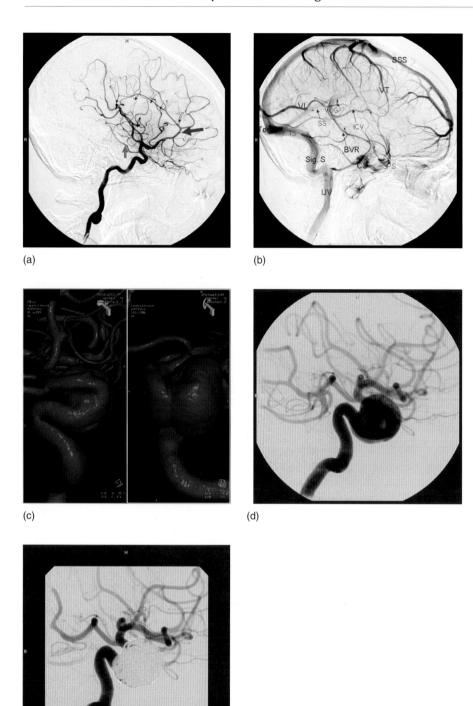

(a)

(b)

Figure 1.21

(a) Lateral carotid angiogram, arterial phase demonstrating anterior cerebral (red arrow), middle cerebral (blue arrows) and posterior cerebral (green arrows) arteries.
(b) Lateral carotid angiogram, venous phase, demonstrating Vein of Trolard (VT), Vein of Labbe (VL), Superior Sagittal Sinus (SSS), Torcula Herophili (Torc), Transverse Sinus (TS) Sigmoid Sinus (Sig S), Cavernous Sinus (CS), and SphenoParietal sinus (SPS). (c) 3D Surface reconstruction of a giant juxta-sellar aneurysm clearly demonstrates aneurysm neck and dome geometries.
(d) Planar angiogram with overlap obscuring aneurysm detail.
(e) Post-endovascular treatment enabled by 3D data.

(c)

(d)

(e)

possible using minimally invasive techniques. Possible limitations relate primarily to uncorrected artifact, which may be magnified by beam hardening (bone) and diminished by improved algorithms and additionally acquired projections.[145,148,150–156]

Summary

Digital imaging techniques afford critical information for the diagnosis and management of cerebrovascular disease.

While much of the information is anatomic, increasingly studies are performed to provide at least relative flow and physiologic insights. CT is widely available and offers the most rapid initial assessment. In the subacute time period (> 6 hours), MRI is extremely helpful in assessing the extent of injury as well as looking for the presence of more chronic hemorrhagic injuries. Ultrasound can be repeatedly transported into the intensive care unit for serial studies in critically ill patients. Nuclear medicine provides insights into complex conditions of cerebral ischemia. Catheter angiography provides increasingly detailed delineation of cerebral vascular anatomy in virtual real time,

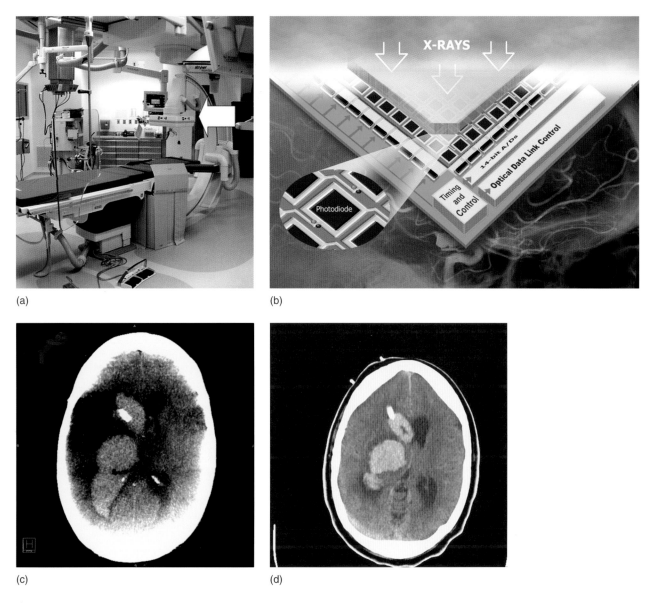

(a)   (b)

(c)   (d)

Figure 1.22
(a) Flat panel (FP) digital detector, single plane unit. Notice low, rectangular profile of detector (white arrow). (b) Detector.
(c) Volumetric, high contrast, 3D acquisition with axial 5 mm sliced displayed demonstrating thalamic hemorrhage with intra-ventricular extension. (d) Corresponding conventional CT scan.

enabling minimally invasive treatments for previously incurable disease states.

References

1. Generalized efficacy of t-PA for acute stroke. Subgroup analysis of the NINDS t-PA Stroke Trial. Stroke 1997; 28: 2119–25.
2. Fisher M, Pessin MS, Furian AJ. ECASS: lessons for future thrombolytic stroke trials. European Cooperative Acute Stroke Study. JAMA 1995; 274: 1058–59.
3. Hacke W, Kaste M, Fieschi C et al. Intravenous thrombolysis with recombinant tissue plasminogen activator for acute hemispheric stroke. The European Cooperative Acute Stroke Study (ECASS). JAMA 1995; 274: 1017–25.
4. Hacke W, Kaste M, Fieschi C et al. Randomised double-blind placebo controlled trial of thrombolytic therapy with intravenous alteplase in acute ischaemic stroke (ECASS II). Second European–Australasian Acute Stroke Study Investigators. Lancet 1998; 352: 1245–51.
5. Marler JR, Tilley BC, Lu M et al. Early stroke treatment associated with better outcome: the NINDS rt-PA stroke study. Neurology 2000; 55: 1649–55.
6. ACR Guidelines and Standards Committee, Applegate KE et al. ACR Practice guideline for communication of diagnostic imaging findings. American College of Radiology, 2005.
7. Cormack AM. Representation of a function by its line integrals, with some radiological applications. J Appl Phys 1963; 34: 2722–7.
8. Cormack AM. Representation of a Function by Its Line Integrals, with Some Radiological Applications.II. J Appl Phys 1964; 35: 2908–13.
9. Hounsfield GN. Nobel Award address. Computed medical imaging. Med Phys 1980; 7: 283–90.
10. Kalender WA, Seissler W, Klotz E, Vock P. Spiral volumetric CT with single-breath-hold technique, continuous transport, and continuous scanner rotation. Radiology 1990; 176: 181–3.

11. Gunnarsson T, Hillman J. Clinical usefulness of bedside intracranial morphological monitoring: mobile computerized tomography in the neurosurgery intensive care unit. Report of three cases. Neurosurg Focus 2000; 9: e5.

12. Gunnarsson T, Theodorsson A, Karlsson P et al. Mobile computerized tomography scanning in the neurosurgery intensive care unit: increase in patient safety and reduction of staff workload. J Neurosurg 2000; 93: 432–6.

13. Kruger RA, Riederer SJ, Mistretta CA. Relative properties of tomography, K-edge imaging, and K-edge tomography. Med Phys 1977; 4: 244–9.

14. von Kummer R, Allen KL, Holle R et al. Acute stroke: usefulness of early CT findings before thrombolytic therapy. Radiology 1997; 205: 327–33.

15. von Kummer R. Effect of training in reading CT scans on patient selection for ECASS II. Neurology 1998; 51: S50–2.

16. von Kummer R, Meyding-Lamade U, Forsting M et al. Sensitivity and prognostic value of early CT in occlusion of the middle cerebral artery trunk. AJNR Am J Neuroradiol 1994; 15: 9–15.

17. von Kummer R, Bourquain H, Bastianello S et al. Early prediction of irreversible brain damage after ischemic stroke at CT. Radiology 2001; 219: 95–100.

18. Lev MH, Farkas J, Gemmete JJ et al. Acute stroke: improved nonenhanced CT detection—benefits of soft-copy interpretation by using variable window width and center level settings. Radiology 1999; 213: 150–5.

19. Coutts SB, Lev MH, Eliasziw M et al. ASPECTS on CTA source images versus unenhanced CT: added value in predicting final infarct extent and clinical outcome. Stroke 2004; 35: 2472–6.

20. Provenzale JM, Jahan R, Naidich TP, Fox AJ. Assessment of the patient with hyperacute stroke: imaging and therapy. Radiology 2003; 229: 347–59.

21. Tomura N, Uemura K, Inugami A et al. Early CT finding in cerebral infarction: obscuration of the lentiform nucleus. Radiology 1988; 168: 463–7.

22. Truwit CL, Barkovich AJ, Gean-Marton A, Hibri N, Norman D. Loss of the insular ribbon: another early CT sign of acute middle cerebral artery infarction. Radiology 1990; 176: 801–6.

23. Tomandl BF, Kehrsbrfhwekf MS. Comprehensive imaging of ischemic stroke with multisection CT. Radiographics 2003; 23: 565–92.

24. Tomsick TA, Brott TG, Chambers AA et al. Hyperdense middle cerebral artery sign on CT: efficacy in detecting middle cerebral artery thrombosis. AJNR Am J Neuroradiol 1990; 11: 473–7.

25. Leys D, Pruvo JP, Godefroy O Rondepierre P, Leclerc X. Prevalence and significance of hyperdense middle cerebral artery in acute stroke. Stroke 1992; 23: 317–24.

26. Barber PA, Demchuk AM, Hudon ME et al. Hyperdense sylvian fissure MCA "dot" sign: A CT marker of acute ischemia. Stroke 2001; 32: 84–8.

27. Coutts SB, Demchuk AM, Barber PA et al. Interobserver variation of ASPECTS in real time. Stroke 2004; 35: e103–5.

28. Pexman JH, Barber PA, Hill MD et al. Use of the Alberta Stroke Program Early CT Score (ASPECTS) for assessing CT scans in patients with acute stroke. AJNR Am J Neuroradiol 2001; 22: 1534–42.

29. Davis KR, New PF, Ojemann RG et al. Computed tomographic evaluation of hemorrhage secondary to intracranial aneurysm. Am J Roentgenol 1976; 127: 143–53.

30. Schriger DL, Kalafut M, Starkman S, Krueger M, Saver JL. Cranial computed tomography interpretation in acute stroke: physician accuracy in determining eligibility for thrombolytic therapy [see comments]. JAMA 1998; 279: 1293–97.

31. Norman D, Price D, Boyd D, Fishman R, Newton TH. Quantitative aspects of computed tomography of the blood and cerebrospinal fluid. Radiology 1977; 123: 335–8.

32. Kistler JP, Crowell RM, Davis KR et al. The relation of cerebral vasospasm to the extent and location of subarachnoid blood visualized by CT scan: a prospective study. Neurology 1983; 33: 424–36.

33. Merten GJ, Burgess WP, Gray LV et al. Prevention of contrast-induced nephropathy with sodium bicarbonate: a randomized controlled trial. JAMA 2004; 291: 2328–34.

34. Rydberg J, Buckwalter KA, Caldemeyer KS et al. Multisection CT: scanning techniques and clinical applications. Radiographics 2000; 20: 1787–806.

35. Kato Y, Katada K, Hayakawa M et al. Can 3D-CTA surpass DSA in diagnosis of cerebral aneurysms. Acta Neurochir (Wien) 2001; 143: 245–50.

36. Kirchner J, Kickuth R, Laufer U, Noack M, Liermann D. Optimized enhancement in helical CT: experiences with a real-time bolus tracking system in 628 patients. Clin Radiol 2000; 55: 368–73.

37. van Hoe L, Marchal G, Baert AL, Gryspeerdt S, Mertens L. Determination of scan delay time in spiral CT-angiography: utility of a test bolus injection. J Comput Assist Tomogr 1995; 19: 216–20.

38. Lev MH, Farkas J, Rodriguez VR et al. CT angiography in the rapid triage of patients with hyperacute stroke to intraarterial thrombolysis: accuracy in the detection of large vessel thrombus. J Comput Assist Tomogr 2001; 25: 520–8.

39. Wildermuth S, Knauth M, Brandt T et al. Role of CT angiography in patient selection for thrombolytic therapy in acute hemispheric stroke. Stroke 1998; 29: 935–8.

40. Shrier DA, Tanaka H, Numaguchi Y et al. CT angiography in the evaluation of acute stroke. AJNR Am J Neuroradiol 1997; 18: 1011–20.

41. Cumming MJ, Morrow IM. Carotid artery stenosis: a prospective comparison of CT angiography and conventional angiography. AJR Am J Roentgenol 1994; 163: 517–23.

42. Chen CJ, Lee TH, Hsu HL et al. Multi-Slice CT angiography in diagnosing total versus near occlusions of the internal carotid artery: comparison with catheter angiography. Stroke 2004; 35: 83–5.

43. Heiss WD. Ischemic penumbra: evidence from functional imaging in man. J Cereb Blood Flow Metab 2000; 20: 1276–93.

44. Derdeyn CP, Grubb RL Jr, Powers WJ. Cerebral hemodynamic impairment: methods of measurement and association with stroke risk. Neurology 1999; 53: 251–9.

45. Latchaw RE, Yonas H, Hunter GJ et al. Guidelines and recommendations for perfusion imaging in cerebral ischemia: A scientific statement for healthcare professionals by the writing group on perfusion imaging, from the council on cardiovascular radiology of the american heart association. Stroke 2003; 34: 1084–104.

46. Reichenbach JR, Rother J, Jonetz-Mentzel L et al. Acute stroke evaluated by time-to-peak mapping during initial and early follow-up perfusion CT studies. AJNR Am J Neuroradiol 1999; 20: 1842–50.

47. Hunter GJ, Hamberg LM, Ponzo JA et al. Assessment of cerebral perfusion and arterial anatomy in hyperacute stroke with three-dimensional functional CT: early clinical results. AJNR Am J Neuroradiol 1998; 19: 29–37.

48. Lev MH, Segal AZ, Farkas J et al. Utility of perfusion-weighted CT imaging in acute middle cerebral artery stroke treated with intra-arterial thrombolysis: prediction of final infarct volume and clinical outcome. Stroke 2001; 32: 2021–28.

49. Klotz E, Konig M. Perfusion measurements of the brain: using dynamic CT for the quantitative assessment of cerebral ischemia in acute stroke. Eur J Radiol 1999; 30: 170–84.

50. Cook AJ. Comparison of contrast injection protocols in CT brain perfusion using two calculation algorithms. Radiology 2001; 221(P): 480.

51. Axel L. Cerebral blood flow determination by rapid-sequence computed tomography: theoretical analysis. Radiology 1980; 137: 679–86.

52. Nabavi DG, Cenic A, Craen RA et al. CT assessment of cerebral perfusion: experimental validation and initial clinical experience. Radiology 1999; 213: 141–9.

53. Wintermark M, Maeder P, Thiran JP, Schnyder P, Meuli R. Quantitative assessment of regional cerebral blood flows by perfusion CT studies at low injection rates: a critical review of the underlying theoretical models. Eur Radiol 2001; 11: 1220–30.

54. Eastwood JD, Engelter ST, MacFall JF, Delong DM, Provenzale JM. Quantitative assessment of the time course of infarct signal intensity

on diffusion-weighted images. AJNR Am J Neuroradiol 2003; 24: 680–7.

55. Wintermark M, Thiran JP, Maeder P, Schnyder P, Meuli R. Simultaneous measurement of regional cerebral blood flow by perfusion CT and stable xenon CT: a validation study. AJNR Am J Neuroradiol 2001; 22: 905–14.

56. Fiorella D, Heiserman J, Prenger E, Partovi S. Assessment of the Reproducibility of Postprocessing Dynamic CT Perfusion Data. AJNR Am J Neuroradiol 2004; 25: 97–107.

57. Mayer TE, Hamann GF, Baranczyk J et al. Dynamic CT perfusion imaging of acute stroke. AJNR Am J Neuroradiol 2000; 21: 1441–9.

58. Koenig M, Klotz E, Luka B et al. Perfusion CT of the brain: diagnostic approach for early detection of ischemic stroke. Radiology 1998; 209: 85–93.

59. Koenig M, Kraus M, Theek C et al. Quantitative assessment of the ischemic brain by means of perfusion-related parameters derived from perfusion CT. Stroke 2001; 32: 431–7.

60. Carr HY PE. Effects of diffusion on free precession in nuclear magnetic resonance experiments. Physiol Rev 1954; 94: 630–8.

61. Leach MO. Nobel Prize in Physiology or Medicine 2003 awarded to Paul Lauterbur and Peter Mansfield for discoveries concerning magnetic resonance imaging. Phys Med Biol 2004; 49: 2.

62. Shellock FG. Reference manual for magnetic resonance safety implants and devices: 2006 Edition. Los Angeles, CA: Biomedical Research Publishing Group; 2006.

63. Atlas SW, Mark AS, Grossman RI, Gomori JM. Intracranial hemorrhage: gradient-echo MR imaging at 1.5 T. Comparison with spin-echo imaging and clinical applications. Radiology 1988; 168: 803–7.

64. Gomori JM, Grossman RI, Goldberg HI, Zimmerman RA, Bilaniuk LT. Intracranial hematomas: imaging by high-field MR. Radiology 1985; 157: 87–93.

65. Ozdoba C, Sturzenegger M, Schroth G. Internal carotid artery dissection: MR imaging features and clinical-radiologic correlation. Radiology 1996; 199: 191–8.

66. Ahlhelm F, Schneider G, Backens M, Reith W, Hagen T. Time course of the apparent diffusion coefficient after cerebral infarction. Eur Radiol 2002; 12: 2322–9.

67. Reith W, Hasegawa Y, Latour LL et al. Multislice diffusion mapping for 3-D evolution of cerebral ischemia in a rat stroke model. Neurology 1995; 45: 172–7.

68. Geijer B, Lindgren A, Brockstedt S, Stahlberg F, Holtas. Persistent high signal on diffusion-weighted MRI in the late stages of small cortical and lacunar ischaemic lesions. Neuroradiology 2001; 43: 115–22.

69. Nagesh V, Welch KM, Windham JP et al. Time course of ADCw changes in ischemic stroke: beyond the human eye! Stroke 1998; 29: 1778–82.

70. Schaefer PW, Hunter GJ, He J et al. Predicting cerebral ischemic infarct volume with diffusion and perfusion MR imaging. AJNR J Neuroradiol 2002; 23: 1785–94.

71. Rodda RA. The arterial patterns associated with internal carotid disease and cerebral infarcts. Stroke 1986; 17: 69–75.

72. Ringelstein EB, Schneider R, Koschorke S. Analysis of patterns of hemispheric brain infarctions on CT: embolic stroke mechanism, territorial infarctions and lacunae. Psychiatry Res 1989; 29: 273–6.

73. Ackerstaff RG, Jansen C, Moll FL et al. The significance of microemboli detection by means of transcranial Doppler ultrasonography monitoring in carotid endarterectomy. J Vasc Surg 1995; 21: 963–9.

74. Tomczak R, Wunderlich A, Liewald F et al. Diffusion-weighted MRI: detection of cerebral ischemia before and after carotid thromboendarterectomy. J Comput Assist Tomogr 2001; 25: 247–50.

75. Muller M, Reiche W, Langenscheidt P et al. Ischemia after carotid endarterectomy: comparison between transcranial Doppler sonography and diffusion-weighted MR imaging. AJNR Am J Neuroradiol 2000; 21: 47–54.

76. van Heesewijk HP, Vos JA, Louwerse ES et al. New brain lesions at MR imaging after carotid angioplasty and stent placement. Radiology 2002; 224: 361–5.

77. Jaeger HJ, Mathias KD, Drescher R et al. Diffusion-weighted MR imaging after angioplasty or angioplasty plus stenting of arteries supplying the brain. AJNR Am J Neuroradiol 2001; 22: 1251–9.

78. Feiwell RJ, Besmertis L, Sarkar R, Saloner DA, Rapp JH. Detection of clinically silent infarcts after carotid endarterectomy by use of diffusion-weighted imaging. AJNR Am J Neuroradiol 2001; 22: 646–9.

79. Wolf O, Heider P, Heinz M et al. Frequency, clinical significance and course of cerebral ischemic events after carotid endarterectomy evaluated by serial diffusion weighted imaging. Eur J Vasc Endovasc Surg 2004; 27: 167–71.

80. Ay H, Buonanno FS, Rordorf G et al. Normal diffusion-weighted MRI during stroke-like deficits. Neurology 1999; 52: 1784–92.

81. Lefkowitz D, LaBenz M, Nudo SR, Steg RE, Bertoni JM. Hyperacute ischemic stroke missed by diffusion-weighted imaging. AJNR Am J Neuroradiol 1999; 20: 1871–5.

82. Lovblad KO, Bassetti C, Schneider J et al. Diffusion-weighted MRI suggests the coexistence of cytotoxic and vasogenic oedema in a case of deep cerebral venous thrombosis. Neuroradiology 2000; 42: 728–31.

83. Keller E, Flacke S, Urbach H, Schild HH. Diffusion- and perfusion weighted magnetic resonance imaging in deep cerebral venous thrombosis. Stroke 1999; 30: 1144–6.

84. Oppenheim C, Stanescu R, Dormont D et al. False-negative diffusion weighted MR findings in acute ischemic stroke. AJNR Am J Neuroradiol 2000; 21: 1434–40.

85. Stadnik TW, Demaerel P, Luypaert RR et al. Imaging tutorial: differential diagnosis of bright lesions on diffusion-weighted MR images. Radiographics 2003; 23: e7.

86. Burdette JH, Elster AD, Ricci PE. Acute cerebral infarction: quantification of spin-density and T2 shine-through phenomena on diffusion-weighted MR images. Radiology 1999; 212: 333–9.

87. Schlaug G, Siewert B, Benfield A et al. Time course of the apparent diffusion coefficient (ADC) abnormality in human stroke. Neurology 1997; 49: 113–9.

88. Atlas SW. MR angiography in neurologic disease. Radiology 1994; 193: 1–16.

89. Nederkoorn PJ, van der GY, Eikelboom BC et al. Time-of-flight MR angiography of carotid artery stenosis: does a flow void represent severe stenosis? AJNR Am J Neuroradiol 2002; 23: 1779–84.

90. Patel MR, Kuntz KM, Klufas RA et al. Preoperative assessment of the carotid bifurcation. Can magnetic resonance angiography and duplex ultrasonography replace contrast arteriography? Stroke 1995; 26: 1753–8.

91. Saloner D. The AAPM/RSNA physics tutorial for residents. An introduction to MR angiography. Radiographics 1995; 15: 453–65.

92. Laub G. Principles of contrast-enhanced MR angiography. Basic and clinical applications. Magn Reson Imaging Clin North Am 1999; 7: 783–95.

93. Back MR, Wilson JS, Rushing G et al. Magnetic resonance angiography is an accurate imaging adjunct to duplex ultrasound scan in patient selection for carotid endarterectomy. J Vasc Surg 2000; 32: 429–38.

94. Borisch I, Horn M, Butz B et al. Preoperative evaluation of carotid artery stenosis: comparison of contrast-enhanced MR angiography and duplex sonography with digital subtraction angiography. AJNR Am J Neuroradiol 2003; 24: 1117–22.

95. Hathout GM, Duh MJ, El Saden SM. Accuracy of contrast-enhanced MR angiography in predicting angiographic stenosis of the internal carotid artery: linear regression analysis. AJNR Am J Neuroradiol 2003; 24: 1747–56.

96. Farb RI, Nag S, Scott JN et al. Surveillance of intracranial aneurysms treated with detachable coils: a comparison of MRA techniques. Neuroradiology 2005; 47: 507–15.

97. Gauvrit JY, Leclerc X, Caron S et al. Intracranial aneurysms treated with Guglielmi detachable coils: imaging follow-up with contrast-enhanced MR angiography. Stroke 2006; 37: 1033–7.

98. Masaryk AM, Frayne R, Unal O, Rappe AH, Strother CM. Utility of CT angiography and MR angiography for the follow-up of experimental aneurysms treated with stents or Guglielmi detachable coils. AJNR Am J Neuroradiol 2000; 21: 1523–31.

99. Tsuruda J, Saloner D, Norman D. Artifacts associated with MR neuroangiography. AJNR Am J Neuroradiol 1992; 13: 1411–22.

100. Anderson CM, Saloner D, Lee RE, Fortner A. Dedicated coil for carotid MR angiography. Radiology 1990; 176: 868–72.

101. Wardlaw JM, Lewis SC, Collie DA, Sellar R. Interobserver variability of magnetic resonance angiography in the diagnosis of carotid stenosis—effect of observer experience. Neuroradiology 2002; 44: 126–32.

102. Villringer A, Rosen BR, Belliveau JW et al. Dynamic imaging with lanthanide chelates in normal brain: contrast due to magnetic susceptibility effects. Magn Reson Med 1988; 6: 164–74.

103. Schaefer PW, Romero JM, Grant PE et al. Perfusion magnetic resonance imaging of acute ischemic stroke. Semin Roentgenol 2002; 37: 230–6.

104. Kluytmans M, van Everdingen KJ, Kappelle LJ et al. Prognostic value of perfusion- and diffusion-weighted MR imaging in first 3 days of stroke. Eur Radiol 2000; 10: 1434–41.

105. Wilkinson ID, Griffiths PD, Hoggard N et al. Short-term changes in cerebral microhemodynamics after carotid stenting. AJNR Am J Neuroradiol 2003; 24: 1501–7.

106. Sorensen AG, Copen WA, Ostergaard L et al. Hyperacute stroke: simultaneous measurement of relative cerebral blood volume, relative cerebral blood flow, and mean tissue transit time. Radiology 1999; 210: 519–27.

107. Sorensen AG, Buonanno FS, Gonzalez RG et al. Hyperacute stroke: evaluation with combined multisection diffusion-weighted and hemodynamically weighted echo-planar MR imaging. Radiology 1996; 199: 391–401.

108. Karonen JO, Partanen PL, Vanninen RL, Vainio PA, Aronen H. Evolution of MR contrast enhancement patterns during the first week after acute ischemic stroke. AJNR Am J Neuroradiol 2001; 22: 103–11.

109. Singer OC, de Rochemont RM, Foerch C et al. Relation between relative cerebral blood flow, relative cerebral blood volume, and mean transit time in patients with acute ischemic stroke determined by perfusion-weighted MRI. J Cereb Blood Flow Metab 2003; 23: 605–11.

110. Wittsack HJ, Ritzl A, Fink GR et al. MR imaging in acute stroke: diffusion weighted and perfusion imaging parameters for predicting infarct size. Radiology 2002; 222: 397–403.

111. Hacke W, Albers G, Al-Rawi Y et al. The Desmoteplase in Acute Ischemic Stroke Trial (DIAS): a phase II MRI-based 9-hour window acute stroke thrombolysis trial with intravenous desmoteplase. Stroke 2005; 36: 66–73.

112. Furlan AJ, Eyding D, Albers GW et al. Dose Escalation of Desmoteplase for Acute Ischemic Stroke (DEDAS): evidence of safety and efficacy 3 to 9 hours after stroke onset. Stroke 2006; 37: 1227–31.

113. Walovitch RC, Cheesman EH, Maheu LJ, Hall KM. Studies of the retention mechanism of the brain perfusion imaging agent 99mTc-bicisate (99mTc-ECD). J Cereb Blood Flow Metab 1994; 14(Suppl): S4–11.

114. Derdeyn CP, Videen TO, Yundt KD et al. Variability of cerebral blood volume and oxygen extraction: stages of cerebral haemodynamic impairment revisited. Brain 2002; 125: 595–607.

115. Derdeyn CP, Gage BF, Grubb RL, Powers WJ. Cost-Effectiveness of PET Screening Prior to EC/IC Bypass in Patients with Carotid Occlusion. Clin Positron Imaging 1999; 2: 341.

116. Derdeyn CP, Videen TO, Grubb RL Jr, Powers WJ. Comparison of PET oxygen extraction fraction methods for the prediction of stroke risk. J Nucl Med 2001; 42: 1195–97.

117. Derdeyn CP, Grubb RL Jr, Powers WJ. Re: Stages and thresholds of hemodynamic failure. Stroke 2003; 34: 589.

118. Edler I, Hertz CH. The use of ultrasonic reflectoscope for the continuous recording of the movements of heart walls. 1954. Clin Physiol Funct Imaging 2004; 24: 118–36.

119. Franklin DL, Schlegel W, Rushmer RF. Blood flow measured by Doppler frequency shift of back-scattered ultrasound. Science 1961; 134: 564–5.

120. Kaneko Z. First steps in the development of the Doppler flowmeter. Ultrasound Med Biol 1986; 12: 187–95.

121. Aaslid R, Huber P, Nornes H. Evaluation of cerebrovascular spasm with transcranial Doppler ultrasound. J Neurosurg 1984; 60: 37–41.

122. de Rochemont RM, Turowski B, Buchkremer M et al. Recurrent symptomatic high-grade intracranial stenoses: safety and efficacy of undersized stents—initial experience. Radiology 2004; 231: 45–9.

123. Ringelstein EB, Droste DW, Babikian VL et al. Consensus on microembolus detection by TCD. International Consensus Group on Microembolus Detection. Stroke 1998; 29: 725–9.

124. Sugimori H, Ibayashi S, Fujii K et al. Can transcranial Doppler really detect reduced cerebral perfusion states? Stroke 1995; 26: 2053–60.

125. White H, Venkatesh B. Applications of transcranial Doppler in the ICU: a review. Intensive Care Med 2006; 32: 981–94.

126. Alexandrov AV, Wojner AW, Grotta JC. CLOTBUST: design of a randomized trial of ultrasound-enhanced thrombolysis for acute ischemic stroke. J Neuroimaging 2004; 14: 108–12.

127. Mahon BR, Nesbit GM, Barnwell SL et al. North American clinical experience with the EKOS MicroLysUS infusion catheter for the treatment of embolic stroke. AJNR Am J Neuroradiol 2003; 24: 534–8.

128. Howard G, Baker WH, Chambless LE et al. An approach for the use of Doppler ultrasound as a screening tool for hemodynamically significant stenosis (despite heterogeneity of Doppler performance). A multicenter experience. Asymptomatic Carotid Atherosclerosis Study Investigators. Stroke 1996; 27: 1951–7.

129. Haschek E, Lindenthal OT. Ein Beitrag zur praktischen Verwertung der Photographie nach Röntgen. Wien Klin Wochensch 1896; 9: 63–4.

130. Moniz E. Die cerebral arteriographie und Phlebographie. Berlin, Germany: Springer-Verlag, 1949.

131. Moniz E. L'encéphalographie artérielle, son importance dans la localisation des tumeurs cérébrales. Rev Neurol (Paris) 1927; 2: 72–90.

132. Littleton JT. For the record: the origin of the rapid serial sheet-film changer. AJR Am J Roentgenol 1994; 163: 282.

133. Kruger RA, Mistretta CA, Houk TL et al. Computerized fluoroscopy in real time for noninvasive visualization of the cardiovascular system. Preliminary studies. Radiology 1979; 130: 49–57.

134. Kruger RA, Mistretta CA, Crummy AB et al. Digital K-edge subtraction radiography. Radiology 1977; 125: 243–5.

135. Mistretta CA, Ort MG, Cameron JR et al. A multiple image subtraction technique for enhancing low contrast, periodic objects. Invest Radiol 1973; 8: 43–9.

136. Serbinenko FA. Balloon catheterization and occlusion of major cerebral vessels. J Neurosurg 1974; 41: 125–45.

137. Gruntzig A. Transluminal dilatation of coronary-artery stenosis. Lancet 1978; 1: 263.

138. Abe T, Hirohata M, Tanaka N et al. Clinical benefits of rotational 3D angiography in endovascular treatment of ruptured cerebral aneurysm. AJNR Am J Neuroradiol 2002; 23: 686–8.

139. Sugahara T, Korogi Y, Nakashima K et al. Comparison of 2D and 3D digital subtraction angiography in evaluation of intracranial aneurysms. AJNR Am J Neuroradiol 2002; 23: 1545–52.

140. Anxionnat R, Bracard S, Macho J et al. 3D angiography. Clinical interest. First applications in interventional neuroradiology. J Neuroradiol 1998; 25: 251–62.

141. Watanabe M, Mochizuki C, Kameshima T et al. Development and evaluation of a portable amorphous silicon flat panel X-ray detector. SPIE 2001; 4320: 1–12.

142. Janesick J. Charge coupled CMOS and hybrid detector arrays. Proceedings of SPIE 5167. 2003.

143. Hamer OW, Volk M, Zorger Z, Feuerbach S, Strotzer M. Amorphous silicon, flat-panel, x-ray detector versus storage phosphor-

based computed radiography: contrast-detail phantom study at different tube voltages and detector entrance doses. Invest Radiol 2003; 38: 212–20.

144. Rapp-Bernhardt U, Roehl FW, Gibbs RC et al. Flat-panel x-ray detector based on amorphous silicon versus asymmetric screen-film system: phantom study of dose reduction and depiction of simulated findings. Radiology 2003; 227: 484–92.

145. Jaffray DA, Siewerdsen JH. Cone-beam computed tomography with a flat-panel imager: initial performance characterization. Med Phys 2000; 27: 1311–23.

146. Groh BA, Siewerdsen JH, Drake DG, Wong JW, Jaffray DA. A performance comparison of flat-panel imager-based MV and kV cone-beam CT. Med Phys 2002; 29: 967–75.

147. Heran NS, Song JK, Namba K et al. The utility of DynaCT in neuroendovascular procedures. AJNR Am J Neuroradiol 2006; 27: 330–2.

148. Ning R, Chen B, Yu R et al. Flat panel detector-based cone-beam volume CT angiography imaging: system evaluation. IEEE Trans Med Imaging 2000; 19: 949–63.

149. Ning R, Tang X, Conover D, Yu R. Flat panel detector-based cone beam computed tomography with a circle-plus-two-arcs data acquisition orbit: preliminary phantom study. Med Phys 2003; 30: 1694–705.

150. Tang X, Ning R, Yu R, Conover D. Cone beam volume CT image artifacts caused by defective cells in x-ray flat panel imagers and the artifact removal using a wavelet-analysis-based algorithm. Med Phys 2001; 28: 812–25.

151. Jaffray DA, Siewerdsen JH, Wong JW, Martinez AA. Flat-panel cone-beam computed tomography for image-guided radiation therapy. Int J Radiat Oncol Biol Phys 2002; 53: 1337–49.

152. Endarterectomy for asymptomatic carotid artery stenosis. Executive Committee for the Asymptomatic Carotid Atherosclerosis Study. JAMA 1995; 273: 1421–8.

153. Siewerdsen JH, Jaffray DA. Cone-beam computed tomography with a flat-panel imager: effects of image lag. Med Phys 1999; 26: 2635–47.

154. Siewerdsen JH, Jaffray DA. A ghost story: spatio-temporal response characteristics of an indirect-detection flat-panel imager. Med Phys 1999; 26: 1624–41.

155. Siewerdsen JH, Jaffray DA. Optimization of x-ray imaging geometry (with specific application to flat-panel cone-beam computed tomography). Med Phys 2000; 27: 1903–14.

156. Siewerdsen JH, Jaffray DA. Cone-beam computed tomography with a flat-panel imager: magnitude and effects of x-ray scatter. Med Phys 2001; 28: 220–31.

2

The angiography suite: diagnostic devices and maneuvers

David Fiorella and Thomas J Masaryk

While the full digitization and post-processing of cerebral angiography has evolved in remarkable ways to create a new repertoire of therapeutic procedures, there are basic elements of the suite that have remained constant. Diligent attention to these fundamental components is required to insure safe delivery of efficacious care.

The endovascular suite: room design and radiation safety

As with many contemporary hospital endeavors, purchasing and siting a dedicated cerebral angiography suite is an inherently expensive and complex proposition. Typical competitors involved in the negotiation for resources and space will include (at a minimum) the departments of radiology, neurosurgery, anesthesia, pharmacy, central supply, nursing, and information technology. As with an operating room, the pivot points about which these accommodations are made are the location of the patient table and the anesthesia machine, gas lines, and suction. Unlike the operating room there are large, mobile, radiation-producing C-arms integral to the configuration, that pose special safety issues (particularly in the era of rotational three-dimensional angiography and flat-panel CT).[1] Co-ordinated efforts to maximize patient access while minimizing the radiation exposure risk to personnel and patients have perhaps been best articulated for pediatric patients (for whom the stochastic effects of radiation are greater) in the form of 'the ALARA concept' (As Low As Reasonably Achievable) (Figure 2.1).[2]

Radiation safety

Rationale

With the advance of endovascular techniques from surgical complement to primary treatment[3] and the introduction of new devices[4] more patients and healthcare workers are being exposed to ever larger doses of radiation. This has led to public expression of concern by numerous healthcare regulatory agencies within the USA.[5–7]

The health hazards inherent in exposure to diagnostic X-rays are produced through the transfer of energy to tissue by indirect ionization. This process can be further subdivided into:

- photoelectric effect
- Compton effect
- coherent scattering.

Photoelectric effect (i.e. the discharge of inner shell electrons from atoms by X-rays) is useful insofar as it creates angiographic image contrast (the effect is proportional to the third power of atomic number) through ready visualization of bone or iodinated contrast. Alternatively, as this occurs with lower energy X-rays, and all of the energy is absorbed by the tissue, it is a substantial contributor to patient dose. (This effect can be minimized by maximizing the energy of the X-rays through increases in voltage, although at the expense of image contrast.)

The Compton effect describes an incident X-ray photon that loses only a fraction of its incident energy by discharging an outer shell target electron, but the X-ray continues, albeit deflected, at a lower energy. These 'scattered' X-Rays result in most of the radiation exposure to healthcare personnel, at energies near those of the incident photon. This can reduced by limiting the amount of X-rays used (i.e. reducing mA), but at the expense of image signal to noise.

Coherent scattering contributes a minimal amount to indirect ionization. The ionizing effects of radiation (i.e. the creation of photoelectrons or recoil electrons) lead to the formation of free radicals, which may interact with, and thus damage, tissue (notably nucleic acid base pairs). It should be noted that different tissues vary in their susceptibility to the ionizing effects of diagnostic X-rays.

Nomenclature and definitions

The effect of tissue damage created by radiation exposure can be subdivided into genetic effects (the effects created by DNA injury to normal germ cells), and somatic effects (local tissue damage and future carcinogenesis). Genetic and carcinogenic effects are often referred to as stochastic effects. Although the tissue response is clearly dose dependent, the severity of the effect is not precisely known at typical levels of exposure seen with diagnostic studies, and it is thus best described in the form of a probability.

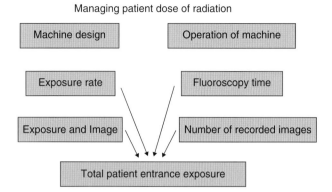

Figure 2.1
As Low As Reasonably Achievable (ALARA) steps to reduce radiation exposure. Reprinted with permission from Radiology.

Non-genetic, non-carcinogenic effects can be described by a dose–response relationship in which the severity beyond a threshold is known, and it is thus termed 'deterministic.' Certain medical conditions may predispose to deterministic effects, these including diabetes mellitus, mixed connective tissue disorders, and hereditary telangiectasia.[8]

The word 'kerma' is an acronymn for 'kinetic energy released in material', 'kinetic energy released in matter', or sometimes 'kinetic energy released per unit mass'. Kerma is the sum of the initial kinetic energies of all the charged particles liberated by uncharged ionizing radiation in a sample of matter, divided by the mass of the sample. The unit for kerma is Joule per kilogram, and the name given it is the gray (Gy), where 1 Gy = 1 J/kg. The amount of ionizing radiation that exists at a position in space (e.g. the output of a fluoroscope) is defined as 'air kerma' and designated as Gy_a. Given that radiation can be distributed over a variable region, the concentration of energy imparted to a cross-sectional area of air (air kerma multiplied by the area of the X-ray beam) is referred to as the dose–area product (DAP). Contemporary X-ray equipment (manufactured on or after June 10, 2006) must display the operator's air kerma rate and cumulative air kerma (equivalent to the estimated cumulative skin dose.)

The concentration of energy actually deposited in tissue, and thus of potential health consequence, is the 'absorbed dose'. Absorbed tissue dose is likewise measured in gray but is designated Gy_t. For the purposes of specifying the risk of skin injury, cataract, and so on (i.e. dose to the patient), absorbed dose is the term most often used. This is often referred in with a temporal reference (e.g. Gy/hour). The absorbed dose rate in the skin from direct beam fluoroscopy is 0.02–0.05 Gy/minute, but may range from 0.01 to more than 0.5 Gy/minute depending on the fluoroscopic mode and the size of the patient. Typical concerns for patients undergoing neuroendovascular procedures include the dose to the skin as well as dose to the lens of the eye and thyroid (Table 2.1.) It is also worth noting that specific procedures (e.g. staged embolization of an arteriovenous malformation) are associated with greater exposure.[4,9] Presently, for the purposes of quality assurance, we document the dose in each plane for every procedure, and we follow up clinically with special attention where cumulative skin exposures dose exceeds 1Gy.

'Equivalent dose' is the tissue dose that accounts for the different ionizing properties of other forms of radiation, and the unit of measure is the Sievert (Sv). When used in the context of gamma-radiation used for fluoroscopy and diagnostic

Table 2.1 Radiation-induced skin injuries

Effect	Dose (Gy)	Time to Onset
Early transient erythema	2	Hours
Temporary epilation	3	3 weeks
Main erythema	6	10 days
Permanent epilation	7	3 weeks
Dry desquamation	10	4 weeks
Invasive fibrosis	10	Varies
Dermal atrophy	11	> 14 weeks
Telangiectasis	12	> 52 weeks
Moist desquamation	15	4 weeks
Late erythema	15	6–10 weeks
Dermal necrosis	18	> 10 weeks
Secondary ulceration	20	> 6 weeks

Adapted from Wagner LK, Eifel PJ, Geise RA. Potential biological effects following high X-ray dose interventional procedures. J Vas Intervent Radiol 1994; 5: 71–84.

Table 2.2 Annual threshold for healthcare workers

Exposure area	Exposure limit (mSv)
Deep (whole body)	50
Lens of eye	150
Shallow (skin)	500
Extremities	500

angiography, the absorbed dose in Gy is the same quantitative value as the equivalent dose (i.e 1 Sv = 1 Gy).

'Effective dose' is the quantitative value designed to account for the fact human exposure is typically non-uniform. The effective dose is that dose that would have to be given to the entire unprotected body to produce the same health effect as a non-uniform dose delivered to a specific tissue. This too is measured in Sievert or milliSievert. As noted previously, different tissues (e.g. bone marrow, neurons, gonads) have varying sensitivities to ionizing radiation. Based on recommendations of the International Commission on Radiological Protection (ICRP), different tissues are assigned weighting factors based on their inherent sensitivity to ionizing radiation.[10] These weighting factors can be used to calculate equivalent whole body exposure. For regulatory and protection purposes of healthcare personnel, exposure limits are given in terms of effective dose.[11] This exposure is serially monitored with film badges worn at the point of highest exposure between the waist and neck. Typical annual threshold occupational doses for healthcare workers are listed in Table 2.2.

Maneuvers to minimize risk to patients

- Monitor dose to patient. Include in quality-assurance program.
- Keep the kVp as high as possible (and mA as low as possible) to achieve the appropriate compromise between image quality and low patient dose. As kVp increases, image

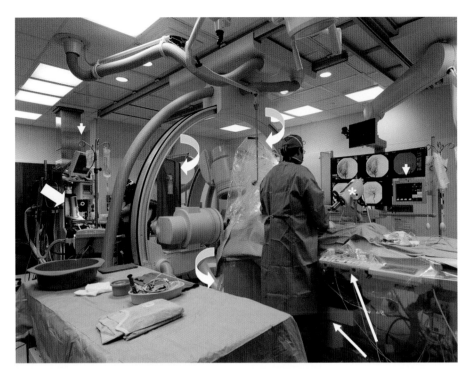

Figure 2.2
Angiography suite with C-arms in place and patient under general anesthesia. Curved arrows identify lead wall, lead skirt (below table), and lead shield (suspended above table) for radiation protection of operator and anesthesiologist. Arrowheads depict distributed physiologic monitors. Thick arrow points to lighted anesthesia machine. Long arrows identify operator controls and table pedestal. Asterisk denotes the power injector mount on the table in close proximity to the vascular access site.

contrast decreases. Patient dose decreases if mA is reduced, and dose to personnel in the room usually decreases.

- Keep the X-ray source as far away from the patient to minimize dose to the skin
- Keep the image intensifier as close to the patient as possible.
- Do not overuse geometric or electronic magnification. Magnification almost always results in increased dose rate to the patient's skin. The least magnification consistent with the goals of the procedure should be used in conjunction with collimation to manage radiation properly.
- Always collimate down to the area of interest. Applying tight collimation improves image quality by reducing scatter, lessens the radiation burden to the patient by reducing the volume of tissue exposed, and reduces dose to personnel in the room by reducing scatter.
- Minimize fluoroscopy time.
- Minimize the number of digital subtraction runs and three-dimensional rotational angiograms.

Maneuvers to minimize risk to personnel

- Monitor dose to staff.
- Wear protective equipment and use shielding. Lead screens, walls or curtains can be particularly helpful not only for the primary operator, but also for ancillary personnel such as the anesthesiologists (Figure 2.2).
- Distance: staff should position themselves (relative to the X-ray source) for minimum dose. The 'inverse square law' applies such that exposure is reduced by a factor of four for every doubling of distance from the source.
- Keep fluoroscopy time to a minimum.
- Pulsed fluoroscopy: use the least number of pulses necessary to perform the procedure – usually 15 pulses/second or less.

- Minimize the number of digital subtraction runs and exposures. The X-ray flux produced by full-image exposure is substantially higher than conventional fluoroscopy or roadmap fluoroscopy. This is the single largest determinant of X-ray dose for endovascular neurosurgical procedures.[9] For complex vascular anatomy, the ability of three-dimensional rotational studies to preclude a multitude of conventional planar exposures (as well as the inherently lower dose technique) may afford a substantial dose savings.[1,12]

The angiography system

As noted previously, the features included in contemporary cerebral angiography systems are ever expanding. Key components and potential features that may play a role in safety, as well as in the ability to complete treatments successfully, include the patient task, the C-arms, and the host computer.

Features of the patient table to consider are:

- weight limit
- tilt (+/− degree Trendelenberg)
- break
- adaptable radiolucent head-holder.

Features of the C-Arms to consider are:

- X-Ray source
- focal spot size
- heat limit
- pulsed fluoroscopy
- X-ray detector (analog II versus digital flat panel, size (area covered), magnification steps, and spatial resolution and matrix)
- mechanization
- arc of rotation
- speed of rotation.

Features of the host computer to consider are:

- disk space
- user interface (tableside or control console)
- image recall and display (for angiography and non-angiographic studies)
- three-dimensionality
- reconstruction time
- display and interface.

Ancillary equipment

As the angiography suite has come to assume a greater therapeutic role in cerebral vascular disease, additional accommodations have become necessary to fulfill this role successfully. Already alluded to is the need for anesthesia gas lines, suction, and the floor space for anesthesia machines, warming and cooling devices, etc. Distributed physiologic monitoring for pulse, blood pressure, heart rhythm, oxygen saturation, and intracranial pressure are available not only to the anesthesiologist but also to the operator and in the control room (see Figure 2.2). For specific cases there may be a need for surgical instruments, electrocautery (e.g. for cut-down vascular access) or for specialized cardiovascular devices (e.g. transvenous pacemaker for high-risk carotid stenting) to be available in the room during the procedure.

There will also need to be some accommodation for a wider spectrum of pharmacologic agents and means for their safe and secure storage (see Chapter 3). Likewise, one may need point-of-service testing to facilitate patient monitoring and therapeutic titration of these agents. This type of testing may include spot serum creatinine, blood sugar, activated clotting time, and even platelet function studies. Use of such testing requires implementation of a documented quality-assurance program to ensure accuracy and precision over time.

Diagnostic angiography devices and maneuvers

The ability to perform and interpret a cerebral angiogram safely and successfully is a function of many variables, not the least of which are:

- a full understanding of the diagnostic goals of the study (including review of previous imaging studies)
- unique patient risk factors (allergies; previous surgery; vascular risk factors (such as smoking, diabetes, and hypertension); and medications (such as warfarin and metformin)
- the experience and training of the operator.

The last-named variable above is perhaps the most important, yet the most difficult to quantify.[13] Although endovascular surgical neuroradiology is now a subspecialty with ACGME-and-RRC-vetted training guidelines, few training programs are formally approved. Even in the context of formal instruction, objective assessment of one's own skill set, judicious planning, conservative management, and willingness to consult colleagues and to participate in continuous quality improvement are characteristics not easily quantified by mere case log numbers.[14–17]

Catheters

Vascular access, while occasionally creative, is most frequently performed utilizing the Seldinger technique via one of the common femoral arteries.[18] Per Amundsen of Norway, working in San Francisco, is often credited with refining and popularizing this technique in the USA, and with good reason. It has the advantage of physically removing the operator from the X-ray beam, allowing for aggressive hemostasis (particularly in cases requiring continuous anticoagulation), and it is more easily tolerated in awake patients.[19] The use of micro-puncture access kits for these maneuvers has greatly minimized the risk of vascular trauma and associated complications. Once obtained, vascular access can be secured with a hemostatic sheath utilizing a one-way valve with side port for pressurized anticoagulant flush solution.

In most adult patients the distance from the lower torso to the neck will necessitate diagnostic catheters (4–5 F diameter) or guiding catheters for therapeutic devices (5–9 F) of 90–100 cm in length. These devices are made from a variety of polymers (e.g. polyurethane, PVC, polyamides, fluoropolymers) with additional enhancements to increase strength and maneuverability (braided reinforcement), increase radio-opacity, resist clotting, reduce friction, and withstand high-volume injection under considerable pressure.

To access the intracranial circulation a coaxial system that routes longer and more flexible micro-catheters (2–3 F) of 150–170 cm in length through the (guide catheter) conduit from the arch is utilized. The development of variable-stiffness micro-catheters represents an infrequently acknowledged, but major, milestone in the advancement of endovascular surgical neuroradiology.[20] Use of these devises in a coaxial configuration requires meticulous attention to potential sources of emboli and the use of pressurized anticoagulant solutions (4000 IU of heparin per liter), with a rotating hemostatic valve (a Tuohy–Borst adapter) to prevent retrograde accumulation of thrombus within the guide (Figure 2.3). The micro-catheters are similarly engineered for a specific purpose (aneurysm or AVM embolization) and are generally limited to hand injection of small volumes under low pressure.

The success of diagnostic and therapeutic cerebral vascular procedures is in large part predicated upon navigation of the aortic arch. In children and young adults the brachiocephalic vessels are relatively straight and aligned with the descending aorta. Under posterior–anterior fluoroscopic guidance the origins of the vessels are engaged by a subtle distal curve of the catheter, and a guiding wire (typically 0.035 in in diameter) is advanced cephalad, and the catheter is then advanced by pushing or stripping the catheter over the wire. These wires are composed of a variety of metal alloys with polymeric coatings, which may limit thrombus formation and reduce friction.[21] These are essentially visual maneuvers, not tactile. As the wire ascends the neck, location (vertebral versus carotid) may often be confirmed by noting the position relative to the lateral mass of sixth cervical vertebra and above in the oblique or lateral projections (the vertebral arteries reside within the transverse foramina at this level whereas carotid arteries lie within the soft tissue).

With age, the aorta may dilate and elongate, the net effect of which may be that the brachiocephalic origins are no longer aligned with the descending aorta, but are positioned more anterior in the mediastinum. As a consequence, cephalad catheter advancement becomes progressively more difficult as the force of stripping or pushing the catheter is no longer directed up,

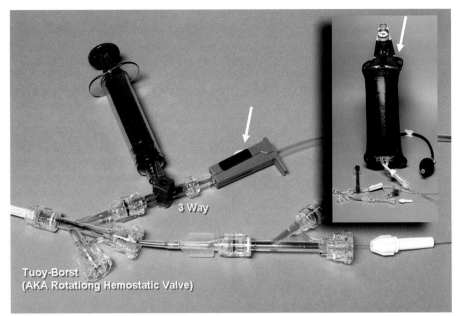

Figure 2.3
Coaxial system with heparinized saline flush driven out the catheter by a color coded (in this case, blue) pneumatic pressure bag (long thin arrows). The blue line control is connected to a three-way stopcock, which allows close regulation of the drip, aspiration or flush of the guide catheter, and contrast injections (pictured here with a red contrast syringe). The stopcock is in turn connected to the rotating hemo-static valve (RHV), which in this case has two valves. Through one of the valves is placed a micro-catheter, likewise connected to a separate RHV with a three-way stopcock, pressurized flush, and contrast (partially obscured).

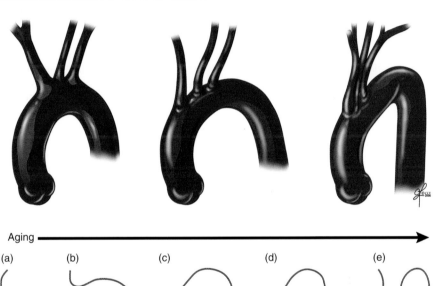

Figure 2.4
As the arch ages, progressively more angulation is required at the catheter tip to engage and advance the devices into the brachiocephalic vessels. Catheters from left to right: a) Hinck Headhunter (H1) catheter, b) Bentson-Hanafee-Wilson (JB1) catheter, c) Bentson-Hanafee-Wilson (JB3) catheter, d) Vitek catheter, and e) Simmons II (Sim2) catheter.

but across the elongated aorta. This may be overcome initially by more robust (i.e. stiffer) guidewires placed more cephalad to anchor the system during advancement. Ultimately, this too may fail and one may need to resort to the use of catheters, with extreme distal curvature. The best examples of these are the Simmons catheters which are shaped like a shepherd's crook. The catheter shape is initially re-formed in the aorta. Subsequently, the distal catheter (i.e. the side-arm) is advanced by pulling the catheter back, or out, at the groin, causing the tip to ascend the brachiocephalic vessels (Figure 2.4).

In extremely difficult cases, and certainly in all cases of intracranial access, one can make use of available digital technology to facilitate catheterization.[22] Contrast injections made in the vascular territory of interest can be recorded and superimposed over real-time fluoroscopy to provide a 'roadmap.' The superimposition is obviously most accurate if the patient remains motionless, a precondition best met by patients who are either remarkably co-operative or anesthetized. Even under these conditions, physiologic cardiac and respiratory motion degrade the map, a scenario obviously more problematic near the aortic arch.

The first attempts at cerebral angiography by Egaz Moniz were characterized by morbidity, mortality and little in the way of angiographic images.[23] Although the morbidity and mortality were very likely a result of the toxicity of the crude halide solutions used as contrast material, these problems serve to emphasize the potentially devastating, and utterly irretrievable, consequences of anything less than the most meticulous technique. Studies using diffusion-weighted MRI suggest that the incidence of silent ischemic injury for diagnostic transarterial catheter studies is approximately 5–25%.[13,24–29]

For diagnostic angiography of the aortic arch and brachiocephalic vessels, an automated power injector is often employed (see Figure 2.2). This has the advantage of operator-selectable parameters for injection (pressure, volume, time, and rate of rise), with the benefit of standardizing the procedure (and thus enhancing reproducibility); injection of larger volumes (20–40 ml for adult aortic studies); and allowing the operator to leave the room and thus reduce his or her radiation exposure. In the context of therapeutic procedures performed through coaxial systems utilizing small volume, low (pressure) tolerance microcatheters, expediency and a theoretical tactile margin of safety often lead operators to inject contrast by hand. (However, rather than watching the fluoroscope screen during the injection, it is wiser to watch the syringe for previously unidentified bubbles or thrombus material moving toward the hub of the catheter: the images can always be recalled and reviewed, but an embolus cannot.)

Other proposed technical nuances to minimize risk include the use of heparin or filters (or both).[25] Repetitive and frequent double flushing and wiping of the wire to minimize the risk of thromboembolism are also useful. Plastic syringes may be color-coded and labeled for local anesthetic, iodinated contrast, heparinized flush solution, vasodilators, and so on to avoid confusion and possible additional risk of emboli (Figure 2.5).[30]

Iodinated contrast

The use of iodinated contrast has been greatly facilitated by the use of non-ionic agents (Table 2.3). Before their use, hyperosmolar ionic material was used and was often unpleasant and more often associated with bizarre symptoms or unusual reactions.[31] Occasionally these materials were associated with histamine release and thus the reactions were generically termed 'allergic reactions.' Although much less common with non-ionic agents injected intra-arterially at body temperature,[32–34] one must be prepared for such a history and have plan for pre-medication as well as treatment of an actual untoward response.[32,35–37] Beyond the rare idiosyncratic reactions to iodinated contrast there is often concern over the impact of these materials on renal function, particularly in patients with pre-existing compromised glomerular filtration rate or those on specific medications.[36,38] These concerns can be addressed by minimizing dose (typically a maximum dose of 150–250 ml or 0.5 ml per kilogram of body weight), by maintaining hydration, and by alkalinization of the urine.[39]

Positioning

With much of diagnostic neuroradiology now commanded by MRI and CT, and with the impressive three-dimensional angiographic displays of those non-invasive modalities, it occasionally seems that the creation of high detail cerebral vascular images is a lost art. But these modalities are static and have little of the dynamic vascular physiology displayed with catheter angiography. Similarly, they cannot match the high contrast (12 bit) or spatial resolution (2000 × 2000) of contemporary digital angiography systems.

Standard angiographic projections and acquisition parameters

Clearly, the limitations lie with either inexperienced or indifferent operators and technologists; however as the 'captain of the ship', the operator carries ultimate responsibility for optimal images. By convention, radiographic projections are named according to the direction of the X-ray beam from source to target. Standard PA and lateral digital subtraction runs are performed at 2 frames

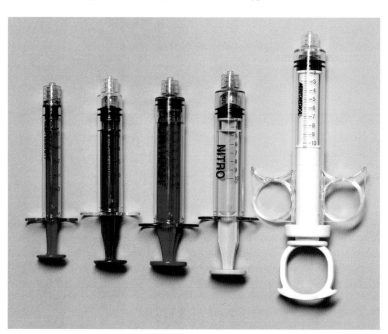

Figure 2.5
Color-coded syringes are invaluable in minimizing mistakes of injection of otherwise identical appearing liquids. For our laboratory, contrast is red, flush solution is white or clear, lidocaine is maroon, and pharmacologic agents (e.g. nitroglycerine) may be blue.

Table 2.3 Intravascular iodinated contrast agents

Class	Generic name	Trade name	Iodine content (mg/ml)	Osmolality (mosm/μg)
High osmolality – ionic	Sodium and/or methylglucamine iothalamate	Conray (Mallinckrodt)	141	633
			282	1415
			370	2016
Low osmolality – ionic – nonionic monomeric	Sodium meglumine ioxaglate	Hexabrix (Mallinckrodt, Guerbet)	320	602
	Ioversol	Optiray (Mallinckrodt)	160	355
			320	680
			350	702
	Iohexol	Omnipaque (Nycomed–Amersham)	240	520
			300	672
			350	844
	Iopamidol	Isovue (Bracco)	200	413
			300	616
			370	796
	Iopromide	Optivist (Berlex, Schering)	300	605
			370	780
	Ioxilan	Oxilan (Cook)	300	585
Nonionic dimer			350	695
	Iodixanol	Visipaque (Nycomed–Amersham)	270	290
			320	290

per second for most disorders. For high-flow lesions (e.g. direct arterial–venous fistulae) the rate may be increased to 6 frames per second; above this level there are often trade-offs in image quality (signal-to-noise, spatial resolution). Injections of contrast 6–8 ml in the carotid artery 3–5 ml in the vertebral artery with 240–300 mg/ml of iodine solution typically produces excellent opacification of the intracranial vessels. Arterial–venous circulation is usually 4.5–6.0 seconds (±1.5 seconds), necessitating exposures lasting approximately 7–10 seconds or between 14 and 20 images.

PA and lateral views are standard for most ischemic stroke studies, which should include the opacified vascular territories centered in the image but magnified just enough to include the draining dural sinuses (Figures 2.6, 2.7). The PA image should be positioned such that the superior orbital rim overlies the petrous ridge (see Figure 2.7). In the lateral projection, the orbital roofs will not overlap (the bony orbit distant to the detector will appear magnified) but should be parallel (see Figure 2.6).

Once the screening dynamic study is claimed, high magnification and angulated views may be obtained to demonstrate the pathology to greatest advantage. For some lesions, such as aneurysms, these runs may be limited to the arterial phase only in order to reduce radiation exposure. Additional views include transorbital obliques (the Reese view) to display anterior circulation aneurysms at the circle of Willis (Figure 2.8). The degree of right–left obliquity (yaw of the C-arm) is defined from midline sagittal.

For projections using cranial–caudal angulation, the degree of pitch is defined according to the zero line drawn from the canthus of the eye to the external auditory meatus (the cantho-meatal line). Caldwell or Waters views can provide cranial–caudal angulation of lesions at the M1 segments of the middle cerebral arteries or those along the basilar trunk (Figures 2.9, 2.10). The Townes view is the optimal means to visualize the distal (P2, P3) posterior cerebral pial vessels (Figure 2.11). Alternatively submental vertex positioning is often an excellent means to visualize complex anatomy at the anterior communicating artery or the M1–M2 junction (Figure 2.12). Often, faithful reproduction and maximum benefit of the submental vertex view will require more than simple gantry angulation: building up of the shoulders and head extension is frequently necessary.

Anticipating and documenting collateral pathways

The dynamic character of catheter angiography provides a unique gauge of collateral circulation to the brain. Cerebrovascular occlusions are often met with near instantaneous recruitment of alternative sources of perfusion. Anticipation of such perfusion pathways is a major key to successful diagnostic angiography and therapeutic endovascular procedures in both ischemic and hemorrhagic cerebral vascular disease. Hence, accurate angiographic documentation is crucial. (Normal vascular anatomy is outlined in Figure 2.13.)

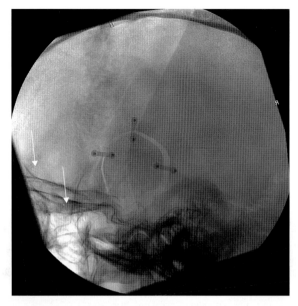

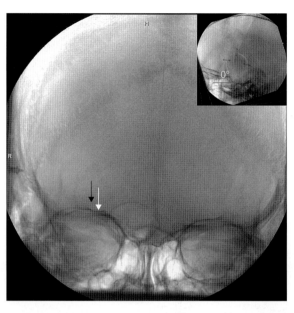

Figure 2.6
Lateral view of the anterior circulation, center just above the ear. Correct positioning can be gauged by the degree of overlap of the orbital roofs, These structures should be parallel, but the side that is away from the detector should be larger and project above the closer side. In the preliminary run it is important to visualize the carotid siphon and the dural sinus at at least 2 frames per second to assess filling patterns, vascular anomalies, and arterial–venous circulation time. Higher frame rates will be necessary to see especially rapid arteriovenous shunting.

Figure 2.7
The AP view is performed with reference to a line drawn from the external auditory meatus to the canthus of the eye (the anatomic baseline: 0° cranial–caudal angulation). A true AP film is performed with zero angulation to this line. If positioning with fluoroscopy, one can appreciated the orbital roof aligning at the level of the petrous ridge in this position. As with the AP view, the field should be collimated for safety; however the carotid siphon, all major pial vessels, the cortical veins, and the dural sinuses should be visible. This is helpful with AVMs and most posterior circulation aneurysms.

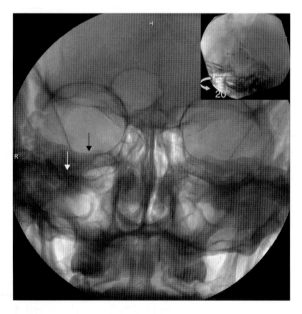

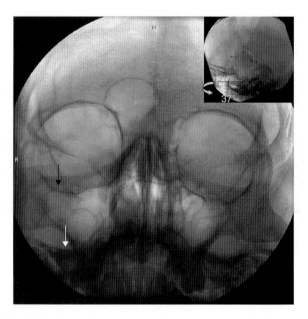

Figure 2.8
The Caldwell view is performed by continuing the forward rotation of the image intensifier (II) to approximately 20° below the canthomeatal line. In this position the petrous ridges should appear within each orbit. It is helpful in cases of AVMs and basilar summit aneurysms.

Figure 2.9
Waters view is a continuation of the angle begun with the Caldwell view, although in this instance the petrous ridge is now in alignment with the orbital floor and the inferior orbital rim. This typically occurs with an angulations of 37°. This view may be useful in cases of middle cerebral artery and basilar terminus aneurysms.

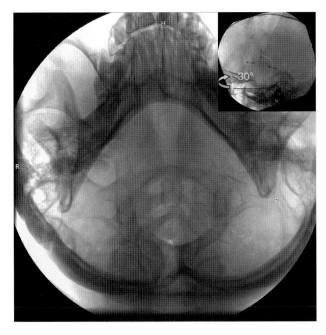

Figure 2.10
The SMV view is the ultimate in forward angulation of the II in the supine, AP-facing, obedient patient. This view can be facilitated by elevating the patient's shoulders, if permitted. This view is often helpful in anterior cerebral artery and middle cerebral artery aneurysms.

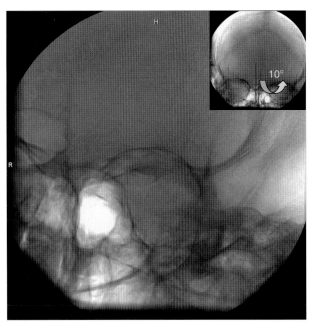

Figure 2.12
Oblique view through the orbit (the Rhese view) is approximately 10° off midline and is excellent for ophthalmic, hypophyseal, posterior communication, anterior choroidal, posterior communicating and carotid terminus lesions.

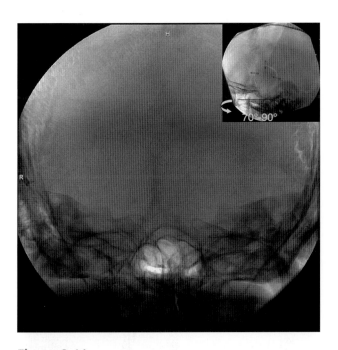

Figure 2.11
The Townes view represents the reverse angulation (to the canthomeatal line) compared with those previously discussed. It is the view best for depicting distal posterior cerebral artery lesions.

Potential collateral cerebral circulation includes:

- congenital collateral circulation (e.g. persistent trigeminal or hypoglossal arteries)
- external–internal collateral circulation (e.g. facial-to-ophthalmic carotid, occipital-to-vertebral)
- circle of Willis (via communicating arteries)
- pial (watershed) collateral circulation
- iatrogenic collateral circulation (e.g. superficial temporal–middle cerebral bypass.)

Congenital deviations of the cerebral circulation are usually obvious but occasionally go unrecognized by the inexperienced operator. Pial collateral routes are often more subtle and require detailed extended filming for adequate documentation. (Figures 2.14 and 2.15.)

Manual compression of non-injected arteries

Side-to-side or front-to-back flow from the communicating arteries can be either obvious or quite subtle. They are often subtle even in the presence of large communicating arteries by virtue of the fact the flow in the circle of Willis is isobaric, and flow through the communicating vessel may be visible only in the setting of a unilateral drop in pressure. This can be facilitated by manual compression of a carotid artery: injection of the contralateral carotid artery will expose the anterior communicating artery, while injection of a dominant vertebral artery will expose the ipsilateral posterior communicating artery. This is the Allcock maneuver (Figure 2.16).[40–42]

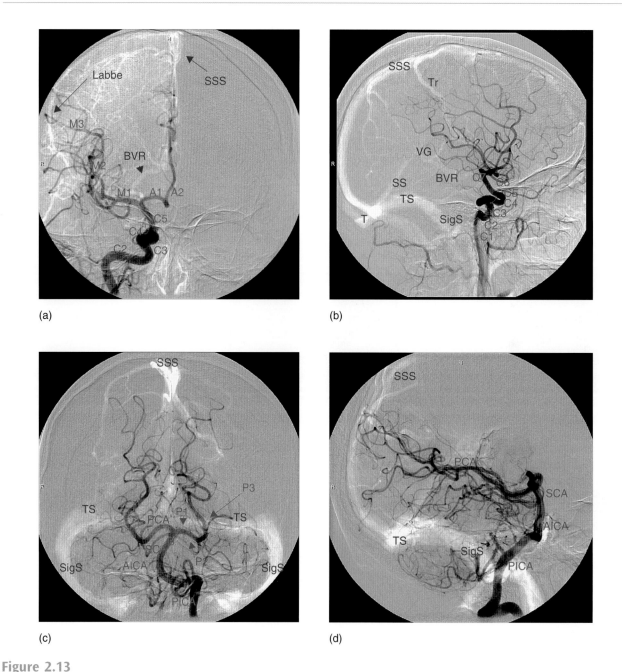

Figure 2.13
Normal vascular anatomy summed arterial (black structures labeled in red) and venous (white structures labeled in blue) phases.
a, b) AP and lateral right internal carotid injection. C1 = cervical carotid, C2 = petrous carotid, C3 = lacerum carotid, C4 = carotid siphon, C5 = clinoid carotid, C6 = opthlamic carotid segment, C7 = communicating carotid segment. M1, M2, M3 = horizontal segment, insular segment, cortical branches of the middle cerebral artery. A1, A2 = horizontal and proximal interhemispheric anterior cerebral branches. c, d) Townes and lateral left vertebral injections. B = basilar artery, PCA = posterior cerebral artery (P1, P2, P3 segments), PICA = posterior inferior cerebellar artery, SCA = superior cerebellar artery, AICA = anerior inferior cerebellar artery. SSS = superior sagiatal sinus, SS = straight sinus, SigS = sigmoid sinus, T = torcula, Tr = vein of Trolard, TS = transverse tinus, BVR = basal vein Of Rosenthal, VG = vein of Galen.

Balloon test occlusion

In the setting of more definitive delineation of collateral support beyond mere anatomy, one can assess the ability of collateral pathways to support normal neurologic function (in anticipation of possible iatrogenic sacrifice) by temporarily occluding a vessel with the patient awake. This procedure has been variously described with much nuance and many permutations, which include some form of perfusion imaging (e.g. SPECT, xenon CT).[43–45] Integral to the accuracy and success of this maneuver is the familiarity of the operator with the patient's baseline neurological examination.

The basic principle is an extension of catheter angiography performed with bilateral vascular access. The second femoral catheterization can be used to access the vessel contemplated for sacrifice with a guide catheter (typically 6 F). Through this

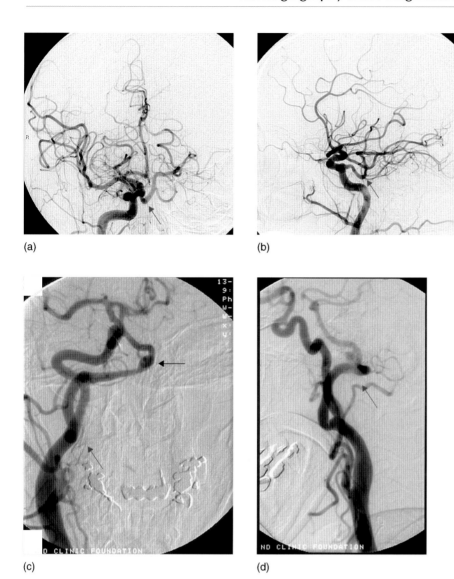

(a)

(b)

(c)

(d)

Figure 2.14

Developmental collateral pathways. a, b) AP and lateral carotid injections demonstrating a persistent trigeminal artery (arrow) arising from the proximal carotid siphon. c, d) AP and lateral carotid injections demonstrating a persistent hypoglossal artery (long arrow) arising from the cervical carotid and coursing to the posterior circulation near the anterior foramen magnum. Note the incidental aneurysm (black arrow).

conduit a soft silicone balloon catheter can be placed distally while the patient is fully anticoagulated (confirmed with in-suite activated clotting time of 250–300 seconds). Potential collateral pathways are catheterized via the alternative access site (Figure 2.17). The sterile field is covered with additional drapes, and the patient's upper extremities are freed to be visible and interactive above the drapes. The balloon is inflated, the diagnostic catheter injected and exposures acquired over the area of interest. The diagnostic catheter is withdrawn and neuro-logical testing is conducted with the balloon inflated. If the patient develops symptoms the balloon is deflated, the patient will rapidly recover, the catheters are withdrawn, and the procedure is discontinued.

If the patient remains asymptomatic occlusion typically continues for 30 minutes with intermittent neurological testing. Often when temporary occlusion is performed in the carotid territory, the patients may become intractably hypertensive, and this may distort what is essentially a functional test of cerebral perfusion.[46] For this reason the examination should be performed

with an arterial line to accurately monitor blood pressure and every effort made to lower the patients blood-pressure to two-thirds of the baseline mean arterial pressure for 15–20 minutes of the examination ('hypotensive challenge'). This may prove challenging, requiring impressive titration of nitrates and intra-venous administration of beta-blockers.[47]

Despite precautions, which include hypotensive challenge or sophisticated imaging, a small percentage of patients may have false-negative examinations such that when treatment is executed and the cerebral vessel is permanently sacrificed, the patient then becomes symptomatic.[45] In the absence of clear imaging evidence of completed infarction, this situation represents a post-operative dilemma of the worst kind. The scenario is often typified by anx-ious attempts to decide if the issue is one of hypoperfusion, requiring emergency surgical bypass, or if there are 'stump emboli' sent downstream of the occluded vessel by the collaterals, requir-ing anti-coagulation of a post-operative patient. When thought-fully considered, this is perhaps the best rationale for careful and conservative interpretation of balloon test occlusion findings.

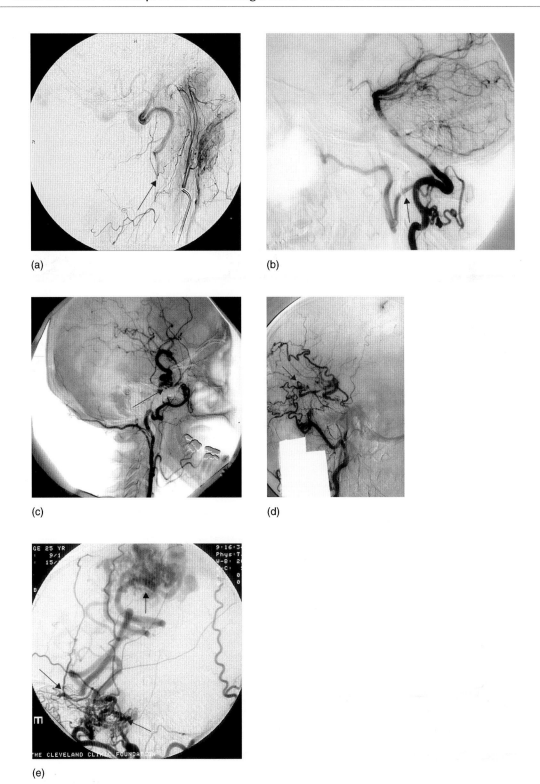

(a)

(b)

(c)

(d)

(e)

Figure 2.15

Acquired collateral pathways. a) Vigorous injection of the ascending pharyngeal branch of the external carotid fills ipsilateral vertebral artery (arrow).
b) Vertebral artery injection with retrograde filling of the ipsilateral occipital and internal maxillary branches of the external carotid (arrow).
c) Internal carotid occluded at the origin with the siphon filling via the artery of the foramen Rotundum via branches of the internal maxillary artery (arrow). d) Proximal internal carotid occlusion with intracranial supply from retrograde flow in the ophthalmic artery (arrow) reconstituted via the internal maxillary, superficial temporal and facial branches of the external carotid. e) Selective external carotid injection with flow through the inferolateral trunk and other small branches of the carotid siphon (arrows) drawn to fill a large Rolandic pial AVM.

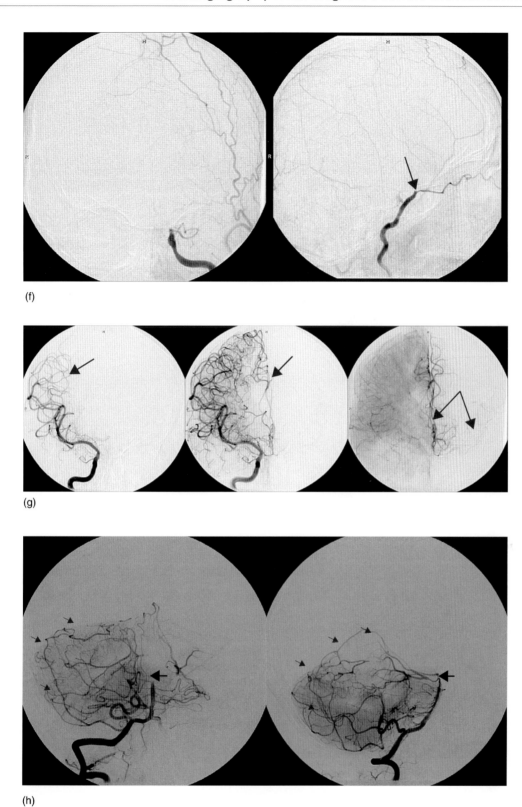

(f)

(g)

(h)

Figure 2.15 (*Continued*)

Acquired collateral pathways. f) Left supra-ophthalmic carotid occlusion (arrow) with g) pial supply partially derived from an isolated right middle cerebral artery which fills the ipsilateral ACA, then the Acom, then the contralateral ACA and PCA via pial watershed anastamotic channels (arrows). h) Mid-Basilar occlusion (black arrow) with compensatory pial watershed collaterals from the inferior vermian to superior vermian branched of the PICA to SCA respectively (red arrows).

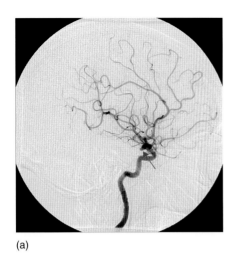

(a)

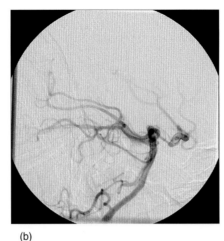

(b)

Figure 2.16
a) Lateral internal carotid injection demonstrates a focal defect arising from the supraclinoid segment, suspicious for possible posterior communicating artery aneurysm. b) Diligent angiography of the vertebrobasilar system with simultaneous manual compression of the same carotid (aka Allcock's Maneuver) demonstrates that this defect is actually an infundibulum of the posterior communicating artery.

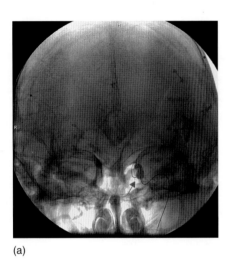

(a)

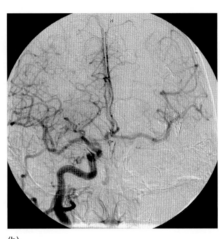

(b)

Figure 2.17
a) Unsubtracted PA right carotid angiogram with a silicone balloon temporarily occluding the left internal carotid artery while the patient is fully awake and fully anticoagulated. This requires vascular access via both femoral arteries. b) Subtracted image better demonstrating collateral support via the anterior communicating artery.

References

1. Schueler BA, Kallmes DF, Cloft HJ. 3D cerebral angiography: radiation dose comparison with digital subtraction angiography. AJNR Am J Neuroradiol 2005; 26: 1898–901.

2. Strauss KJ, Kaste SC. The ALARA (as low as reasonably achievable) concept in pediatric interventional and fluoroscopic imaging: striving to keep radiation doses as low as possible during fluoroscopy of pediatric patients: a white paper executive summary. Radiology 2002; 240: 621–2.

3. Molyneux AJ, Kerr R, Stratton I et al. International subarachnoid aneurysm trial of neurosurgical clipping versus endovascular coiling in 2143 patients with ruptured intracranial aneurysms: a randomised trial. Lancet 2002; 360: 1267–74.

4. van Rooij WJ, Sluzewski M, Beute GN. Brain AVM embolization with onyx. AJNR Am J Neuroradiol 2007; 28: 172–7.

5. US Food and Drug Administration. Med Bullet 1994; 24: 2–6.

6. US Food and Drug Administration. FDA public health advisory: avoidance of serious x-ray-induced skin injuries to patients during fluoroscopically guided procedures. Washington, DC: 1994.

7. The National Cancer Institute. Interventional Fluoroscopy: Reducing Radiation Risks for Patients and Staff. NIH Publication No. 05-5286. National Cancer Institute Division of Cancer Epidemiology and Genetics/Radiation Epidemiology Branch, 2005.

8. Wagner LK, McNeese MD, Marx MV, Siegel EL. Severe skin reactions from interventional fluoroscopy: case report and review of the literature. Radiology 1999; 213: 773–6.

9. Layton KF, Kallmes DF, Cloft HJ et al. Radiation exposure to the primary operator during endovascular surgical neuroradiology procedures. AJNR Am J Neuroradiol 2006; 27: 742–3.

10. Lee C, Lee C, Han EY, Bolch WE. Consideration of the ICRP 2006 revised tissue weighting factors on age-dependent values of the effective dose for external photons. Phys Med Biol 2007; 52: 41–58.

11. Vano E, Faulkner K. ICRP special radiation protection issues in interventional radiology, digital and cardiac imaging. Radiat Prot Dosimetry 2005; 117: 13–17.

12. Sugahara T, Korogi Y, Nakashima K et al. Comparison of 2D and 3D digital subtraction angiography in evaluation of intracranial aneurysms. AJNR Am J Neuroradiol 2002; 23: 1545–52.

13. Krings T, Willmes K, Becker R et al. Silent microemboli related to diagnostic cerebral angiography: a matter of operator's experience and patient's disease. Neuroradiology 2006; 48: 387–93.

14. Croskerry P. The cognitive imperative: thinking about how we think. Acad Emerg Med 2000; 7: 1223–31.

15. Higashida RT, Hopkins LN, Berenstein A et al. Program requirements for residency/fellowship education in neuroendovascular surgery/interventional neuroradiology: a special report on graduate medical education. AJNR Am J Neuroradiol 2000; 21: 1153–9.

16. Barr JD, Connors JJ III, Sacks D et al. Quality improvement guidelines for the performance of cervical carotid angioplasty and stent placement: developed by a collaborative panel of the American Society of Interventional and Therapeutic Neuroradiology, the American Society of Neuroradiology, and the Society of Interventional Radiology. AJNR Am J Neuroradiol 2003; 24: 2020–34.

17. Fox AJ. Technical aspects of neuroangiography: are risks and safeguards understood in the same way? AJNR Am J Neuroradiol 2001; 22: 1809–10.

18. Seldinger SI. Catheter replacement of the needle in percutaneous arteriography; a new technique. Acta Radiol 1953; 39: 368–76.

19. Rosenbaum AE, Petter Eldevik O, Mani JR et al. In Re: Amundsen P. Cerebral angiography via the femoral artery with particular reference to cerebrovascular disease. Acta Neurol Scand 1967; 115. AJNR Am J Neuroradiol 2001; 22: 584–9.

20. Engelson E. Catheter for guide-wire tracking. United States patent: Application number: 06/869597. Publication date: April 26, 1988.

21. Pinto RS, Robbins E, Seidenwurm D. Thrombogenicity of Teflon versus copolymer-coated guidewires: evaluation with scanning electron microscopy. AJNR Am J Neuroradiol 1989; 10: 407–10.

22. Lee TH, Choi CH, Park KP et al. Techniques for intracranial stent navigation in patients with tortuous vessels. AJNR Am J Neuroradiol 2005; 26: 1375–80.

23. Wolpert SM. Neuroradiology classics moniz: pioneer in cerebral angiography. AJNR Am J Neuroradiol 1999; 20: 1752–3.

24. Bendszus M, Koltzenburg M, Burger R et al. Silent embolism in diagnostic cerebral angiography and neurointerventional procedures: a prospective study. Lancet 1999; 354: 1594–7.

25. Bendszus M, Koltzenburg M, Bartsch AJ et al. Heparin and air filters reduce embolic events caused by intra-arterial cerebral angiography: a prospective, randomized trial. Circulation 2004; 110: 2210–5.

26. Bendszus M, Stoll G. Silent cerebral ischaemia: hidden fingerprints of invasive medical procedures. Lancet Neurol 2006; 5: 364–72.

27. Busing KA, Schulte-Sasse C, Fluchter S et al. Cerebral infarction: incidence and risk factors after diagnostic and interventional cardiac catheterization: prospective evaluation at diffusion-weighted MR imaging. Radiology 2005; 235: 177–83.

28. Hamon M, Gomes S, Oppenheim C et al. Cerebral microembolism during cardiac catheterization and risk of acute brain injury: a prospective diffusion-weighted magnetic resonance imaging study. Stroke 2006; 37: 2035–8.

29. Kato K, Tomura N, Takahashi S et al. Ischemic lesions related to cerebral angiography: evaluation by diffusion weighted MR imaging. Neuroradiology 2003; 45: 39–43.

30. Ginsberg LE, Stump DA, King JC, Deal DD, Moody DM. Air embolus risk with glass versus plastic syringes: in vitro study and implications for neuroangiography. Radiology 1994; 191: 813–6.

31. Katayama H, Ishida O, Osawa T et al. Clinical survey on adverse reaction of contrast media (final report). Nippon Igaku Hoshasen Gakkai Zasshi 1988; 48: 423–32.

32. Bush WH, Swanson DP. Acute reactions to intravascular contrast media: types, risk factors, recognition, and specific treatment. AJR Am J Roentgenol 1991; 157: 1153–61.

33. Cohan RH, Dunnick NR. Intravascular contrast media: adverse reactions. AJR Am J Roentgenol 1987; 149: 665–70.

34. Rydberg J, Charles J, Aspelin P. Frequency of late allergy-like adverse reactions following injection of intravascular non-ionic contrast media. A retrospective study comparing a non-ionic monomeric contrast medium with a non-ionic dimeric contrast medium. Acta Radiol 1998; 39: 219–22.

35. Halpern JD, Hopper KD, Arredondo MG, Trautlein JJ. Patient allergies: role in selective use of nonionic contrast material. Radiology 1996; 199: 359–62.

36. Namasivayam S, Kalra MK, Torres WE, Small WC. Adverse reactions to intravenous iodinated contrast media: a primer for radiologists. Emerg Radiol 2006; 12: 210–15.

37. Vergara M, Seguel S. Adverse reactions to contrast media in CT: effects of temperature and ionic property. Radiology 1996; 199: 363–6.

38. Rasuli P, French GJ, Hammond DI. Metformin hydrochloride all right before, but not after, contrast medium administration. Radiology 1998; 209: 586–7.

39. Merten GJ, Burgess WP, Gray LV et al. Prevention of contrast-induced nephropathy with sodium bicarbonate: a randomized controlled trial. JAMA 2004; 291: 2328–34.

40. Allcock JM, Drake CG. Postoperative Angiography in cases of ruptured intracranial aneurysm. J Neurosurg 1963; 20: 752–9.

41. Allcock JM. Vertebral angiography: its accuracy in the diagnosis of intra-cranial space-occupying lesions. J Can Assoc Radiol 1962; 13: 65–9.

42. Fox AJ. John Allcock, MD, 1920-2001. AJNR Am J Neuroradiol 2001; 22: 1973.

43. Barker DW, Jungreis CA, Horton JA, Pentheny S, Lemley T. Balloon test occlusion of the internal carotid artery: change in stump pressure over 15 minutes and its correlation with xenon CT cerebral blood flow. AJNR Am J Neuroradiol 1993; 14: 587–90.

44. Linskey ME, Jungreis CA, Yonas H et al. Stroke risk after abrupt internal carotid artery sacrifice: accuracy of preoperative assessment with balloon test occlusion and stable xenon-enhanced CT. AJNR Am J Neuroradiol 1994; 15: 829–43.

45. Mathis JM, Barr JD, Jungreis CA et al. Temporary balloon test occlusion of the internal carotid artery: experience in 500 cases. AJNR Am J Neuroradiol 1995; 16: 749–54.

46. Shaibani A, Khawar S, Bendok B et al. Temporary balloon occlusion to test adequacy of collateral flow to the retina and tolerance for endovascular aneurysmal coiling. AJNR Am J Neuroradiol 2004; 25: 1384–6.

47. Standard SC, Ahuja A, Guterman LR et al. Balloon test occlusion of the internal carotid artery with hypotensive challenge. AJNR Am J Neuroradiol 1995; 16: 1453–8.

3

Therapeutic options: pharmacology

David Fiorella and Vivek A Gonugunta

Historically, in both surgery and interventional radiology, emphasis has always been placed on devices, instrumentation, routes of access, and means of exposure. However, in recent years there has been a growing awareness of the importance of intraprocedural pharmacology in the success of endovascular treatments for cerebrovascular disease. This chapter is an introductory primer on these critical therapeutic adjuncts.

Anticoagulants

The vast majority of neurologic complications encountered during neuroendovascular procedures are thromboembolic. This holds true whether the lesion being treated is a hemorrhagic entity (an aneurysm or an arterial–venous malformation) or a thrombotic entity (a carotid atherostenosis). Correspondingly, a successful approach to the management of coagulation is paramount for minimizing complications and maximizing the risk–benefit profile of all neuroendovascular interventions. Given the broad spectrum of disease processes addressed, multiple different regimens of anticoagulation are required. To adequately construct a rational treatment plan for each individual patient and scenario, the operator must possess a thorough knowledge of the available pharmacological agents.

Antithrombotic agents

Heparin

Unfractionated heparin is a collection of glycosaminoglycans, which range widely in molecular size and anticoagulant activity. The anticoagulant activity of heparin is derived from a pentasaccharide component with a high-affinity binding site for antithrombin III (ATIII). However, only one-third of the molecules possess this activity. Heparin binds ATIII and thrombin to form a ternary complex. The bound ATIII undergoes a conformational change that greatly enhances its ability to inactivate thrombin, factor Xa and factor IXa.

Heparin has a unique pharmacokinetic profile. Heparin is removed from the circulation by two mechanisms:

- surface receptors on endothelial cells and macrophages binding and internalizing the heparin; and
- first-order renal clearance.

Because the first mechanism can be saturated, the half-life of heparin varies with dosage, ranging from 30 minutes with a dose of 25 IU per kilogram up to 150 minutes with doses of 400 IU per kilogram. The heparin doses used in neuroendovascular therapeutics are entirely dependent on the clinical setting.

Because of the variable effects of the same heparin dose on different patients, monitoring the anticoagulant effect is ultimately more important than the recommended starting dose. After the initial dose is given, the measured effect governs further therapy. When administered in lower doses, such as those prescribed for deep venous thrombosis or acute coronary syndromes, the activated partial thromboplastin time (aPTT) may be used, with the typical goal of achieving a ratio of 1.5 times the normal value. However, at higher concentrations, such as those used during angioplasty and stenting, the aPTT becomes prolonged beyond measurable levels. In these cases, an activated clotting time (ACT) is used with a target of 250–300 seconds (Figure 3.1).

Direct thrombin inhibitors

Bivalirudin

Despite a growing literature supporting the application of direct thrombin inhibitors in percutaneous coronary intervention (PCI), the application of these agents in neuroendovascular therapeutics remains limited. Currently, only bivalirudin is commercially available as an approved alternative to heparin for PCI.

Bivalirudin has a number of important therapeutic advantages:

- it acts directly on thrombin and does not require a cofactor interaction (e.g. AT-III);
- it does not bind plasma proteins and has a predictable dose – response relationship;
- it does not bind platelet factor 4 and thereby does not induce or perpetuate heparin-induced thrombocytopenia;
- it has no potential for activating platelets; and
- it binds both bound fibrin as well as fluid-phase thrombin.

Bivalirudin has a short half-life (25 minutes) in comparison with heparin. PCI studies indicate that it is at least as effective as heparin with respect to the prevention of procedural thrombosis

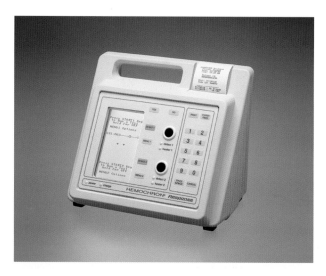

Figure 3.1
Hemochron Response for point of service testing of activated clotting time (ACT). (With premission from International Technidyne Corporation (ITC).)

and that it has a lower risk of associated peri-procedural bleeding complications.[1–3] In the REPLACE-2 trial, bivalirudin was administered as a 0.75 mg per kilogram bolus followed by an at 1.75 mg per kilogram per hour infusion (with the provisional administration of a IIb–IIIa antagonist allowed).[3] This regimen was found not to be inferior to heparin administered with a IIb–IIIa antagonist. ACTs were monitored and tended to be significantly higher in patients given bivalirudin in comparison with those given unfractionated heparin with a IIb/IIIa antagonist.[4]

Like heparin, bivalirudin may be used safely in conjunction with the IIb–IIIa inhibitors. In the CACHET trial, provisional abciximab therapy was required in 24% of the patients treated with bivalirudin.[2] These patients experienced a 4.7% incidence of major bleeding, a rate that was no statistically different from that observed in patients receiving heparin with abciximab (6.3%).

Antiplatelet agents

Platelets represent the predominant component of arterial thrombi that form in response to stimuli such as endothelial injury, turbulent blood flow with associated high wall shear stress, and the introduction of an intravascular foreign body. Correspondingly, it follows that platelet inhibition represents the cornerstone of antithrombotic therapy in cerebrovascular intervention.

Mechanism of Platelet Aggregation

Platelets are anucleate blood cells with a tremendous capacity for interaction with their surrounding vascular environment. Platelets contain storage granules, which hold multiple chemokines, cytokines and growth factors. In addition, platelets can synthesize bioactive prostaglandins from membrane phospholipids.

In the resting state, the intact endothelium releases inhibitory factors, such as prostaglandin (PG)-I$_2$ (= prostacyclin) and nitric

oxide, which function to maintain platelets in a nonactivated state (Figure 3.2a). Following the introduction of a stimulus, a cascade of events begins that ultimately results in thrombus formation. This cascade consists of platelet adhesion, activation, secretion, and finally aggregation (see Figure 3.2). The most common and best understood stimulus is endothelial injury. However, high wall shear stress and the introduction of an intravascular foreign body both represent additional stimuli that can also activate the process of platelet aggregation.

When an endothelial injury exposes thrombogenic collagen and subendothelial matrix, platelets adhere to the injured surface primarily via the interactions between the platelet surface Ib receptor with von Willebrand's Factor (vWF) bound to the exposed collagen (Figure 3.2b). These adherent platelets spread to form a monolayer along the surface of the injured endothelium. The adherent platelets become activated after adhesion. Endothelial injury also exposes tissue factor (TF) to the blood stream. TF is expressed exclusively by cells that are not in contact with the blood under normal circumstances (e.g. fibroblasts). Exposed TF binds factor VIIa, leading to the activation of the intrinsic and extrinsic coagulation pathways that ultimately result in thrombin formation. Thrombin, in addition to converting fibrinogen to fibrin monomers, also functions as a potent platelet agonist, resulting in further platelet activation. The activated platelets secrete additional soluble agonists including adenosine diphosphate (ADP), calcium and serotonin (5-HT), which are prepackaged in storage granules, and the platelets synthesize and secrete thromboxane A$_2$ (TXA$_2$). These substances all result in the further amplification of platelet activation (Figure 3.2c). Platelet activation by this myriad of agonists results in the stimulation of multiple different intracellular signaling pathways. These pathways all ultimately converge to induce a conformational change in the platelet surface glycoprotein (GP) IIb–IIIa receptor. This conformational change converts the IIb–IIIa receptor from a quiescent, low-affinity state to an activated, high-affinity binding site for fibrinogen and vWF. The stronger platelet agonists (i.e. thrombin and collagen) also recruit additional GPIIb–IIIa receptors from the intracellular storage pool to the platelet surface.

The binding of the active platelet IIb–IIIa receptor to fibrinogen (and vWF) results in the formation of platelet–platelet and platelet–matrix adhesive interactions and the formation of stable, larger platelet aggregate at the site of injury (Figure 3.2d). While there is a significant level of redundancy built into the cascade of platelet activation, the binding of the IIb–IIIa receptor to fibrinogen (or vWF) represents the final common pathway to platelet aggregation and thus the formation of stable thrombus. As this stable platelet aggregate forms, insoluble fibrin monomers begins precipitating around the aggregated platelets and eventually become cross-linked to form a more permanent thrombus.

Aspirin

The initial activation of platelets results in the activation of phospholipase A2 (PLA$_2$), leading to the liberation of arachidonic acid (AA) from membrane phospholipids. AA is immediately converted by cylco-oxygenase (COX)-1 to PGG$_2$ and PGH$_2$ and then by thromboxane synthase (TS) to thromboxane A2 (TXA-2). TXA-2 is then released from the platelet to participate in a platelet-receptor-mediated positive feedback loop, which plays a critical role in the further amplification of regional platelet activation. TXA$_2$ also functions to recruit additional platelets to the site of

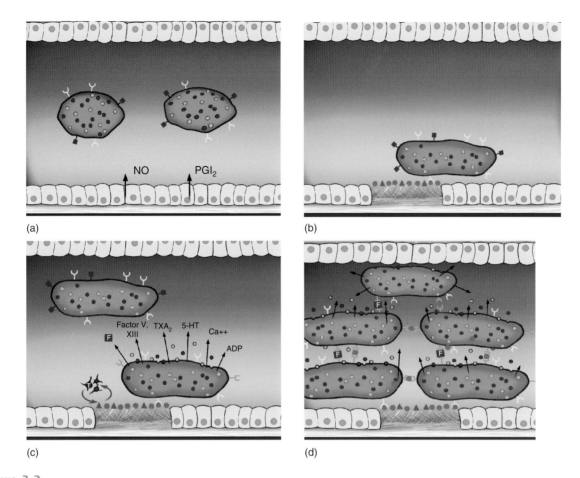

Figure 3.2

a) Intact endothelium releases inhibitory factors, such as prostacyclin (PGI$_2$) and nitric oxide (NO), which function to maintain platelets in a non-activated state. b) Endothelial injury exposes the thrombogenic collagen and subendothelial matrix; platelets adhere to the injured surface primarily via the interactions between the platelet surface Ib receptor (yellow) with von Willebrand's Factor (vWF, red) bound to the exposed collagen. Injury to the endothelium also exposes tissue factor (green triangles). Note Glycoprotein Ib (yellow) and inactivated glycoprotein IIbIIIa (dark blue). c) Activated platelets secrete additional soluble agonists which are prepackaged in storage granules (including adenosine diphosphate [ADP], calcium and serotonin [5-HT]) and synthesize and secrete thromboxane A$_2$ (TXA$_2$). These substances all result in the further amplification of platelet activation. Fibrinogen (F) activated IIbIIa (light blue). Also, exposed TF (green) binds factor VIIa leading to the activation of the intrinsic and extrinsic coagulation pathways that ultimately result in thrombin (T) formation. Thrombin, in addition to converting fibrinogen to fibrin monomers, also functions as a potent platelet agonist, resulting in further platelet activation. d) Platelet activation by myriad agonists results in the stimulation of multiple different intracellular signaling pathways which induce a conformational change in the platelet surface glycoprotein IIb/IIIa receptor (light blue). This conformational change converts the IIb/IIIa receptor from a quiescent low-affinity state to an activated high-affinity binding site for fibrinogen (F) and vWF (red). The binding of the active platelet IIb/IIIa receptor (light blue) to fibrinogen (and vWF) results in the formation of platelet-platelet and platelet-matrix adhesive interactions and the formation of a stable, larger platelet aggregate at the site of injury. Reprinted with permission.

thrombus formation and induces local vasoconstriction. Aspirin irreversibly inactivates COX-1 through the acetylation of a serine residue at position 529, thus blocking the conversion of AA to PGG$_2$ and PGH$_2$ and ultimately therefore the production of TXA-2. Platelets lack the synthetic machinery to generate new COX-1. Therefore this inhibition of TXA-2 synthesis persists for the lifetime of the platelet.[5]

Aspirin also has effects on vascular endothelial cells, in which the blockade of COX activity inhibits the synthesis of prostacyclin, a prostaglandin that functions to decrease platelet activation. These effects are typically seen only at higher aspirin doses, at which the activity of both COX-1 and COX-2 are inhibited. This phenomenon has been termed the 'aspirin dilemma' and has led to the hypothesis that an optimal aspirin dose could provide maximal inhibition of TXA-2 synthesis with minimal disruption of the production of PGI$_2$. In addition, this phenomenon may explain the relatively decreased efficacy of aspirin administered in

higher doses.[6] Unlike platelets, vascular endothelial cells have the synthetic machinery to generate new COX enzyme, so the inhibition of PGI$_2$ synthesis is likely to be fully reversed within the interval between the once per day doses of aspirin administered for platelet inhibition.[7]

The onset of antiplatelet activity following an oral dose of aspirin is remarkably fast. Serum levels of thromboxane B2 (a marker of TXA$_2$ production) are significantly reduced as early as 5 minutes after oral administration, with the maximum effect occurring within 30–60 minutes and remaining stable for 24 hours. The rapid rate of onset has been attributed to the acetylation of COX-1 in platelets within the pre-systemic portal circulation.[7,8]

Aspirin has a myriad of effects in addition to its antiplatelet activity, functioning as it does as an analgesic, an antipyretic, and an anti-inflammatory. These effects all exhibit different dose – response relationships, with the lowest doses required to achieve platelet inhibition. Ex-vivo studies of platelet inhibition have demonstrated that similar levels of inhibition can be achieved with daily aspirin doses ranging from 30 mg to 325 mg.[7,8] In a large meta-analysis, the Anti-Platelet Trialists Collaboration found no evidence to support high-dose aspirin therapy. The meta-analysis demonstrated that doses of 75–150 mg (a 32% decrease), 160–325 mg (26%) and 500–1500 mg (19%) produced similar reductions in vascular events.[9] In this same meta-analysis, doses of less than 75 mg (13%) demonstrated a significantly smaller beneficial effect. In the ASA and Carotid Endarterectomy Trial, lower doses of aspirin (81 mg or 325 mg) resulted in lower rates of stroke, death and myocardial infarction than higher dosing regimens (625–1300 mg) at 3 months.[6]

Taken together, the available data would suggest that an aspirin dose between 81 mg and 325 mg would provide an optimal risk profile. If the lower range is to be used (i.e. 81 mg per day), the operator should consider the administration of a 160–325 mg loading dose so that a therapeutic level of antiplatelet activity can be achieved immediately.

Aspirin resistance is a significant problem that has been recognized recently as tests for the adequacy of platelet blockade have become more available (see below). Between 5 and 40% of patients are resistant to the antiplatelet effects of standard doses of aspirin.[10,11] The incidence of aspirin resistance has been found to be related to aspirin dose, with 56% resistance observed at an 81 mg daily dose and 28% resistance at a 325 mg dose.[12] The same authors reported that 65% of patients taking enteric-coated aspirin had normal platelet function tests. In addition, aspirin resistance may progressively develop over time with long-term therapy. Pulcinelli et al.[13] observed a significant reduction in platelet sensitivity to aspirin therapy over a 24-month period.

A growing volume of data suggests that aspirin resistance has significant clinical implications. Gum et al.[10] reported a three times higher risk of death, myocardial infarction, and cerebrovascular accident over an approximately 2-year period. Chen et al.[11] found that aspirin-resistant patients had a three times greater risk of having creatine kinase-MB elevations following non-emergent percutaneous coronary intervention. In patients with a previous stroke, those with aspirin resistance were 89% more likely to have a recurrent cerebrovascular accident within 2 years.[14] After peripheral intervention, an increase in arterial re-occlusion has been observed in a cohort of aspirin non-responders.[15]

Although no studies currently exist, similar implications should be anticipated for neuroendovascular patients undergoing procedures requiring stent deployment or angioplasty. A knowledge of previous aspirin resistance could have a significant impact on the treatment plan, particularly in those cases in which other reasonable therapeutic options exist (e.g. carotid endarterectomy versus carotid stenting, balloon assisted versus stent-assisted aneurysm embolization). This is the rationale for pre- and intraprocedure monitoring of platelet function.[16]

Thienopyridines (Clopidogrel)

Clopidogrel and ticlopidine are the two commercially available thiopyridines that have been routinely used as antiplatelet agents. Both agents have no activity *in vitro*, as because they require hepatic transformation to active metabolites, which mediate the antiplatelet effect. The active metabolites irreversibly inhibit ADP from binding to its platelet surface P2Y12 receptor. This blockade prevents the soluble platelet agonist ADP from stimulating activation of the intracellular second-messenger (adenylate

cyclase) system, which functions to amplify regional platelet activation by stimulating secretion and ultimately modulates the conversion of the GP IIb–IIIa receptor to its high-affinity state.

Ticlopidine usage has declined substantially over the past decade, owing to the associated side-effect of bone marrow depression, with neutropenia occurring in 2.4% of patients, and the emergence of clopidogrel as an adequate substitute.[17] In CLASSICS (a direct comparison of ticlopidine and clopidogrel administered in combination with aspirin), clopidogrel demonstrated a superior safety profile and comparable efficacy in preventing thrombotic complications after coronary stenting.[18] Studies of the pharmacokinetics of both agents indicate that clopidogrel also demonstrates a prompter onset of maximal platelet inhibition in comparison with ticlopidine.[19] Currently, the use of ticlopidine is largely restricted to patients who are intolerant of clopidogrel. For this reason, the remainder of this section focuses on the pharmacology of clopidogrel.

Clopidogrel is rapidly absorbed and quickly metabolized, with very low plasma concentrations of the drug measured in patients on daily therapy.[20] The active metabolites produce an irreversible alteration of the ADP binding site, and subsequently the effect persists for the duration of the platelet's lifespan, with 7 days required for return of normal platelete function after therapeutic levels are have been attained.

The time required to establish maximally therapeutic levels of platelet inhibition with clopidogrel is dependent on the dosing regimen employed.[21] If a standard daily dose of 75 mg is administered without a loading dose, only 25–30% inhibition at 48 hours. An average of 5 days (range of 3–7 days) is required to achieve maximal steady state levels (50–60%) of platelet inhibition at this dose.[22,23] However, if a loading dose (300–600 mg) is administered, maximal levels of inhibition are achieved within 2–6 hours and remain relatively stable for up to 48 hours.[22,24,25] In the CREDO study, patients who received the 300 mg loading dose of clopidogrel 6 hours or more before their procedure had a 38.6% reduction in death, myocardial infarction or urgent target vessel revascularization at 1 month, whereas no benefit was observed in patients receiving the loading dose before the 6 hour time point.[26]

The efficacy of clopidogrel differs between patients, with a significant incidence of resistance described in the literature. Unlike aspirin, clopidogrel resistance has been classified as both a binary and a graded phenomenon by different investigators. Resistance is measured by determining the degree of reduction in ADP-induced platelet aggregation. Gurbel et al.[27] observed resistance in 31% of patients at 24 hours and 5 days, decreasing to 15% at 30 days, following a 300 mg loading dose of clopidogrel and a dose of 75 mg per day dose after that. When resistant patients were subcategorized, Muller et al.[28] reported that 5–11% were non-responders and 9–26% were semi-responders, depending on the dose of ADP employed to stimulate platelet aggregation. Lau et al.[29] reported rates of clopidogrel resistance in 22% of patients and 16% of volunteers, with an additional 23% of patients and 12% of volunteers categorized as 'low' responders.

As with aspirin, clopidogrel resistance has been demonstrated to have significant clinical implications. For example, individual variability in response to clopidogrel in the setting of percutaneous coronary intervention after myocardial infarction was found to predict an increased risk of recurrent cardiovascular events.[30]

Unlike aspirin, clopidogrel resistance does not appear to develop with time. Thus, if a patient is confirmed to be responsive to clopidogrel initially, a durable antiplatelet effect can be anticipated with long-term administration.[31] This durability may

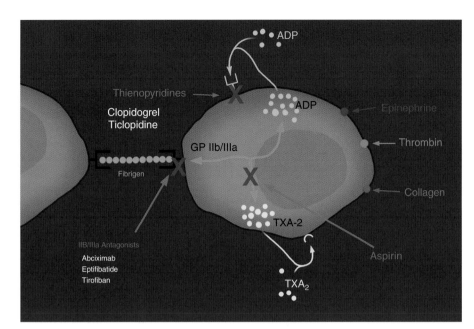

Figure 3.3
Points of attack of various platelet inhibitors: aspirin, thienopyridines, and IIb-IIIa inhibitors. Because their mechanisms of action are different, the effects of each class of drug are believed to be additive. ADP, adenosine diphosphate, TXA-2, thromboxane A2.

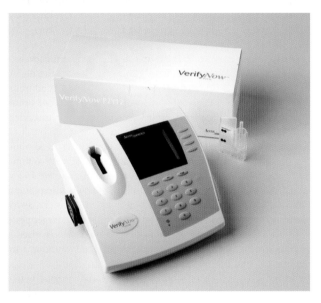

Figure 3.4
Accumetrics 'Verify Now' point-of-service testing for platelet function. This device has seperate cartridges, which test for sensitivity to IIb-IIIa inhibitors, aspirin, and clopidigrel. (With permission from Accumetrics.)

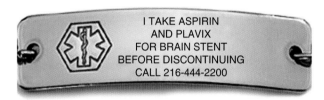

Figure 3.5
Medical bracelet reinforcing the importance of dual antiplatelet therapy in patients in whom a cerebral stent has been placed.

account for the added benefit observed when clopidogrel is added to supplement long-term aspirin therapy (see below).

The mechanisms of clopidogrel resistance are incompletely understood. The leading hypothesis is that individual differences in hepatic metabolism result in variable rates of conversion of the clopidogrel to its active metabolite.[29]

As with aspirin, platelet inhibition by the theinopyridines is durable for the lifetime of the platelet. Platelet function gradually returns to normal, via platelet turnover, over a period of 7 days after the last dose of clopidogrel is administered. (Correspondingly, immediate reversal can be achieved only with a platelet transfusion.) In an effort to ensure patient compliance and reduce delayed thromboembolic effects, patients requiring oral platelet inhibition following intervention are encouraged to wear a medical bracelet (Figure 3.5).

Glycoprotein IIb–IIIa inhibitors

The IIb–IIIa inhibitors block platelet aggregation by preventing fibrinogen and other adhesion molecules such as vWF from binding to the IIb–IIIa integrin on platelets. There are two general classes of antagonists: the irreversible antagonist, abciximab, and the reversible antagonists, eptifibatide and tirofiban.

Abciximab is a monoclonal antibody that binds irreversibly to the IIb–IIIa receptor at the beta-chain of the integrin. Eptifibatide and tirofiban are peptides that mimic the naturally occurring arginine–glycine–aspartic acid (RGD) sequence, which is avidly bound by the IIb–IIIa receptor. This RGD binding site mediates the binding of vWF, vitronectin, fibronectin, and fibrinogen to platelets. Eptifibatide and tirofiban compete with these factors for binding at the RGD site, functioning as reversible, competitive inhibitors of the IIb–IIIa receptor. By eliminating the function of the IIb–IIIa receptor, these agents block the final common pathway of platelet function and platelet aggregation. At approximately 80% IIb–IIIa receptor blockade, platelet aggregation is nearly completely abolished, and at levels greater than 90%, platelet function is ablated to the point that bleeding times become markedly elevated.[32]

In addition to its effects at the platelet IIb–IIIa receptor, abciximab also binds to the vitronectin receptor (on vascular smooth muscle and endothelial cells) and the integrin MAC1 (on activated neutrophils and monocytes). The consequences of these additional receptor interactions remain to be elucidated; however, some researchers have hypothesized that these interactions may play a role in decreasing the inflammatory reaction that follows angioplasty and stenting, thus limiting subsequent intimal hyperplasia.

All three IIb–IIIa inhibitors have the potential to induce thrombocytopenia. This occurs at a slightly higher rate with abciximab (up to 6.5%) than with the competitive antagonists.[33] Thrombocytopenia induced by IIb–IIIa inhibitors is usually quickly reversed by stopping the drug. Typically, a complete recovery evolves over several days.

Abciximab

Abciximab, a monoclonal antibody, is a large molecule with very high affinity for platelet IIb–IIIa receptors. Correspondingly, the plasma half-life of the free drug is short, approximately 10 minutes, as the agent binds immediately to circulating platelets. The agent not bound to platelet receptors is quickly cleared from the circulation. Once bound to platelets, the dissociation time is very long and the molecule remains biologically active on the surface of platelets for 12–14 hours. These characteristics result in a rapid onset of action and a slow reversal of activity after cessation of administration.[34] After the administration of a bolus and an infusion of abciximab, 28% occupation of the IIb–IIIa receptors is sustained at 8 days, declining to 13% at 15 days.

Abciximab is typically administered as a loading dose of 0.25 mg per kilogram, followed by an infusion at 0.125 μg per kilogram per minute (maximum 10 μg per minute) for 12 hours.[35] If the bolus is given alone, bleeding times and platelet function recover to near-normal values by 12 hours, with platelet aggregation returning to greater than 50% of baseline within 24–48 hours in almost all patients. If the infusion is administered, platelet inactivation is maintained throughout the duration of the infusion.

Eptifibatide and tirofiban

Eptifibatide, a synthetic peptide, is a structural analog of barbourin, a snake venom disintegrin polypeptide. Tirofiban is non-peptide tyrosin derivative that is also based on the structure of a known disintegrin polypeptide. These agents have less affinity than abciximab for the IIb–IIIa receptor and their binding to the receptor is reversible.[35] Eptifibatide, in particular, is a low-affinity agonist for the IIb–IIIa receptor. Both compounds demonstrate a very rapid dissociation (in seconds) from the receptor. Correspondingly, after cessation of administration, platelet function returns rapidly to normal. Both agents are cleared through the kidneys and, as such, the effects of these agents may persist for longer in patients with renal failure. The plasma half-time of both agents is approximately 1.5 hours in

patients with normal renal function. Bleeding times begin to return toward normal shortly (within 15 minutes) after the discontinuation of eptifibatide, with return to greater than half of the normal platelet aggregation response within 4 hours. Bleeding times also return to normal within approximately 4 hours after the discontinuation of tirofiban infusion, with platelet aggregation inhibition declining to levels >50% at this time point.

The PRIDE (Platelet Aggregation and Receptor Occupancy with Integrillin) study demonstrated that a 180 μg per kilogram bolus of eptifibatide followed by an infusion at 2.0 μg per kilogram per minute for 12 hours consistently resulted in >90% platelet inhibition within 5 minutes.[36] However, this effect decreased at 1 hour and did not return to the targeted therapeutic level until a steady state was reached at 8–24 hours. For this reason, it is currently recommended that two boluses (180 μg per kilogram) be administered 10 minutes apart, followed by a continuous infusion at 2.0 μg per kilogram per minute to achieve a more stable therapeutic effect.[36,37] Tirofiban is administered as a 10 μg per kilogram bolus, followed by an infusion at 0.15 μg per kilogram per minute for 12 hours. This regimen results in a mean inhibition of platelet aggregation (5 μmol/l ADP) of 96% at 5 minutes, 100% at 2 hours, and 95% at the end of the infusion.[38]

Dosage and use of glycoprotein II–IIIa inhibitors

When IIb–IIIa receptor inhibitors are used in conjunction with heparin, the dose of heparin should be decreased (50–70 IU/kg) slightly, as the existing literature indicates an increased risk of bleeding without a significantly increased efficacy.[39,40]

The therapeutic window for these agents is narrow, as the occupation of approximately 80% of IIb–IIIa receptors is required for clinically effective inhibition of platelet aggregation, however, greater than 90% inhibition may result in excessive bleeding complications.[35] The number of platelet receptors available for binding varies with the relative state of platelet activation.[41] In addition, the actual platelet counts and consequently the number of receptors vary quite substantially across patients.[42] As such, determining a universal dose of IIb–IIIa inhibitors is challenging.

In a study directly comparing the efficacy of all three IIb–IIIa inhibitors in the setting of high-risk PCI, it was determined that only 52% of patients achieved targeted levels of platelet inhibition after administration of the recommended bolus dose of IIb–IIIa inhibitor (41%, 66%, and 49% with tirofiban, eptifibatide and abciximab, respectively). The remaining 48% of patients required a second half-bolus to achieve the target levels.[43] In the GOLD study,[16] 25% of all patients administered the recommended bolus doses of IIb–IIIa inhibitors did not achieve adequate platelet inhibition and experienced a significantly higher incidence of adverse cardiac events.

Thus, as with aspirin and the thiopyridines, there is substantial variability in the level of platelet function inhibition achieved with standard regimens of GP IIb–IIIa antagonist therapy, and the level of platelet function inhibition is an independent predictor for the risk of complications during PCI.

Abciximab has a protracted duration of action and, as such, reversal requires platelet transfusion. The antiplatelet effects of the competitive antagonists will abate over a relatively short period of time if the infusion is discontinued. While platelet transfusions will hasten the return of normal function, they are less effective in this setting, as the competitive antagonists have a very short dissociation time and maintain higher plasma concentrations. Fibrinogen supplementation, in the form of cryoprecipitate or fresh frozen plasma, represents a useful means by which to achieve reversal of these agents. The increasing concentration of fibrinogen tips the balance of competition at the IIb – IIIa receptor in the favor of fibrinogen, counteracting the effects of the circulating IIb/IIIa inhibitors.[44]

In a direct comparison, abciximab was superior to tirofiban for the prevention of ischemic events after percutaneous coronary angiography (PTCA).[45] However, in a comparison of all three agents in high risk patients undergoing PTCA, no difference in major cardiac events was detected at 30 days.[43]

Thrombolytics

Thrombolytic agents function by converting plasminogen (which is inactive) to plasmin. Plasmin functions to cleave fibrin enzymatically, fibrin being the primarily constituent of clot. These agents fall into two general categories:

- fibrin-specific agents – alteplase (rt-PA), reteplase (r-PA), and tenecteplase (TNK); those which preferentially activate fibrin-bound plasminogen; and
- non-fibrin-specific agents – urokinase (UK) and streptokinase (SK); which non-specifically activate plasminogen.

The fibrin-specific agents, primarily rt-PA, are preferred in neuroendovascular therapeutics. The remainder of this section pertains to rt-PA.

Alteplase

rt-PA has a relatively short half-life, requiring a bolus and continuous infusion technique to maintain steady-state plasma concentrations. The plasma concentrations decrease in a biphasic pattern, which is dominated by a very short alpha-phase half-life (3.5 minutes). The beta-phase is somewhat longer, at 72 minutes. Despite the rapid clearance of the agent from plasma, rt-PA induces a fibrinolytic state, which persists for hours in the region of the thrombus. Measurable elevations of fibrin degradation products and peripheral markers of plasmin activity remain elevated for more than 7 hours after the initiation of rt-PA therapy.[46,47] This is attributable to the continued activity of both fibrin-bound rt-PA and plasmin long after measurable rt-PA is cleared from the systemic circulation.

rt-PA dosing is covered in more detail in Chapter 5. While there is no officially recommended dosing for intra-arterial therapy, doses of up to 40 mg have been used.[48] The tendency is to use much lower doses for direct intra-arterial stroke therapy, ranging between 2 mg and 15 mg. In most cases rt-PA is administered in conjunction with small doses of intra-arterial abciximab (2–10 mg). The synergistic combination of the two agents is supported by the coronary thrombolysis literature[49] as well as by observations during intra-arterial stroke thrombolysis.[50,51] If intra-arterial pharmacological thrombolysis is anticipated or if intravenous thrombolysis has already been initiated, half of the typical heparin dose is given (30–40 IU/kg) as a bolus after femoral access is achieved. In cases where intravenous lytic therapy has been initiated in the interim before neuroendovascular

intervention, we generally have stopped the intravenous rt-PA infusion while the patient is being prepped for angiography and the table is being prepared.

rt-PA may also be administered as a continuous infusion in cases of venous sinus thrombosis. In these cases, the infusion is typically preceded by catheterization of the occluded sinus with subsequent mechanical or rheolytic thrombolysis and/or local pharmacological thrombolysis (1–2 mg aliquots delivered through the microcatheter directly into the clotted sinus, up to a total of 10 mg rt-PA). We then prepare a solution of 1–5 mg rt-PA per 10 ml of normal saline and run the infusion through a microcatheter hooked up to an infusion pump at a rate of 1–5 mg per hour for 12–24 hours, with control angiography performed after at least 12 hours of therapy. During the infusion, therapeutic heparinization is maintained (aiming at an aPTT 1.5 times normal).[52]

Vasodilators

The vasodilators are primarily applied during neuroendovascular interventions for medically refractory cerebral vasospasm involving segments of the cerebrovasculature that are not amenable to compliant balloon angioplasty. Occasionally, these agents are also required for the treatment of persistent or severe catheter-induced vasospasm.

Nimodipine, a calcium-channel blocker, is prophylactically administered orally to patients after subarachnoid hemorrhage to decrease the risk of cerebral vasospasm.

Papaverine

Papaverine is a benzylisoquinolone derivative of opium. It functions as a vasodilator, probably via the inhibition of phosphodiesterase. Since the early 1990s, papaverine infusions have been employed as a treatment for cerebral vasospasm after aneurysmal subarachnoid hemorrhage, with varying degrees of success. When effective, the vasodilatory effects of papaverine are typically short-lived, often lasting less than a few hours.[53,54] During the intra-arterial infusion, intracranial pressure (ICP) monitoring is essential, as the agent may produce significant elevations in ICP.[55] Recently Smith et al.[56] have documented a direct neurotoxic effect of papaverine.

For these reasons, we have completely abandoned papaverine as an agent for the management of cerebral vasospasm in favor of the calcium-channel blocker nicardipine (see below).

Calcium-channel blockers

There are five major classes of calcium channel blockers:

- bensothazepines (diltiazem)
- dihydropyridines (nicardipine, nifedipine, nimodipine)
- phenylalkylamines (verapamil)
- diarylaminopropylamine ethers (bepridil)
- benzimidazole-substituted tetralines (midefradil).

Three of these agents – nicardipine, nimodipine and verapamil – are applied frequently in neuroendovascular therapeutics.

All of the calcium-channel blockers decrease coronary vascular resistance and increase coronary blood flow, decrease peripheral vascular resistance via vasodilatation of arterioles, and are without significant effect on venous tone at normal doses. The relative inotropic and chronotropic effects of the different classes of calcium-channel blockers are related to the class of calcium channels that they block. Negative inotropic effects dominate in those agents that preferentially block L-type channels. Dihydropyridines (nimodipine and nicardipine) have minimal negative inotropic effects and do not directly effect the atrioventricular (AV) conduction system or the sinoatrial (SA) node (and therefore do not effect conduction or automaticity). In fact, these agents may cause a reflex tachycardia in response to their potent vasodilating effects. In addition, any weak negative inotropic effects that these agents may possess are overcome by the reflex sympathetic response that they engender. Overall, they typically produce a drop in blood pressure, an increase in heart rate and contractility, and an increase in cardiac output.

Verapamil, in comparison to the dihydropyridines, has greater negative chronotropic and inotropic effects and also slows cardiac conduction. The effects of the drug are generally more than sufficient to overcome the reflex sympathetic response stimulated by peripheral vasodilation, resulting in a lower blood pressure and lower heart rate. The negative inotropic effects may be particularly important in patients with underlying left ventricular dysfunction either from 'cardiac stunning' (frequently seen in the setting of aneurysmal subarachnoid hemorrhage) or ischemic coronary disease. In addition, verapamil is specifically contraindicated in combination with beta-blockers, or in patients with SA node or AV conduction abnormalities because of the possibility of AV block or severe ventricular dysfunction. For these reasons, we have chosen not to use verapamil for the treatment of cerebral vasospasm.

In addition to having a favorable cardiac pharmacological profile, the dyhydropyridines (whether administered orally or intravenously) have been shown to reduce delayed ischemic injury after subarachnoid hemorrhage.[57] Intravenous nicardipine has been demonstrated to have efficacy as a prophylactic agent for the prevention of angiographic and clinical vasospasm.[58–60] Nimodipine (60 mg orally every 4 hours) has been demonstrated to improve patient outcome at 3 months. One meta-analysis demonstrated a 27% relative risk reduction (95% CI, 13–39%) with only 13 patients (8–30) needing to be treated with oral nimodipine to avoid one poor outcome.[57]

Nicardipine is metabolized primarily by the liver, with a half-life of approximately 3–4 hours. Drug levels can be significantly prolonged in patients with challenged liver function.

For catheter-induced vasospasm, nicardipine (10 mg in 25 ml) may be diluted in sterile water to a concentration of 0.25–0.5 mg/ml. A dose of 2–3 mg can be administered through the guiding catheter over 5 minutes. Typically this results in complete resolution of catheter-induced spasm, and it the resolution is usually maintained throughout the case.

For cerebral vasospasm, nicardipine is diluted in normal saline to a concentration of 0.1–0.2 mg/ml and administered through a diagnostic catheter, a guiding catheter or a microcatheter at a rate of 3–6 mg over 10 minutes using a mechanical power injector. After each 10-minute infusion, control angiography is performed. Additional infusions are performed (as tolerated by the patient's hemodynamic status) until angiographic resolution of vasospasm is achieved. In our experience, the primary limiting factor is the induction of hypotension. To counter this, we routinely begin a phenylephrine drip simultaneously with the nicardipine infusion, titrating the drip to maintain the mean arterial pressure. We have administered up to 27 mg of nicardipine into a single vascular distribution during one session.

Preliminary experience with nicardipine has been favorable with respect to its efficacy in producing angiographic improvement in cerebral vasospasm.[61] However, the durability of the observed effects and its impact on patient outcome remain unknown.

Nitroglycerine

Nitroglycerine, a paste preparation, represents an inexpensive, readily accessible, and relatively efficacious means by which to treat catheter-induced vasospasm. In the setting of spasm, 2.5–5.0 cm of topical nitropaste can be applied to the patient's chest. This is often effective in resolving the spasm. However, it is critical that the operator remembers to remove the nitropaste at the conclusion of the intervention.

Neuroprotective agents

Despite extensive translational research, currently no pharmacological agents have been proven effective for peri-procedural neuroprotection. While hypothermia has been demonstrated to improve neurological outcome after cardiac arrest[62] and perinatal asphyxia,[63] no beneficial effect has been demonstrated during aneurysm surgery.[64] Some studies have suggested a beneficial effect of barbiturates,[65] but other studies have indicated no benefit.[66–68] Although the evidence for a beneficial effect of barbiturates is conflicting, there is general agreement that the application of these agents results in myocardial depression, increased need for vasopressors, and prolonged time to tracheal extubation.[65,68] Several animal studies have suggested that propofol, which has a superior pharmacologic profile to barbiturates, may also have additional, unique neuroprotective properties. However, these benefits were not manifest in a human investigation of neurological outcomes after open cardiac surgery.[69]

Encouraging pre-clinical data exist for the alpha-2 adrenoreceptor agonist dexmedetomidine;[70] however, it has yet to be tested clinically.

Statins

Statins are among the most commonly prescribed medications, ranking second after hydrocodone. Statins are competitive inhibitors of 3-hydroxy-3-methylglutaryl coenzyme A (HMG-CoA) reductase, which catalyzes an early, rate-limiting step in cholesterol biosynthesis. Decreased cholesterol synthesis in the liver results in increased expression of the low-density lipoprotein (LDL) receptor gene. The greater number of LDL receptors on the surface of hepatocytes results in increased removal of LDL from the blood, thereby lowering the LDL-cholesterol levels. Although the most pronounced effect of the statins is reduction of LDL cholesterol, there is also a reduction in the cholesterol content of very low-density lipoprotein particles, while high-density lipoprotein cholesterol may increase slightly. As a result, statins are the most effective and best tolerated agents available for treating dyslipidemias.

Statin pleiotropy is defined as the effects of statin therapy that extend beyond lipid modification and are independent of reduction in levels of LDL cholesterol.[71–76] These pleiotropic effects may be mediated through improving or restoring endothelial function, enhancing the stability of atherosclerotic plaques, and decreasing oxidative stress and vascular inflammation.[77] These effects are reported as directly benefiting coronary and cerebrovascular tissue, bone, and kidney and glucose metabolism, and decreasing the incidence of dementia, allograft rejection, and osteoporosis.

Statins have limited oral bioavailability. These are subject to extensive (50–80%) first-pass hepatic metabolism, and as a result drug concentrations in the systemic circulation are low. Plasma elimination half-life varies from approximately 2 hours (for pravastatin and fluvastatin) to 14 hours (for atorvastatin). Hence atorvastatin can be given at any time of the day, whereas others should be taken at bed time, since steroid synthesis is more active at night. All the statins are administered as the active lactone form except simvastatin and lovastatin, which are very lipophilic pro-drugs requiring metabolism in the liver by CYP3A4; therefore these latter agents can induce adverse drug interactions. CYP3A4 (a subset of cytochrome P450 system) is also important to the biotransformation of atorvastatin.

Statin selection should be based on the goals of therapy, efficacy, and cost – as most of the agents currently available have been used safely in clinical trials involving thousands of subjects for 5 or more years. Once drug treatment is initiated, it is almost always lifelong. It is advisable to start patients on a low dose that will achieve the patient's target goal for lowering LDL cholesterol levels. Each statin has a low recommended starting dose (10–20 mg usually), which reduces LDL cholesterol by 20–30%.

Myopathy is the only major adverse effect of clinical significance associated with statin use. Cerivastatin caused hundreds of cases of rhabdomyolysis before its withdrawal from the market in 2001. The incidence of myopathy is low (<0.1%) in patients taking statins without concomitant administration of drugs that enhance the risk of myopathy. Fibrates (gemfibrozil and clofibrate) and niacin are lipid-lowering agents that cause myopathy by themselves, but when used with statins, the risk is increased, owing to enhanced inhibition of skeletal muscle sterol synthesis. CYP3A4 inhibitors like itraconazole, cyclosporin, erythromycin, clarithromycin, verapamil, and diltiazem can increase the levels of statins in the blood, contributing to myopathy.

Myopathy syndrome is characterized by intense myalgia associated with fatigue. Serum creatinine kinase (CK) levels in affected patients are typically 10 times higher than normal. However, routine CK monitoring is not recommended unless statins are used with one of the predisposing drugs, and, moreover, patients receiving combined therapy may develop myopathy months to years after starting the therapy. The statin and any other drug suspected of contributing to myopathy should be discontinued if true myopathy is suspected even if CK levels are unavailable to document the presence of myopathy. Rhabdomyolysis should also be excluded and renal function monitored in appropriate patients.

Hepatotoxicity resulting from statin use has an incidence of less than 1%, and it appears to be dose related. Baseline measurement of alanine transaminase (ALT) and repeat testing at 3–6 months are recommended. If ALT is normal initially, it need not be repeated more than once every 6–12 months.

Atorvastatin (and not pravastatin) may reduce the effects of clopidogrel by inhibiting the formation of the active metabolite (clopidogrel itself is an inactive pro-drug), which is metabolized mainly by CYP3A4 isozyme. This decreases the inhibitory effect of clopidogrel on platelet aggregation.[78] However, the clinical importance of this interaction is unclear, and the post-hoc analysis of the CREDO trial demonstrated that there was no difference in clinical outcomes.[79]

Many landmark lipid-lowering trials have shown that treatment with statins is associated with a significant decrease in risk of stroke and transient ischemic attack (TIA) in patients with symptomatic coronary artery disease or multiple risk factors for atherosclerosis.[80] Statins have been shown to be efficacious in secondary prevention of stroke as well; in the Heart Protection Study, major vascular event rates were reduced from 30% to 25% (p=0.001) in a cohort of 3280 patients with a history of stroke or TIA.[81] The national guidelines produced by the American Stroke Association and the American Heart Association recommend that a statin should be initiated during hospitalization for first ischemic stroke caused by atherosclerosis of small and or large vessels.[82] The target cholesterol level is < 100 mg/dL for patients at low risk and <70 mg/dL for patients at high risk.

It has been shown that intracellular adhesion molecule (ICAM)-1-mediated leukocyte extravasation contributes to the pathogenesis of cerebral vasospasm.[83] Experimental evidence suggests that statins competitively inhibit leukocyte function antigen (LFA)-1 binding to endothelium and also decrease ICAM-1 expression, and hence they may play an important role in alleviating vasospasm.[73] A phase 2 randomized placebo controlled study by Tseng et al.[76] demonstrated that acute treatment with pravastatin after a subarachnoid hemorrhage ameliorates cerebral vasospasm, improves cerebral autoregulation, and reduces vasospasm-related delayed ischemic deficits. Statins may up-regulate endothelial NO synthetase to improve cerebral vasomotor reactivity, increase cerebral blood flow, and potentially modulate the development of cerebral proliferative vasculopathy.[76]

Less well defined, but equally compelling, is the protective effect that statins appear to convey in ischemic cerebrovascular disease, not only in acute stroke syndromes but also during elective cerebral revascularization.[71,75,76,84,85]

References

1. Bittl JA, Chaitman BR, Feit F, Kimball W, Topol EJ. Bivalirudin versus heparin during coronary angioplasty for unstable or postinfarction angina: final report reanalysis of the Bivalirudin Angioplasty Study. Am Heart J 2001; 142: 952–9.

2. Lincoff AM, Kleiman NS, Kottke-Marchant K et al. Bivalirudin with planned or provisional abciximab versus low-dose heparin and abciximab during percutaneous coronary revascularization: results of the Comparison of Abciximab Complications with Hirulog for Ischemic Events Trial (CACHET). Am Heart J 2002; 143: 847–53.

3. Lincoff AM, Bittl JA, Harrington RA et al. Bivalirudin and provisional glycoprotein IIb/IIIa blockade compared with heparin and planned glycoprotein IIb/IIIa blockade during percutaneous coronary intervention: REPLACE-2 randomized trial. JAMA 2003; 289: 853–63.

4. Maroo A, Lincoff AM. Bivalirudin in PCI: an overview of the REPLACE-2 trial. Semin Thromb Hemost 2004; 30: 329–36.

5. Schafer AI. Antiplatelet therapy. Am J Med 1996; 101: 199–209.

6. Taylor DW, Barnett HJ, Haynes RB et al. Low-dose and high-dose acetylsalicylic acid for patients undergoing carotid endarterectomy: a randomised controlled trial. ASA and Carotid Endarterectomy (ACE) Trial Collaborators. Lancet 1999; 353: 2179–84.

7. Patrono C. Aspirin as an antiplatelet drug. N Engl J Med 1994; 330: 1287–94.

8. Awtry EH, Loscalzo J. Aspirin. Circulation 2000; 101: 1206–18.

9. Collaborative overview of randomised trials of antiplatelet therapy–I: prevention of death, myocardial infarction, and stroke by prolonged antiplatelet therapy in various categories of patients. Antiplatelet Trialists' Collaboration. BMJ 1994; 308: 81–106.

10. Gum PA, Kottke-Marchant K, Welsh PA, White J, Topol EJ. A prospective, blinded determination of the natural history of aspirin resistance among stable patients with cardiovascular disease. J Am Coll Cardiol 2003; 41: 961–65.

11. Chen WH, Lee PY, Ng W, Tse HF, Lau CP. Aspirin resistance is associated with a high incidence of myonecrosis after non-urgent percutaneous coronary intervention despite clopidogrel pretreatment. J Am Coll Cardiol 2004; 43: 1122–26.

12. Alberts MJ, Bergman DL, Molner E et al. Antiplatelet effect of aspirin in patients with cerebrovascular disease. Stroke 2004; 35: 175–8.

13. Pulcinelli FM, Pignatelli P, Celestini A et al. Inhibition of platelet aggregation by aspirin progressively decreases in long-term treated patients. J Am Coll Cardiol 2004; 43: 979–84.

14. Grotemeyer KH, Scharafinski HW, Husstedt IW. Two-year follow-up of aspirin responder and aspirin non responder. A pilot-study including 180 post-stroke patients. Thromb Res 1993; 71: 397–403.

15. Mueller MR, Salat A, Stangl P et al. Variable platelet response to low-dose ASA and the risk of limb deterioration in patients submitted to peripheral arterial angioplasty. Thromb Haemost 1997; 78: 1003–7.

16. Steinhubl SR, Talley JD, Braden GA et al. Point-of-care measured platelet inhibition correlates with a reduced risk of an adverse cardiac event after percutaneous coronary intervention: results of the GOLD (AU-Assessing Ultegra) multicenter study. Circulation 2001; 103: 2572–8.

17. Quinn MJ, Fitzgerald DJ. Ticlopidine and clopidogrel. Circulation 1999; 100: 1667–72.

18. Bertrand ME, Rupprecht HJ, Urban P, Gershlick AH. Double-blind study of the safety of clopidogrel with and without a loading dose in combination with aspirin compared with ticlopidine in combination with aspirin after coronary stenting : the clopidogrel aspirin stent international cooperative study (CLASSICS). Circulation 2000; 102: 624–9.

19. Muller I, Seyfarth M, Rudiger S et al. Effect of a high loading dose of clopidogrel on platelet function in patients undergoing coronary stent placement. Heart 2001; 85: 92–3.

20. A randomised, blinded, trial of clopidogrel versus aspirin in patients at risk of ischaemic events (CAPRIE). CAPRIE Steering Committee. Lancet 1996; 348: 1329–39.

21. Patrono C, Bachmann F, Baigent C et al. Expert consensus document on the use of antiplatelet agents. The task force on the use of antiplatelet agents in patients with atherosclerotic cardiovascular disease of the European society of cardiology. Eur Heart J 2004; 25: 166–81.

22. Savcic M, Hauert J, Bachmann F et al. Clopidogrel loading dose regimens: kinetic profile of pharmacodynamic response in healthy subjects. Semin Thromb Hemost 1999; 25: 15–19.

23. Gurbel PA, Cummings CC, Bell CR et al. Onset and extent of platelet inhibition by clopidogrel loading in patients undergoing elective coronary stenting: the Plavix Reduction Of New Thrombus Occurrence (PRONTO) trial. Am Heart J 2003; 145: 239–47.

24. Cadroy Y, Bossavy JP, Thalamas C et al. Early potent antithrombotic effect with combined aspirin and a loading dose of clopidogrel on experimental arterial thrombogenesis in humans. Circulation 2000; 101: 2823–8.

25. Patrono C. Pharmacology of antiplatelet agents. In: Loscalzo J SA, ed. Thrombosis and Hemorrhage. Baltimore: William and Wilkins; 1998; 261–91.

26. Steinhubl SR, Berger PB, Mann JT III et al. Early and sustained dual oral antiplatelet therapy following percutaneous coronary intervention: a randomized controlled trial. JAMA 2002; 288: 2411–20.

27. Gurbel PA, Bliden KP, Hiatt BL, O'Connor CM. Clopidogrel for coronary stenting: response variability, drug resistance, and the effect of pretreatment platelet reactivity. Circulation 2003; 107: 2908–13.

28. Muller I, Besta F, Schulz C et al. Prevalence of clopidogrel non-responders among patients with stable angina pectoris scheduled for elective coronary stent placement. Thromb Haemost 2003; 89: 783–7.

29. Lau WC, Gurbel PA, Watkins PB et al. Contribution of hepatic cytochrome P450 3A4 metabolic activity to the phenomenon of clopidogrel resistance. Circulation 2004; 109: 166–71.

30. Matetzky S, Shenkman B, Guetta V et al. Clopidogrel resistance is associated with increased risk of recurrent atherothrombotic events in patients with acute myocardial infarction. Circulation 2004; 109: 3171–5.

31. Gurbel PA, Bliden KP. Durability of platelet inhibition by clopidogrel. Am J Cardiol 2003; 91: 1123–5.

32. Coller BS. Platelet GPIIb/IIIa antagonists: the first anti-integrin receptor therapeutics. J Clin Invest 1997; 99: 1467–71.

33. Gawaz M, Neumann FJ, Schomig A. Evaluation of platelet membrane glycoproteins in coronary artery disease: consequences for diagnosis and therapy. Circulation 1999; 99: E1–11

34. Brener SJ, Barr LA, Burchenal JE et al. Randomized, placebo-controlled trial of platelet glycoprotein IIb/IIIa blockade with primary angioplasty for acute myocardial infarction. ReoPro and Primary PTCA Organization and Randomized Trial (RAPPORT) Investigators. Circulation 1998; 98: 734–41.

35. Neumann FJ, Hochholzer W, Pogatsa-Murray G et al. Antiplatelet effects of abciximab, tirofiban and eptifibatide in patients undergoing coronary stenting. J Am Coll Cardiol 2001; 37: 1323–28.

36. Tcheng JE, Talley JD, O'Shea JC et al. Clinical pharmacology of higher dose eptifibatide in percutaneous coronary intervention (the PRIDE study). Am J Cardiol 2001; 88: 1097–102.

37. Novel dosing regimen of eptifibatide in planned coronary stent implantation (ESPRIT): a randomised, placebo-controlled trial. Lancet 2000; 356: 2037–44.

38. Effects of platelet glycoprotein IIb/IIIa blockade with tirofiban on adverse cardiac events in patients with unstable angina or acute myocardial infarction undergoing coronary angioplasty. The RESTORE Investigators. Randomized Efficacy Study of Tirofiban for Outcomes and Restenosis. Circulation 1997; 96: 1445–53.

39. Smith SC Jr, Dove JT, Jacobs AK et al. ACC/AHA guidelines for percutaneous coronary intervention (revision of the 1993 PTCA guidelines)-executive summary: a report of the American College of Cardiology/American Heart Association task force on practice guidelines (Committee to revise the 1993 guidelines for percutaneous transluminal coronary angioplasty) endorsed by the Society for Cardiac Angiography and Interventions. Circulation 2001; 103: 3019–41.

40. Platelet glycoprotein IIb/IIIa receptor blockade and low-dose heparin during percutaneous coronary revascularization. The EPILOG Investigators. N Engl J Med 1997; 336: 1689–96.

41. Kleiman NS, Raizner AE, Jordan R et al. Differential inhibition of platelet aggregation induced by adenosine diphosphate or a thrombin receptor-activating peptide in patients treated with bolus chimeric 7E3 Fab: implications for inhibition of the internal pool of GPIIb/IIIa receptors. J Am Coll Cardiol 1995; 26: 1665–71.

42. Renda G, Rocca B, Crocchiolo R, Cri8stofaro RD, Landolfi R. Effect of fibrinogen concentration and platelet count on the inhibitory effect of abciximab and tirofiban. Thromb Haemost 2003; 89: 348–54.

43. Kini AS, Richard M, Suleman J et al. Effectiveness of tirofiban, eptifibatide, and abciximab in minimizing myocardial necrosis during percutaneous coronary intervention (TEAM pilot study). Am J Cardiol 2002; 90: 526–9.

44. Li YF, Spencer FA, Becker RC. Comparative efficacy of fibrinogen and platelet supplementation on the in vitro reversibility of competitive glycoprotein IIb/IIIa receptor-directed platelet inhibition. Am Heart J 2002; 143: 725–32.

45. Topol EJ, Moliterno DJ, Herrmann HC et al. Comparison of two platelet glycoprotein IIb/IIIa inhibitors, tirofiban and abciximab, for the prevention of ischemic events with percutaneous coronary revascularization. N Engl J Med 2001; 344: 1888–94.

46. Agnelli G, Buchanan MR, Fernandez F, Van RJ, Hirsh J. Sustained thrombolysis with DNA-recombinant tissue type plasminogen activator in rabbits. Blood 1985; 66: 399–401.

47. Tanswell P, Tebbe U, Neuhaus KL et al. Pharmacokinetics and fibrin specificity of alteplase during accelerated infusions in acute myocardial infarction. J Am Coll Cardiol 1992; 19: 1071–5.

48. Qureshi AI, Suri MF, Shatla AA et al. Intraarterial recombinant tissue plasminogen activator for ischemic stroke: an accelerating dosing regimen. Neurosurgery 2000; 47: 473–6.

49. de Lemos JA, Gibson CM, Antman EM et al. Abciximab and early adjunctive percutaneous coronary intervention are associated with improved ST-segment resolution after thrombolysis: Observations from the TIMI 14 Trial. Am Heart J 2001; 141: 592–8.

50. Mangiafico S, Cellerini M, Nencini P, Gensini G, Inzitari D. Intravenous glycoprotein IIb/IIIa inhibitor (tirofiban) followed by intra-arterial urokinase and mechanical thrombolysis in stroke. AJNR Am J Neuroradiol 2005; 26: 2595–601.

51. Deshmukh VR, Fiorella DJ, Albuquerque FC et al. Intra-arterial thrombolysis for acute ischemic stroke: preliminary experience with platelet glycoprotein IIb/IIIa inhibitors as adjunctive therapy. Neurosurgery 2005; 56: 46–54.

52. Kim SY, Suh JH. Direct endovascular thrombolytic therapy for dural sinus thrombosis: infusion of alteplase. AJNR Am J Neuroradiol 1997; 18: 639–45.

53. Milburn JM, Moran CJ, Cross DT III et al. Increase in diameters of vasospastic intracranial arteries by intraarterial papaverine administration. J Neurosurg 1998; 88: 38–42.

54. Vajkoczy P, Horn P, Bauhuf C et al. Effect of intra-arterial papaverine on regional cerebral blood flow in hemodynamically relevant cerebral vasospasm. Stroke 2001; 32: 498–505.

55. Cross DT III, Moran CJ, Angtuaco EE et al. Intracranial pressure monitoring during intraarterial papaverine infusion for cerebral vasospasm. AJNR Am J Neuroradiol 1998; 19: 1319–23.

56. Smith WS, Dowd CF, Johnston SC et al. Neurotoxicity of intra-arterial papaverine preserved with chlorobutanol used for the treatment of cerebral vasospasm after aneurysmal subarachnoid hemorrhage. Stroke 2004; 35: 2518–22.

57. Feigin VL, Rinkel GJ, Algra A, Vermeulen M, van GJ. Calcium antagonists in patients with aneurysmal subarachnoid hemorrhage: a systematic review. Neurology 1998; 50: 876–83.

58. Flamm ES, Adams HP Jr, Beck DW et al. Dose-escalation study of intravenous nicardipine in patients with aneurysmal subarachnoid hemorrhage. J Neurosurg 1988; 68: 393–400.

59. Haley EC Jr, Kassell NF, Torner JC. A randomized controlled trial of high-dose intravenous nicardipine in aneurysmal subarachnoid hemorrhage. A report of the Cooperative Aneurysm Study. J Neurosurg 1993; 78: 537–47.

60. Haley EC Jr, Kassell NF, Torner JC. A randomized trial of nicardipine in subarachnoid hemorrhage: angiographic and transcranial Doppler ultrasound results. A report of the Cooperative Aneurysm Study. J Neurosurg 1993; 78: 548–53.

61. Badjatia N, Topcuoglu MA, Pryor JC et al. Preliminary experience with intra-arterial nicardipine as a treatment for cerebral vasospasm. AJNR Am J Neuroradiol 2004; 25: 819–26.

62. Mild therapeutic hypothermia to improve the neurologic outcome after cardiac arrest. N Engl J Med 2002; 346: 549–56.

63. Whitelaw A, Thoresen M. Clinical trials of treatments after perinatal asphyxia. Curr Opin Pediatr 2002; 14: 664–8.

64. Todd MM, Hindman BJ, Clarke WR, Torner JC. Mild intraoperative hypothermia during surgery for intracranial aneurysm. N Engl J Med 2005; 352: 135–45.

65. Nussmeier NA, Arlund C, Slogoff S. Neuropsychiatric complications after cardiopulmonary bypass: cerebral protection by a barbiturate. Anesthesiology 1986; 64: 165–70.

66. Ward JD, Becker DP, Miller JD et al. Failure of prophylactic barbiturate coma in the treatment of severe head injury. J Neurosurg 1985; 62: 383–88.

67. Randomized clinical study of thiopental loading in comatose survivors of cardiac arrest. Brain Resuscitation Clinical Trial I Study Group. N Engl J Med 1986; 314: 397–403.

68. Zaidan JR, Klochany A, Martin WM et al. Effect of thiopental on neurologic outcome following coronary artery bypass grafting. Anesthesiology 1991; 74: 406–11.

69. Roach GW, Newman MF, Murkin JM et al. Ineffectiveness of burst suppression therapy in mitigating perioperative cerebrovascular dysfunction. Multicenter Study of Perioperative Ischemia (McSPI) Research Group. Anesthesiology 1999; 90: 1255–64.

70. Hoffman WE, Kochs E, Werner C, Thomas C, Albrecht RF. Dexmedetomidine improves neurologic outcome from incomplete ischemia in the rat. Reversal by the alpha 2-adrenergic antagonist atipamezole. Anesthesiology 1991; 75: 328–32.

71. Kennedy J, Quan H, Buchan AM, Ghali WA, Feasby TE. Statins are associated with better outcomes after carotid endarterectomy in symptomatic patients. Stroke 2005; 36: 2072–76.

72. O'Neil-Callahan K, Katsimaglis G, Tepper MR et al. Statins decrease perioperative cardiac complications in patients undergoing non-cardiac vascular surgery: the Statins for Risk Reduction in Surgery (StaRRS) study. J Am Coll Cardiol 2005; 45: 336–42.

73. McGirt MJ, Pradilla G, Legnani FG et al. Systemic administration of simvastatin after the onset of experimental subarachnoid hemorrhage attenuates cerebral vasospasm. Neurosurgery 2006; 58: 945–51.

74. Tseng MY, Czosnyka M, Richards H, Pickard JD, Kirkpatrick PJ. Effects of acute treatment with statins on cerebral autoregulation in patients after aneurysmal subarachnoid hemorrhage. Neurosurg Focus 2006; 21: E10

75. Groschel K, Ernemann U, Schulz JB et al. Statin therapy at carotid angioplasty and stent placement: effect on procedure-related stroke, myocardial infarction, and death. Radiology 2006; 240: 145–51.

76. Tseng MY, Hutchinson PJ, Czosnyka M et al. Effects of acute pravastatin treatment on intensity of rescue therapy, length of inpatient stay, and 6-month outcome in patients after aneurysmal subarachnoid hemorrhage. Stroke 2007; 38: 1545–50.

77. Crisby M, Nordin-Fredriksson G, Shah PK et al. Pravastatin treatment increases collagen content and decreases lipid content, inflammation, metalloproteinases, and cell death in human carotid plaques: implications for plaque stabilization. Circulation 2001; 103: 926–33.

78. Lau WC, Waskell LA, Watkins PB et al. Atorvastatin reduces the ability of clopidogrel to inhibit platelet aggregation: a new drug-drug interaction. Circulation 2003; 107: 32–7.

79. Saw J, Steinhubl SR, Berger PB et al. Lack of adverse clopidogrel-atorvastatin clinical interaction from secondary analysis of a randomized, placebo-controlled clopidogrel trial. Circulation 2003; 108: 921–4.

80. Sanossian N, Ovbiagele B. Multimodality stroke prevention. Neurologist 2006; 12: 14–31.

81. Collins R, Armitage J, Parish S, Sleight P, Peto R. Effects of cholesterol-lowering with simvastatin on stroke and other major vascular events in 20536 people with cerebrovascular disease or other high-risk conditions. Lancet 2004; 363: 757–67.

82. Adams HP Jr, del ZG, Alberts MJ et al. Guidelines for the early management of adults with ischemic stroke: a guideline from the American Heart Association/American Stroke Association Stroke Council, Clinical Cardiology Council, Cardiovascular Radiology and Intervention Council, and the Atherosclerotic Peripheral Vascular Disease and Quality of Care Outcomes in Research Interdisciplinary Working Groups: The American Academy of Neurology affirms the value of this guideline as an educational tool for neurologists. Circulation 2007; 115: e478–534.

83. Sills AK Jr, Clatterbuck RE, Thompson RC, Cohen PL, Tamargo RJ. Endothelial cell expression of intercellular adhesion molecule 1 in experimental posthemorrhagic vasospasm. Neurosurgery 1997; 41: 453–60.

84. Ovbiagele B, Saver JL, Starkman S et al. Statin enhancement of collateralization in acute stroke. Neurology 2007; 68: 2129–31.

85. Cakmak A, Yemisci M, Koksoy C et al. Statin pre-treatment protects brain against focal cerebral ischemia in diabetic mice. J Surg Res 2007; 138: 254–8.

4

Embolic agents and materials, stents, delivery systems, and retrieval devices

David Fiorella and Raymond D Turner IV

The field of endovascular surgical neuroradiology is predicated upon the development of minimally invasive techniques and implantable devices. While freely borrowing from the fields of cardiology and interventional radiology, the seminal innovation of devices and procedures for specific neurological disorders has been in many ways the defining milestone of the specialty; certainly Serbinenko's detachable balloons, Engleson's variable stiffness microcatheter, and the Guglielmi detachable coil system rank among them.[1–4] Less conspicuous, but no less influential, has been the role of the government regulatory agencies charged with ensuring the safety and efficacy of such products.

In the USA, regulatory oversight is provided by the Food and Drug Administration (FDA). The FDA is a dynamic organization, which continually changes and adapts to the vagaries of politics, public opinion, the marketplace, and the technological and scientific advances in healthcare. The FDA possesses federal authority to regulate medical devices via the secretary of the Department of Health and Human Services (DHHS), a cabinet-level position within the executive branch of government.[5] There is also legislative oversight via the Senate and House of Representatives, as well as judicial checks and balances, via the Department of Justice, in the US attorneys.

The FDA came into being with the Food and Drug Act of 1906, primarily in response to public outcry over contaminated food.[6] In 1938, the Food and Drug Act was amended, mentioning for the first time oversight of medical devices.[5] Nevertheless, this legislation focused primarily on pharmaceuticals and thus had numerous shortcomings and limitations. A major regulatory watershed came with the passage of the Medical Devices Amendment of 1976[5] (coincidentally, this was about the time that Serbinenko began using balloons to treat cerebrovascular disease). This amendment clearly defined oversight for new or high-risk medical devices and it attempted to 'grandfather' those known to be safe and efficacious by previous experience. With the passage of this amendment, the FDA was charged with categorizing all medical devices into a three-tier classification and regulatory system on the basis of their risk. It specified two types of pre-marketing procedures for 'approval.' A detailed submission, called a pre-market approval (PMA) was implemented for new and high-risk devices. A less thorough submission was implemented for devices that were substantially equivalent to those marketed before the amendment (and deemed safe). This submission was called a pre-market notification, or '510(K)' in reference to the section of the Act specifying this approach.

Another milestone came with the Medical Devices Act of 1990, which was primarily concerned with user and manufacturer medical device reporting and with post-marketing surveillance and tracking for safety.[5]

The FDA's Center for Devices and Radiological Health has primary responsibility for regulating medical devices. As noted above, the Center divides these into three classes (the higher the class, the higher the risk):[7,8]

- class I – those devices that do not support human life, and are not important in preventing impairment of human health, and do not pose significant risk of illness or injury. Examples would include dental filling, daily-wear contact lenses, and tongue depressors. These devices are regulated by 'general controls', which are primarily post-marketing and meant to ensure safety, purity, and accurate labeling.
- class II – those devices that require performance standards to assure safety and efficacy for the intended use, as well as standards for the manufacturing and operation of the device. In addition to general controls of class I, these devices are also subject to 'special controls' concerned with performance and design standards, post-market surveillance, patient registries, guidelines, and other actions. Examples would include lead wires and cables to medical devices.
- class III – those devices with potential for serious risk to health, safety, and welfare and are intended as an implant, used in sustaining or supporting human life, or are of substantial importance in diagnosing, curing, mitigating, or treating disease or preventing impaired health.

Commercial interstate marketing and sale of medical devices in the USA typically involves successful 510(K) or PMA. However, medical devices may also be obtained for use with an investigational device exemption (IDE), humanitarian device exemption (HDE) – custom device and emergency device mechanisms prior to any approval.[7] These latter mechanisms are highly regulated to ensure patient safety with strict oversight by an independent Investigational Review Board under guidelines established by the FDA and the DHHS. Key to this process is intimate familiarity with state and local common law regarding informed consent standards (which may vary).[7,9–12] If a device is already approved for another marketed indication but is used in a non-approved fashion, this may be acceptable medical practice (assuming this use is not marketed). This is termed 'off-label' use, and it should be employed when such practice is widely recognized in the specialty, and the operator is trained and familiar with the use as well as its limitations. Informed consent may also be an issue in these cases, although it may be reasonable to assume the 'prudent patient doctrine.' Much more detailed discussions of these complex topics may be found in the bibliography references at the end of this chapter.[7–9,13–17]

This chapter is not meant to be a compendium of neuroendovascular devices, rather it is meant as a broad overview, with special attention focusing on implantable, therapeutic devices. The use of guide catheters, sheaths, connectors, torque devices, and the like, (while the basic substrate and foundation of cerebral endovascular access) is often defined by training, familiarity, and subjective impressions of success (not to mention luck), and they are thus excluded from this discussion.

Liquid embolic agents

Liquid embolic agents are primarily used for the embolization of arterial–venous shunts [arterial–venous malformations (AVMs) and dural arteriovenous fistulae (dAVF)]. On occasion, these agents can be employed for tumor embolization as well.[18]

Cyanoacrylates

These liquid adhesive polymer agents offer several important advantages:

- they have the potential for penetration deep into an AVM nidus, as well the potential for transarterial-to-venous pouch penetration for a dAVF.
- they can achieve permanent embolization with durable occlusion of the vessel or pedicle being embolized.
- they can be delivered through small, flexible, flow-directed catheters, which can be safely and atraumatically manipulated into the most distal and tortuous locations within the cerebral vasculature.
- they can be easily and quickly delivered into the pedicle, with infusions generally requiring less than 1 minute (unlike particulate embolization, which can require numerous prolonged injections from a given catheter position).

Several different polymers have been employed. The first agent available was iso-butyl-2-cyanoacrylate (IBCA): however, this was discontinued after studies demonstrated that it possessed some carcinogenic potential in animals. Currently, n-butyl-cyanoacrylate (nBCA) (Cordis Neurovascular, Miami Lakes, Florida) is the cyanoacrylate of choice for AVM embolization.

These agents are introduced as liquid monomers that subsequently polymerize to form a stable solid when they come into contact with a solution that contains anions, such as the hydroxyl groups in blood. The rate of polymerization and the rate of injection determine how far the agent will travel within the cerebral vasculature before solidifying. nBCA itself is radiolucent and must be mixed with a radio-opaque agent, typically ethiodized oil (e.g., lipiodol, ethiodol) – we employ a 1.5:1–3:1 oil–nBCA mixture for most applications (Figure 4.1). In addition to imparting radio-opacity to the nBCA, the oil acts as a retardant, slowing the rate of polymerization and acting to allow the nBCA to travel

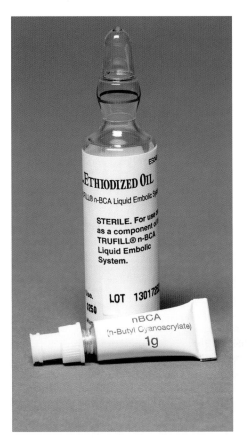

Figure 4.1
n-butyl-2-cyanoacrylate (nBCA) supplied with ethiodol used to radiographically opacify this liquid embolic agent, as well as prolong polymerization time.

further in the vessel before solidifying. Several investigators have observed that increasing the volume of ethiodized oil increases the time to polymerization.[19,20] Glacial acetic acid may also be added in small quantities to the mixture to retard further the rate of polymerization.[21]

nBCA is, for all intents and purposes, a permanent embolic agent. Once solidified, the cyanoacrylates (if a sufficient volume has been injected) create an immediate occlusion of the embolized pedicle. An intense inflammatory reaction follows, which leads to fibrous in-growth, which in turn produces a durable occlusion.[22] Although recanalization can occur, it is rare after an adequate embolization.

Disadvantages of the liquid adhesives include:

- the high level of expertise required to control safely the injection in order to achieve adequate nidal penetration without allowing the agent to extend into the vein; and
- the risk of nBCA adhering to the catheter, making withdrawal traumatic or impossible.

Ethylene-vinyl alcohol copolymer in dimethyl sulfoxide solvent

Ethylene-vinyl alcohol (EVOH) is a polymeric agent recently approved by the FDA for the preoperative embolization of brain

AVMs (EV3 Neurovascular, Irvine, California). EVOH is an insoluble co-polymer, which is dissolved in dimethyl sulfoxide (DMSO) to form a viscous suspension (Onyx). After the DMSO solvent dissipates from the solution, the EVOH precipitates to form a coherent embolus.

As a liquid embolic agent, EVOH is in many respects similar to nBCA. However, EVOH is non-adhesive, reducing the possibility of the catheter adhering to the injected polymer. This allows the operator a much greater degree of flexibility with respect to the volume and rate of the injection. The operator may even temporarily halt an EVOH–DMSO infusion in progress to perform control angiography and assess the status of the AVM nidus and draining veins before continuing the infusion. In addition, the behavior of the agent during the injection is vastly superior to that of nBCA. The EVOH precipitates from the outside in, forming a 'skin' around the outside of a centrally liquid core (Figure 4.2a). This phenomenon allows the continued forward flow of the embolic agent after an initially occlusive proximal cast is created. The 'plug-and-push' technique takes advantage of this property of EVOH. After reflux is observed, the infusion may be temporarily suspended for 30 seconds and then resumed. Not infrequently, the agent will then progress through the fluid center of the pre-existing, proximally occlusive embolic cast to penetrate antegrade further into the AVM nidus. Using this technique, very large volumes of the agent (>1 ml) can be routinely infused safely into the AVM nidus, yielding much deeper nidal penetration and much more complete occlusion of the AVM nidus.

Two different preparations of Onyx are commercially available in the USA, Onyx-18 and Onyx-34, to accommodate differences in pedicle flow characteristics. The Onyx-18 preparation is less viscous and is recommended for most injections. The Onyx-34 is more viscous and is recommended for high-flow pedicles and fistulae. A third, yet more viscous, preparation has been developed for treatment of aneurysms, but is not yet widely available.[23–25]

Initial studies demonstrated that the DMSO component of the mixture induced vasospasm and angionecrosis.[26,27] Subsequent investigations indicated that these effects could be largely eliminated by limiting the volume of DMSO injected and limiting the rate at which it was introduced.[28] Jahan et al[29] did report one complication (proximal reflux) related to distal vasospasm that developed during an injection. To avoid problems with spasm, Onyx is injected at a slow, steady rate of approximately 0.15 ml per minute. In addition, the total volume of DMSO used to purge the catheter before the injection should be limited to the dead space of the microcatheter, a feature emphasized through the use of separate, color-coded syringes (Figure 4.2b). At the current time, only the Marathon (0.23 ml dead space, EV3), UltraFlowHPC (0.26 ml EV3), Rebar 10 (0.27 ml, EV3) and Rebar 14 (0.29 ml, EV3) are approved for use with Onyx.

In the US AVM IDE trial, a multi-center, randomized study in pre-surgical AVM patients, Onyx was demonstrated to be non-inferior to nBCA in achieving >50% AVM volume reduction when all patients entered into the study were considered ($p=0.00002$) and it was significantly better if only those patients who were evaluable ($p<0.04$) were considered. It is important to note that at the time this study was conducted, the injection techniques that are currently employed with EVOH were not yet fully refined. Thus, it is possible that the true extent of the superiority of EVOH was underestimated in this initial trial. Whether the widespread application of Onyx using the current infusion techniques results in substantially higher angiographic cure rates and improved patient outcomes after surgery remains to be seen.

The EVOH–DMSO mixture itself is radiolucent. Commercially available EVOH–DMSO comes pre-packaged as a suspension containing micronized tantalum. The tantalum is maintained in suspension by placing the agent on a mechanical shaker, Vortex Genie-2 (Figure 4.2c), which provides continuous agitation of the mixture to avoid sedimentation during the procedure. The suspension must be agitated on the shaker for a minimum of 20 minutes prior to use. Additionally, it is important to note that the use of electrocautery on tantalum containing Onyx may produce sparks and at least one instance of spontaneous intra-operative combustion has been reported.[30]

Although long-term data are lacking, EVOH is, like nBCA, for all intents and purposes, a permanent agent. Jahan et al.[29] reported no recanalization in a small number of patients imaged up to 20 months after embolization. Murayama et al.[28] demonstrated no recanalization in swine rete at 6 month follow-up.

Ethyl alcohol

On the basis of their success using ethanol to eradicate peripheral vascular malformations, Yakes et al.[31] have advocated the use of undiluted absolute ethyl alcohol (ETOH) (98% dehydrated alcohol injection USP) for the embolization of central nervous system AVMs. They reported their initial results in a series of 17 patients. They were able to cure seven patients with ETOH alone, three additional patients were cured after surgery, and one after radiotherapy. Despite this impressive cure rate, it is important to note that two patients with partially treated lesions died and eight patients suffered complications related to the therapy. No other similar case series describing the application of ethanol has been reported to date.

ETOH is a sclerosant, functioning to dehydrate and denude the endothelium, creating fractures within the vessel wall that extend to the level of the internal elastic lamina. These changes result in acute thrombosis of the vessel.[32]

ETOH causes significant brain edema, necessitating treatment with high doses of corticosteroids immediately before and for 2 weeks after the procedure. In some cases, brain edema and increases in intracranial pressure necessitate mannitol therapy. In high doses, ETOH has been also found to induce pulmonary pre-capillary vasospasm, which can lead to cardiopulmonary collapse. This effect has been reported in humans after the embolization of peripheral AVMs with ETOH. It is critical that the appropriate anesthesia and critical care resources are alerted to this possibility. Given these risks, the high level of experience required to perform ETOH embolization safely, and the relatively widespread experience and comfort level with the cyanoacrylates, there has been a general reluctance amongst most endovascular neurointerventionalists to use ETOH for the embolization of brain AVMs.

Particulate embolic agents

Many different particulate embolysates have been employed for the embolization of vascular malformations, tumors, and miscellaneous sources of uncontrolled head and neck bleeding.

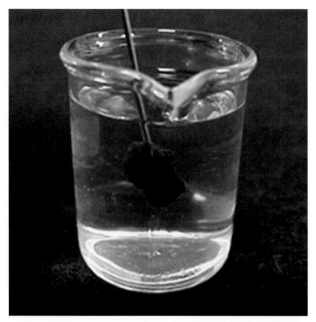

(a)

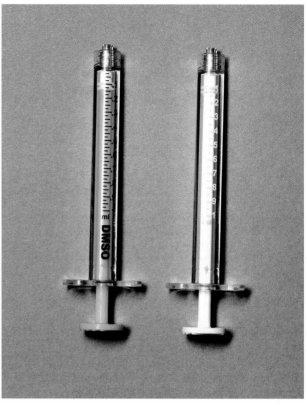

(b)

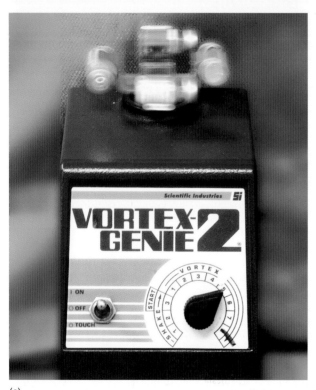

(c)

Figure 4.2
(a) Ethylene-vinyl alcohol (EVOH) copolymer radiographically opacified with tantalum powder (Onyx) suspended in saline.
(b) Onyx is dissolved in dimethyl sulfoxide (DMSO) which must be injected precisely and slowly to avoid toxicity. This is facilitated through the use of color-coded syringes.
(c) Tantalum remains suspended in the EVOH solution through continuous, vigorous agitation prior to injection. (Provided by ev3 with permission.)

These agents initially included such items as silk sutures and microfibrillar collagen material, eventually evolving to more refined materials including polyvinyl alcohol (PVA) and embolization microspheres. The application of particulate embolysates for the pre-operative embolization of vascular malformations has gradually declined with the increasing use of the liquid embolic agents (see above), which can be delivered through lower-profile microcatheter systems and provide a more complete and permanent occlusion. Currently, we do not employ particulate embolysates for the embolization of AVMs or AVF.

Polyvinyl alcohol and embospheres

Embolization with particulate agents is fundamentally different from embolization with liquid agents.

Durability

Vessels embolized with particulate agents recanalize over time (i.e. these are temporary embolic materials). Sorimachi et al.[33]

reported a 43% rate of nidal recanalization after particulate embolization with PVA. Mathis et al.[34] reported a 12% recanalization rate for AVMs embolized with PVA in preparation for radiosurgery when portions of the AVM were not included in the radiation field. With the exception of preoperative embolization in anticipation of a prompt and complete resection to follow, particulate agents are relatively contraindicated given the availability of more permanent embolysates.

Microcatheter selection

To perform particulate embolization, a microcatheter with an internal diameter (ID) large enough to accept the particulate agent without clumping and clogging must be employed [Rapid Transit (Cordis Neurovascular, Miami, Florida), Prowler Plus (Cordis Neuromuscular), Excelsior 1018 (Boston Scientific, Natick, Massachusetts), Renegade (Boston Scientific)]. These catheters are of higher profile and are considerably less flexible than the smaller diameter flow-directed catheters [Elite 1.5F or 1.8F (Boston Scientific), Marathon (EV3, Irvine California)]. Correspondingly, an over-the-wire technique must be employed to negotiate the micro-catheter into the targeted vessel. These technical factors make superselective catheterization of pedicles that feed the target more labor-intensive and, in the case of an intracranial AVM, more hazardous, with a greater potential for vascular perforation.[35]

Particle size selection

Particulate embolysates are available in a variety of size ranges. Choice of embolysate type (PVA or Embospheres) and size is critical and varies to some extent with the targeted lesion.

PVA particles (Cordis Neurovascular) and Embospheres (Biosphere Medical, Rockland, Massachusetts) come in a wide variety of sizes ranging from 40 µm to 1200 µm. Although mechanistically similar, the application of the particles are fundamentally different, owing to differences in their respective properties. PVA particles are irregularly shaped and tend to clump together within the vessel, creating an occlusion. The PVA particles also elicit an inflammatory response, eventually inciting a foreign-body giant-cell reaction and necrotizing vasculitis. Embospheres are spherical, hydrophilic and compressible. For these reasons, similarly sized particles of the two agents produce markedly different types of occlusions, with the Embospheres achieving much more distal penetration and a more complete obliteration of the targeted vascular bed. When substituting Embospheres for PVA, a substantial increase in particle size selection is required to avoid tissue excessive tissue necrosis (when this is not the goal of the procedure, e.g. in treating epistaxis by embolization), cranial nerve damage, and unintentional embolization through small non-visualized artery-to-artery collaterals.

It is important to keep in mind that the types of procedures requiring particulate embolization are typically non-life-threatening (e.g. epistaxis embolization, preoperative tumor embolization) and the clinical difference between a very distal embolization with very small particles and a standard embolization is usually minimal. At the same time, as the size of the embolization particles decrease, the risk of significant complications (including blindness, stroke, tissue necrosis, and cranial nerve injury) increase substantially. For this reason, for almost all tumor and head and neck embolizations, we use PVA 250–350 µm particles.

Preparation

PVA particles are mixed with high-density non-ionic contrast (Ultravist-300, Visipaque-320). The volume of contrast (typically 30–35 ml per bottle of PVA particles) should produce a suspension that can be injected without producing excessive clogging at the microcatheter hub. Periodically between particulate injections, the hub should be cleared of particles using a saline syringe with an attached needle. Injections of particles should be periodically followed with an injection of saline to keep the microcatheter clear. Whenever the micro-catheter is being injected, whether with particles or with saline, the operator should be conscious of watching on fluoroscopy to avoid an unintended, unobserved injection of embolysate.

Embospheres come pre-loaded in a syringe into which contrast is aspirated. The suspension is prepared within the pre-loaded syringe and injected using a three-way stopcock and an additional 1 ml or 3 ml syringe.

Detachable balloons

The use of catheter-delivered, inflated, detached, and implanted embolic balloons is regarded by many as marking the beginning of endovascular surgical neuroradiology, and most credit Serbinenko as the first user.[2,36] This work was followed by the contributions of Debrun and Heishima in North America, where the use of such devices became popular: for endovascular occlusion of direct carotid cavernous fistulae; Hunterian occlusion of skull base aneurysms following test occlusion; and finally, with the adaptation of variable stiffness micro-catheters, balloon occlusion of intracranial aneurysms.[37–39] This last-mentioned application has been supplanted by detachable coil embolization, which affords much more control over subarachnoid aneurysm treatment; it is consequently also much safer.

The devices themselves are characterized by the composition of the shell (latex or silicon) in a variety of sizes and shapes; by the valve mechanism, whose function is to sustain inflation over time and to occlude permanently large cranial vessels (from 3–10 mm in diameter); by the radio-opaque, compatible material used to inflate the balloon; and by the mechanism of detachment. In today's practice, the advantage of detachable silicon balloons is conferred by their ability to create large vessel occlusions rapidly and economically. The disadvantages reside in their limited availability and relatively limited control for placement and detachment.

Debrun's initial balloons were latex, fixed to the catheter by a manually tied string of latex thread, which would tighten as a result of elastic tension when the balloon was detached, in effect serving as a valve. These are no longer widely used.

Heishima introduced a simple, elegant silicon balloon with a more standardized silicon mitral valve that was open when mounted on the catheter (Figure 4.3). Silicon is semi-permeable so that contrast used to opacify the embolus needs be mixed to an osmolality that closely approximates that of blood, to avoid the risk of the device changing its size (and hence, secondarily, its position) after it had been implanted. Originally produced by a small company (International Therapeutics Corporation,

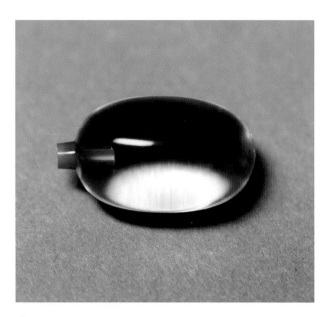

Figure 4.3
Detachable silicon balloon, no longer commercially available.

Fremont, California) but later produced by Boston Scientific (Natick, Massachusetts), these devices were painted with the same broad brush as silicon gel breast implants in the 1990s. Negative press, the small market, and the arrival of detachable coils designed expressly for aneurysms ultimately led to their removal from the marketplace. The lone remaining commercially produced detachable balloon is the latex Gold Valve Balloon (Nycomed, Paris; Acta Vascular, Santa Clara, California), which at present is not FDA-approved for use in the USA.

Once the target vessel has been catheterized with an 8F guide (or larger) with a double tuoy, the balloon is mounted on a micro-catheter and all air is purged. Valve competency should be test on the bench top. The catheter-mounted balloon may be positioned for deployment by successive inflation and deflation, which will cause the device to 'sail' with the flow of the vessel to the target point. A second balloon may be used to provide stability (by inflating it immediately proximal to the first balloon) so that, during traction on the initial balloon catheter, there is no movement during deployment. The second balloon may then be similarly deployed; in the event that one of these lesions fails, the alternate balloon continues to cede flow and thus precludes downstream embolization.[40]

Detachable coils

The introduction of detachable embolization coils has been the single largest advance in the field of neuroendovascular intervention. These coils greatly facilitate the safe percutaneous endovascular treatment of cerebral aneurysms. The available shapes, stiffness, and composition of the coils have changed dramatically over the past two decades.

Sizes

The weave of the platinum fibers that ultimately constitute the coil and define its outer diameter is referred to as the primary helix. The majority of aneurysm embolization coils are of either 0.010 inch (0.25 mm) outer diameter (OD) (e.g. GDC-10 Guglielmi detachable coils (GDC-10)) or 0.015 inch (0.38 mm) OD (e.g. GDC-18). Some manufactures have recently introduced coils with intermediate ODs (Orbit, Cordis Neurovascular: 0.012 inch (0.3 mm) OD). The coils also have a secondary helix, which defines the diameter that the coil would take if delivered unconstrained, measuring between 2 mm and 20 mm. Finally, coils have a defined length, which varies between 1 cm and 50 cm.

Shapes

In general, there are two varieties of coil shapes used for aneurysm embolization. Framing coils (three-dimensional or complex coils) are designed to emerge from the microcatheter in a configuration that results in the formation of a 'basket' distributed about the periphery of the aneurysm (Figure 4.4a). This basket then functions to contain the subsequent filling coils (standard, two-diameter or helical aneurysm coils of varing diameter, length and softness) within the central portion of the aneurysm (Figure 4.4b). Recently, several vendors have developed systems which are designed to fill the aneurysm via the successive use of multiple, complex framing-type coils, which are introduced in successively smaller sizes to form concentric baskets (Orbit, Cordis Neurovascular; GDC-360, Boston Scientific).

Detachment mechanism

Detachable coils are manipulated via an extended radiolucent 'pusher' segment, which extends from the proximal end of the radio-opaque platinum embolization coil. Once the coil has been introduced into the aneurysm and is in an acceptable position, the coil may be permanently detached from the pusher wire. Complete extrusion of the embolization coil from the micro-catheter is signaled in a variety of ways. All micro-catheters employed for aneurysm embolization have two markers, one indicating the distal tip of the micro-catheter and another 3 cm proximal to the distal tip marker. The pusher wires for embolization coils likewise have a radio-opaque proximal marker. The orientation of the proximal markers of the coil and micro-catheter serves to indicate that the coil has completely exited the microcatheter and may be detached (Figure 4.4c,d). Different vendors use different proximal marker configurations to indicate adequate coil introduction. The operator must remain cognizant of the appropriate configuration for the coil being used to avoid over- or under-deployment before attempted detachment.

The mechanisms for coil detachment also differ quite substantially between vendors. GDCs are deployed by passing a 9 volt current through the coil, which results in electrolysis of the distal segment of the radiolucent stainless steel pusher wire (Figure 4.4e). The initial generation of this technology was associated with prolonged detachment time, typically ranging between 4 and 12 minutes, but sometimes becoming substantially prolonged as the current was dissipated within a large coil mass. Further iterations of the detachment system with insulation added at the junction between the pusher wire and coil resulted in decreased dissipation of current and improved rapidity of detachment, which now typically requires less than

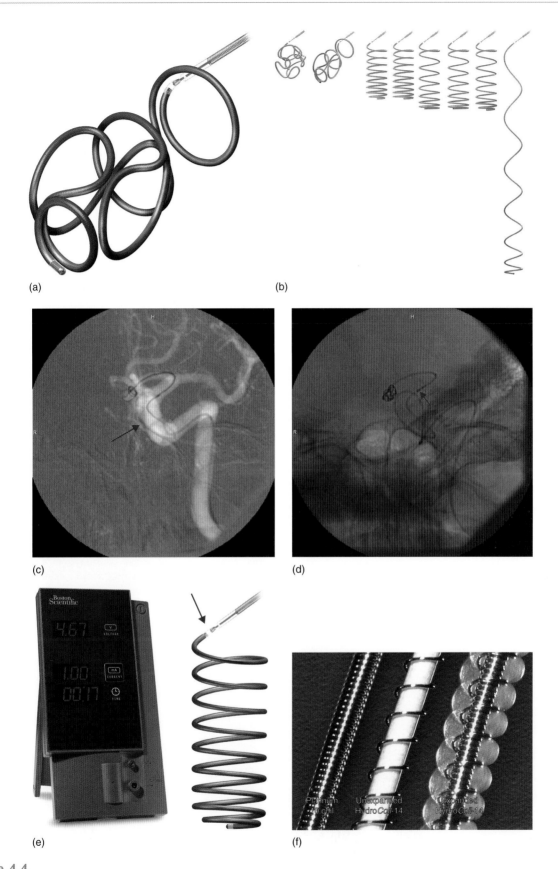

Figure 4.4

(a) Boston Scientific detachable framing coil. (b) Framing and packing coils (Left to right). The packing coils have variable degrees of 'softness', which is reflected by their ability to maintain shape when they are extended from the stylet (with permission from Boston Scientific). (c) Placement of coils under roadmap guidance within an anterior communicating artery aneurysm via the left internal carotid artery. Arrow indicates the coil marker along the stylet. (d) Fully placed framing coil. The arrow indicates the coil stylet marker 'T'd' at the proximal catheter marker. (e) Power pack and soldered junction used to detach coils. (f) Bare platinum, unexpanded hydrocoil, expanded hydrocoil. (Courtesy of Terumo.)

2 minutes. Other systems employ different pusher wire–coil detachment schemes; these alternative systems are all substantially faster then the initial GDC electrolytic detachment mechanism. Hydraulic detachment mechanisms used by Microvention-Terumo (Aliso Viejo, California) and Cordis Neurovascular are nearly instantaneous. ACT MicroCoils (Micrus Corp, Sunnyvale, California) use resistive heat-induced fracture of a tensioned polyester fiber that connects the platinum coil and pusher wire in Mircus coils, a process that takes approximately 5 seconds.

Stretch Resistance

During the repositioning of coils within an aneurysm, friction between the coils and within the microcatheter can result in a loss of coil integrity, with stretching or even breaking of the coil. To avoid this problem, some coils are designed with an internal 9.0 polypropylene thread, which confers some additional tensile strength and increases the tolerance of the coil to stretching.

Composition

Detachable embolization coils were initially composed purely of platinum.[41] Later, detachable coils with bound Dacron fibers were provided to augment thrombogenicity. However, these coils are significantly less compliant than bare platinum coils and are used primarily for vessel sacrifice and fistula occlusion.[42]

Studies of aneurysms treated with platinum embolization coils have demonstrated recurrence rates ranging between 20% and 35%, with a significant percentage of those patients requiring re-treatment.[43,44] Correspondingly, histological studies of explanted aneurysms after endovascular coil embolization have demonstrated that intra-aneurysmal clot organization is typically delayed and incomplete, with tiny open spaces left between coils – even in aneurysms that appear completely occluded angiographically. In addition, there is frequently incomplete or absent endothelialization of the aneurysm neck.[45] For these reasons, newer generations of detachable coils were developed in an attempt to promote more complete and durable aneurysm occlusion.

Polyglycolic polylactic coils

Polyglycolic polylactic acid (PGPLA) has been used extensively as suture material. The co-polymer undergoes hydrolysis over a period of several months, resulting in an inflammatory reaction that stimulates a more rapid organization of intra-aneurysmal thrombus and eventually a durable intra-aneurysmal scar. Three different preparations of PGPLA coils are currently available. The Matrix Detachable Coil System (MDC, Boston Scientific) is composed of a central platinum coil coated with PGPLA. The Cerecyte coil (Micrus, Sunnyvale, California) is composed of an outer platinum coil with an inner polyglycolic acid (PGA) filament. The Nexus coil (Microtherapeutics, Irvine, California) is composed of a platinum coil with numerous tiny PGPLA filaments, which extend from the inside of the coil outward. The durability advantages of these coils have yet to be demonstrated in humans.

Hydrocoil

The Hydrocoil Embolic System (HES Microvention-Terumo, Tokyo, Japan) contains an inner platinum core coil that is coated with a dehydrated hydrogel. When exposed to blood, the hydrogel expands over 20 minutes, substantially increasing the volume of the coils (Figure 4.4f) and thereby significantly augmenting packing density. The long-term durability of these coils, as well the full short-term impact upon the biology of subarachnoid aneurysms, is only beginning to be realized with clinical experience.[46–50]

Pushable or injectable coils

Pushable or injectable coils are relatively inexpensive and can be delivered quickly in large numbers. As such, they are most useful in situations in which a large volume of embolic material is required to achieve the desired therapeutic effect. However, because these coils are not detachable, they can only be safely applied in those situations in which precise control of coil positioning is not absolutely required.

Berenstein liquid coils

This unique product is made in two ODs – 0.008 inch (0.2 mm) and 0.016 inch (0.4 mm) outer and in various lengths up to 30 cm. These coils are pre-loaded in a clear plastic launching tube, which is flushed and then used to load the coils into a microcatheter. The coils are then injected using a 3 ml saline syringe with fluoroscopic observation, usually under blank fluoroscopic roadmap control. These small, long coils are excellent for filling space and achieving a dense packing over a long segment. They are very useful for parent vessel occlusion and fistula embolization (i.e. cases in which a large embolic coil mass is typically required).

Pushable Coils

There are numerous available fibered and non-fibered pushable coils available in a wide range of sizes (0.010–0.035 inches; 0.25–0.9 mm) and shapes (straight, complex or helical, and conical). These coils are loaded into the micro-catheter and either injected with saline or pushed out of the micro-catheter or diagnostic catheter with a coil pusher or wire. These coils can be quickly deployed and are very thrombogenic; again, they are most useful in achieving parent vessel occlusion and fistula embolization.

Stents

The term stent refers to an appliance used to correct a stenosis, (which derives from the Greek "to narrow.") It is believed to have arisen from a dentist, Charles Thomas Stent (1807–1885), who gained notoriety through the introduction of a substance that became known as Stent's compound used to form molded dental appliances or obturators (Stent's Dressing) in the 1800's. Ultimately this was commercialized in London and became widely used by English speaking oral and plastic surgeons. It has been posited that in the generalized training of surgeons, principles and applications of one specialty merged into another with ultimate use of the term to other applications and new technologies.[51]

In the context of endovascular therapeutics, the term refers flexible mesh tubes used primarily to preserve the luminal diameter of arteries. Typically these begin as solid metal of a given diameter which is precision cut and finished to a desired pattern of varying cell size and cross-linking.[52] Vascular stents can be characterized by size, shape, alloy (e.g. stainless steel, cobalt chromium, nitinol), delivery mechanism and the presence or absence of coating polymer or mesh covering.

Balloon expandable stents

Large (> 4 mm) stents

The larger available balloon expandable stents are useful primarily for stenting the proximal extracranial vessels as they arise from the aortic arch, usually the subclavian or innominate arteries. In these cases, precise stent delivery is absolutely essential. These segments of the vessels are within the thorax and are therefore protected from significant deformation. As such, a self-expanding stent is not required. A variety of balloon-mounted stent systems are available, such as the Herculink [Abbott Vascular Devices, Santa Clara, CA, 4–7 mm diameter, 12–18 mm length, 0.014 inch (0.36 mm) microwire system], Omnilink [Abbott Vascular Devices, 4–10 mm diameter, 12–58 mm length, 0.035 inch (0.9 mm) guidewire system), Express (Boston Scientific, 4–7 mm, 15–19 mm), Racer (Medtronic, 4–7 mm, 12–18 mm), Palmaz Genesis (Cordis Neurovascular, 5–12 mm, 12–59 mm), and Palmaz Blue Cobalt Chromium (Cordis Neurovascular, 4–7 mm, 12–24 mm).

Small (2.25–4.0 mm) stents

Non-drug-eluting stents

The non-drug eluting or 'bare metal', stainless steel stents were originally introduced as an inflexible 'slotted tube' design (Palmaz, Cordis Neurovascular). Progressive iterations of balloon-mounted stents were increasingly flexible and much better suited to intracranial delivery and deployment. These stents and the balloon catheters upon which they are mounted have continued to evolve, increasing the ease with which they can be used for neuroendovascular applications. The currently available devices include Driver and S660 (Medtronic), Multilink Vision, Minivision, Zeta, and Pixel (Abbott); Express-2 and Liberte (Boston Scientific). The only balloon-expandable stent specifically designed for use in the cerebrovasculature for the treatment of atherostenoses was the Neurolink (Guidant), which is no longer manufactured.

Drug-eluting stents

Delayed in-stent re-stenosis (ISR), attributable to intimal hyperplasia, has been noted to occur in up to 35% of patients after coronary stenting. A newer generation of drug-eluting stents has been developed, which, over time, release antiproliferative drugs (e.g. paclitaxel) or antineoplastic drugs (e.g, sirolimus, tacrolimus, everolimus), drugs which prevent smooth muscle cell in-growth and proliferation. These stents have led to a dramatic reduction in the rate and severity of ISR. To date, only balloon-mounted coronary drug-eluting stents are commercially available – Taxus Express-2 (Boston Scientific, which releases paclitaxel) and Cypher (Cordis, which releases sirolimus).

Self-expanding stents

Large self-explanding stents

Balloon-expandable stents are prone to kinking with normal physiologic neck motion, which can result in the stents being crushed or permanently deformed with subsequent occlusion or in-stent stenosis. For this reason, self-expanding devices are used almost exclusively for extracranial carotid stenting. A number of different carotid stent systems are available. The first FDA-approved stent was the Guidant Acculink system (Figure 4.5a), which may be used with or without a distal protection device (Accunet). The Acculink stent comes in diameters between 5 mm and 10 mm, including two tapered sizes (Figure 4.5b), which graduate from 6 mm to 8 mm from 7 mm to 10 mm over their length. The stents come in sizes from 20 mm to 40 mm. Other available self expanding stent systems include the Magic WallStent (Boston Scientific, 3.5–6 mm in diameter, 11–43 mm in length, reconstrainable), WallStent (Boston Scientific, 5–12 mm diameter, 20–90 mm in length, reconstrainable), Precise (Cordis Neurovascular, 5–10 mm, 20–40 mm, non-reconstrainable).

Small self-expanding stents

Neuroform

The Neuroform (Boston Scientific), a small (2.5–4.5 mm) self-expanding, flexible, micro-catheter-delivered, nitinol stent was introduced in 2002 for the treatment of wide-necked cerebral aneurysms (Figure 4.6). This very low radial force stent is composed of very thin (60 μm) struts separating large (2Fch) interstices, through which a microcatheter can be passed. The stent is deployed across the neck of a cerebral aneurysm, functioning to support aneurysm embolization by preventing the prolapse of coils from the aneurysm into the parent vessel.[53] Flexibility of these devices is afforded by the open-cell design and variable cross-linking (Figure 4.6b). Recently available is the Enterprise Stent (Cordis Neurovascular), which has a tear-drop-shaped, closed-cell design.

Wingspan

The Wingspan (Boston Scientific) is a small, self-expanding stent, which is very similar in design to the Neuroform. As opposed to Neuroform, Wingspan has been engineered to have a significantly greater radial force, and it is designed for the treatment of intracranial atheromatous disease. Following pre-dilation with a companion balloon (Gateway PTA Balloon Catheter, Boston Scientific), the lesion is crossed with the Wingspan delivery

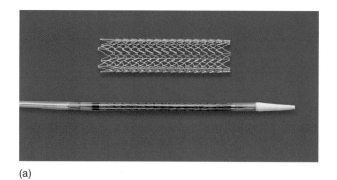

(a)

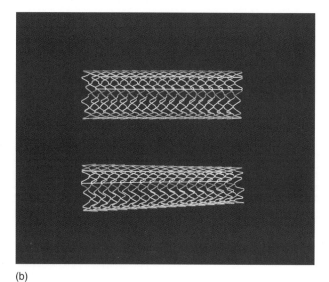

(b)

Figure 4.5
(a) Unexpanded and expanded nitinol, Acculink carotid stent.
(b) Non-tapered and tapered carotid stents. (Courtesy of Abbott Vascular.)

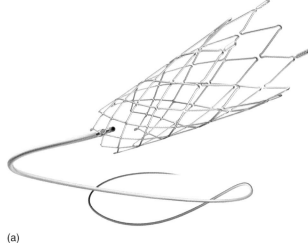

(a)

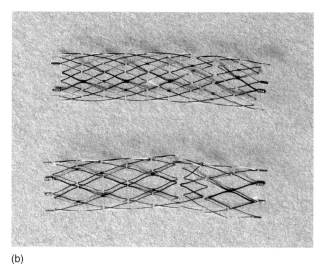

(b)

Figure 4.6
(a) Neuroform Boston Scientific self-expanding micro-stent (Courtesy of Boston Scientific). (b) Neuroform III (above) and Neuroform II stents. Notice the difference in strut cross-linking.

system and the self-expanding stent is delivered, functioning to prevent post-angioplasty re-coil and to secure any post-angioplasty dissection or endothelial injury.

Covered stent grafts

Metal stents covered with a membrane were introduced in the late 1990s for the treatment of coronary atheromatous disease, coronary artery aneurysms, and pseudoaneurysms and for the management of iatrogenic vessel perforation. The neuroendo-vascular applications of these devices has been limited to the exclusion of extracranial and proximal intracranial aneurysms and pseudoaneurysms.

The Jostent Graftmaster (9–26 mm in length, 3–5 mm in diameter; Abbott Vascular Devices, Santa Clara, California) is a balloon-mounted system that consists of two coaxially aligned, stainless steel stents which encompass a microporous polytetra-fluoro-ethylene (PTFE) membrane that sits between the two stents. Several self-expanding, covered stents are also available, including the Symbiot (Boston Scientific, made of PTFE),

Wallgraft (7–14 mm in diameter, 20–70 mm in length; Boston Scientific, made of polyethyelene teraphthalate), and Viabahn (Figure 4.7) (5–13 mm in billion, 25–150 mm in length; WL Gore and Associates, made of expanded PTFE).

Smith et al.[54] reported in-stent stenosis or occlusion in three of four Wallgraft stents implanted for the management of carotid pseudoaneurysms. This was attributed to an inflammatory response caused by the polyethyelene teraphthalate material. The durability and rates of in-stent stenosis for these devices has not yet been established, and their application in the cerebrovascula-ture remains off-label and should probably be reserved for des-perate situations in which few other options exist (e.g., carotid blowout).

Emboli protection and retrieval devices

Although technically not 'implantables' devices, emboli protec-tion and retrieval devices are often used in the course of device

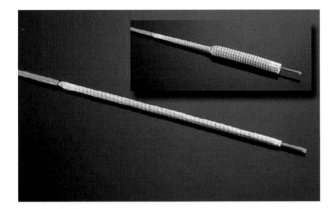

Figure 4.7
Nitinol stent covered in expanded polytetrafluoroethylene.
(Viabahn, WL Gore and Associates.)

implantation in order to prevent or reverse catastrophe. Increasingly, such devices are being specifically designed for use in acute stroke (e.g. the Merci Retriever) in an effort to mitigate the time constraints imposed by thrombolytic therapy alone.

Embolic protection

In the infancy of endovascular treatment of cerebral atherosclerotic disease, angioplasty and stent implantation were simply conducted over a guidewire. Perhaps in recognition of the formidable competition of relatively low risk carotid endarterectomy, the procedure evolved with implementation devices to limit embolization of atherosclerotic debris. There are essentially three strategies to such devices:

- filtration using modified quidewires
- cessation of antegrade flow utilizing a balloon-mounted guidewire, followed by vigorous flushing
- reversal of antegrade flow with temporary proximal occlusion utilizing a balloon-mounted guide catheter.

Filter wires

There are a variety of distal embolic protection devices that also serve as the guidewire for angioplasty and stent placement in the cervical carotid arteries. These include Angioguard (Cordis Neurovascular) Filterwire EX (Boston Scientific), Trap (Microvena, White Bear Lake, Minnesota), Neuroshield and Accunet (Abbott) (Figure 4.8a) and the Spider Fx (Ev3, Plymouth, Minnesota). The simple concept behind these devices is similar, although they do differ in important ways such as the materials, they are made of and the mechanism of deployment and recapture. It is important to emphasize that while emboli protection devices may be useful, they are not fool-proof, and emboli do occur despite their routine use.[55] Likewise, depending upon the local anatomy (tortuosity of the aortic arch and target vessel, the presence of atherosclerotic plaque) these devices also have the potential to produce significant vascular trauma, and in some circumstances they may be contraindicated.[56–58]

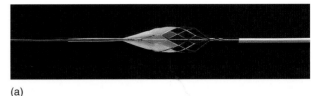

(a)

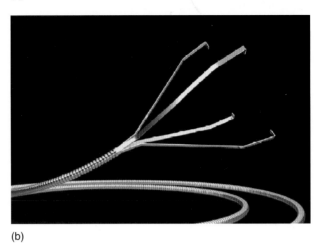

(b)

Figure 4.8
(a) Accunet embolic protection device/ filter. (Courtesy of Abbott Vascular). (b) Alligator retrieval device. (Courtesy of Chestnut Medical.)

Distal occlsion

An alternative approach to the use of filtration is complete distal occlusion utilizing a low-profile balloon on a 0.014 inch (0.36 mm) guidewire (GuardWire, Medtronic, Santa Rosa, California). Immediately prior to angioplasty and stenting the balloon is inflated. Afterward, the area is cleaned by aspiration and flushed via an aspiration catheter (Export XT Catheter, Medtronic Vascular, Santa Rosa, California) advanced over the wire.[59] Limited comparisons suggest that this may have success similar to that of other embolic protection techniques.[60]

Proximal occlusion

A third approach to limiting distal embolization during cervical intervention is the use of a proximal occluding balloon on the guide catheter to suspend antegrade flow. The Parodi antiembolization catheter (ArteriA, San Francisco, California) is a guiding catheter with an occlusion balloon attached at the distal end of the catheter. The main lumen has an inner diameter of 7F, which allows the passage of balloons and stents. When the Parodi catheter is inserted in the common carotid artery, a Parodi external balloon is inserted and inflated in the artery. Then, the occlusion balloon, attached on the outer surface of the Parodi catheter, is inflated, thereby occluding inflow to the carotid bifurcation while maintaining access to the carotid bifurcation lesion through the main lumen. The side port of the Parodi catheter may then connected to a sheath that is percutaneously inserted into the femoral vein to create a temporary arterial – venous shunt. This shunt, along with the Parodi catheter, will create reversal of flow in the internal carotid artery. One might presume that the ease of use and success of the device is predicated on a functional circle of Willis; however, the technique appears to be quite robust.[61,62] A similar rationale underlies the use of balloon-mounted guide catheters (Concentric Medical, Mountain View, California) for mechanical thrombectomy in the setting of acute stroke.[63,64]

Retrieval devices

Although fortunately a rare occur, the vagaries of anatomy, pathology, device malfunction or operator error may conspire against optimal or safe implantation of a neurovascular device. After such incidents one is often reminded of Hippocrates: 'Life is short, the art is long. Opportunity is fleeting, experiment dangerous, judgment difficult. Desperate cases need desperate remedies.[65]

The decision to retrieve a foreign body or embolus mechanically, and the selection of the appropriate device, is dictated by multiple factors, including the clinical presentation (e.g. hemorrhagic or ischemic), the need for adjunctive pharmacologic therapy (e.g. thrombolysis or anticoagulation), and the projected risk and clinical consequences of failure (*primum non nocere*–first, do no harm).[64]

Devices for foreign body removal

Gooseneck snare

A simple wire loop [e.g. the Anplatz Goose Neck Snare (Microvena Corporation, White Bear Lake, Minnesota)] may be advanced through a micro-catheter in an effort to ensnare and retrieve a foreign object.[67] This maneuver is best accomplished when the object has a free edge projecting to the lumen of the vessel and the snare loop approximates the diameter of the lumen. The device can be tightened to the target by advancing the delivery catheter and thus closing the loop. Occasionally this maneuver can be performed over an existing catheter, delivering the loop directly to the target.[68]

Alligator retrieval device

The Alligator retrieval device (Chestnut Medical Technologies, Menlo Park, California) operates under a similar strategy as the snare; however, rather than lassoing the target object, the device has four arched prongs that close or grasp an object when the delivery microcatheter is advanced distally (Figure 4.8b). This device is capable of retrieving small stents and aneurysm coils as well as large thrombotic emboli.[69]

Baskets

The Neuronet or In-Time retrieval devices (Boston Scientific and Target Therapeutics) are the natural engineering extension of the Microsnare and the Alligator: a miniature wire basket deployed through a microcather, which can be engaged and tightened upon a foreign body for retrieval.[68,70]

Mechanical thrombectomy

Merci retriever

The Merci retriever system of devices (Concentric Medical, Mountain View, California) have undergone multiple iterations

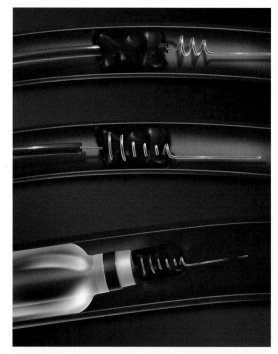

(a)

(b)

(c)

Figure 4.9
(a) Merci balloon guide catheter permits reversal of flow and facilitates intracerebral thrombectomy. (Courtesy of Concentric Medical.) (b) Original Merci retriever (model X5) used to ensnare intracerebral vascular emboli. (c) Merci L5 retriever.

since their initial introduction to clinical practice. Optimally, each is introduced through a balloon-occluding guide catheter, which facilitates retrieval of emboli by reversing flow (or at least limiting antegrade flow) in the carotid or vertebral arteries. (Figure 4.9a) The retriever itself began as a simple 0.014 inch (0.36 mm) nitinol corkscrew (models X5, X6, Figure 4.9b), but has since evolved to a more complex configuration with filaments meant to ensure a greater yield in securing distal embolic material (Model L5) (Figure 4.9c). The obvious advantage of these devices is the potential for rapid re-canalization relative to pharmacologic therapy.

AngioJet

If the Merci retriever is the 'hand vacuum' for small distal emboli, the AngioJet (Possis Medical, Minneapolis, Minnesota) is the 'industrial shop vacuum'. The AngioJet is actually a variety of

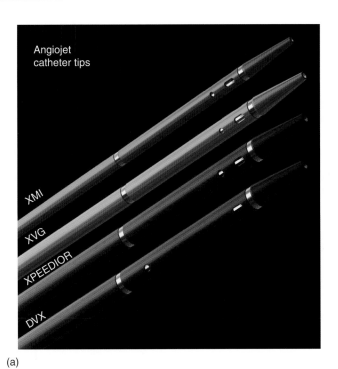

(a)

Figure 4.10
(a) AngioJet rheolytic catheters (b) AngioJet pump and drive unit (Courtesy of Possis Medical.).

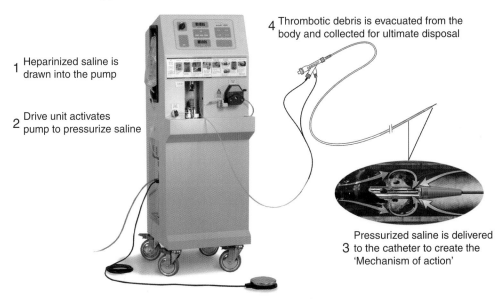

(b)

mechanical thrombectomy catheters (Figure 4.10a) connected to a high-pressure, pulsed saline pump (Figure 4.10b) to create a low-pressure Venturi effect that fragments and 'sucks' thrombus into the catheter lumen. The device also aspirates effluent from the catheter and pump circuit (see Figure 4.10b).[71,72] Originally used for coronary revascularization and lower extremity occlusive disease, it has also been applied to the cerebral circulation. While reports of use in the carotid and vertebral arteries are limited,[73,74] there are multiple reports of successful revascularization of large clot burden in cases of extensive dural sinus thrombosis.[75–77]

Closure devices

A number of devices are available for arteriotomy closure, including the Angioseal STS Platform (St Jude Medical, St Paul,

Minnesota), Vasoseal (Datascope Corp, Montvale, New Jersey), Perclose or Starclose (Abbott Vascular, Santa Clara, California), and Duett (Vascular Solutions, Minneapolis, Minnesota). Although no sufficiently powered study currently exists to demonstrate the superiority of these devices over mechanical compression, they do allow a shorter time to hemostasis and patient ambulation, particularly when patients are anticoagulated or on antiplatelet medications. The available devices employ a variety of different mechanisms, including delivery of sealant [e.g. Bovine collagen (Angioseal) or collagen plus thrombin (Duett), suture (Perclose), or hemostatic clip placement (Starclose). Some devices can also be classified as intravascular (Angioseal, Perclose) or extravascular (Duett, Starclose).

Angioseal achieves hemostasis by anchoring an exovascular bovine collagen plug to the arteriotomy site via an intravascular bioabsorbable anchor (Figure 4.11). Both components of the sealing device are absorbed in 8–12 weeks. This device comes in

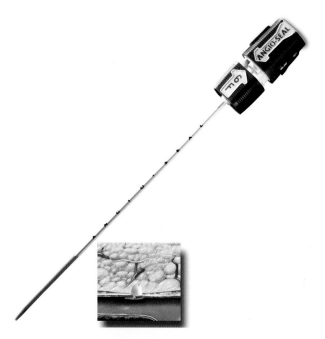

Figure 4.11
Angioseal closure system for arterial puncture and access.
(Courtesy of St Jude Medical.)

6 F and 8 F sizes. The Vasoseal system delivers an extraluminal purified collagen plug over the arteriotomy site. The Duett system delivers an extravascular pro-coagulant mixture of collagen and thrombin into the soft tissues around the arteriotomy site. The Perclose system delivers a suture at the arteriotomy site, providing immediate hemostasis when effective, while the Starclose system uses a circular, crenated nitinol clip.

References

1. Strother CM. Interventional Neuroradiology. AJNR Am J Neuroradiol 2000; 21: 19–24.
2. Teitelbaum GP, Larsen DW, Zelman V, Lysachev AG, Likhterman LB. A tribute to Dr Fedor A Serbinenko, founder of endovascular neurosurgery. Neurosurgery 2000; 46: 462–9.
3. Engelson E. Catheter for guide-wire tracking. United States patent: [4739768]. Application number: 06/869 597. Publication date. April 26, 1998.
4. Guglielmi G. Historical note. AJNR Am J Neuroradiol 2002; 23: 342.
5. Monsein LH. Primer on medical device regulation. Part I. History and background. Radiology 1997; 205: 1–9.
6. Schlosser E. Has politics contaminated the food supply? The New York Times; 2006.
7. Monsein LH. Primer on medical device regulation. Part II. Regulation of medical devices by the US Food and Drug Administration. Radiology 1997; 205: 10–18.
8. Sherertz RJ, Streed SA. Medical devices. Significant risk vs non significant risk. JAMA 1994; 272: 955–6.
9. Smith JJ, Berlin L. Informed consent when using medical devices for indications not approved by the Food and Drug Administration. AJR Am J Roentgenol 1999; 173: 879–82.
10. Cooper JA. Responsible conduct of radiology research. Part III. Exemptions from regulatory requirements for human research. Radiology 2005; 237: 3–7.
11. Cooper JA. Responsible conduct of radiology research: part II. Regulatory requirements for human research. Radiology 2005; 236: 748–52.
12. Cooper JA. Responsible conduct of radiology research: part I. The regulatory framework for human research. Radiology 2005; 236: 379–81.
13. Smith JJ, Berlin L. Off-label use of interventional medical devices. AJR Am J Roentgenol 1999; 173: 539–42.
14. Smith JJ, Berlin L. Informed consent when using medical devices for indications not approved by the Food and Drug Administration. AJR Am J Roentgenol 1999; 173: 879–82.
15. Smith JJ. Physician modification of legally marketed medical devices: regulatory implications under the federal Food, Drug, and Cosmetic Act. Food Drug Law J 2000; 55: 245–54.
16. Smith JJ. Regulatory and legal implications of modifying FDA-approved medical devices. J Vasc Interv Radiol 2000; 11: 19–23.
17. Smith JJ. Regulation of medical devices in radiology: current standards and future opportunities. Radiology 2001; 218: 329–35.
18. Deshmukh VR, Fiorella DJ, McDougall CG, Spetzler RF, Albuquerque FC. Preoperative embolization of central nervous system tumors. Neurosurg Clin N Am 2005; 16: 411–32.
19. Brothers MF, Kaufmann JC, Fox AJ, Deveikis JP. n-Butyl 2-cyanoacrylate: substitute for IBCA in interventional neuroradiology: histopathologic and polymerization time studies. AJNR Am J Neuroradiol 1989; 10: 777–86.
20. Spiegel SM, Vinuela F, Goldwasser JM, Fox AJ, Pelz DM. Adjusting the polymerization time of isobutyl-2 cyanoacrylate. AJNR Am J Neuroradiol 1986; 7: 109–12.
21. Gounis MJ, Lieber BB, Wakhloo AK et al. Effect of glacial acetic acid and ethiodized oil concentration on embolization with N-butyl 2-cyanoacrylate: an in vivo investigation. AJNR Am J Neuroradiol 2002; 23: 938–44.
22. Wikholm G, Lundqvist C, Svendsen P. The Goteborg cohort of embolized cerebral arteriovenous malformations: a 6-year follow-up. Neurosurgery 2001; 49: 799–805.
23. Cekirge HS, Saatci I, Geyik S et al. Intrasaccular combination of metallic coils and onyx liquid embolic agent for the endovascular treatment of cerebral aneurysms. J Neurosurg 2006; 105: 706–12.
24. Molyneux AJ, Cekirge S, Saatci I, Gal G. Cerebral Aneurysm Multicenter European Onyx (CAMEO) trial: results of a prospective observational study in 20 European centers. AJNR Am J Neuroradiol 2004; 25: 39–51.
25. Weber W, Siekmann R, Kis B, Kuehne D. Treatment and follow-up of 22 unruptured wide-necked intracranial aneurysms of the internal carotid artery with Onyx HD 500. AJNR Am J Neuroradiol 2005; 26: 1909–15.
26. Chaloupka JC, Vinuela F, Vinters HV, Robert J. Technical feasibility and histopathologic studies of ethylene vinyl copolymer (EVAL) using a swine endovascular embolization model. AJNR Am J Neuroradiol 1994; 15: 1107–15.
27. Sampei K, Hashimoto N, Kazekawa K et al. Histological changes in brain tissue and vasculature after intracarotid infusion of organic solvents in rats. Neuroradiology 1996; 38: 291–4.
28. Murayama Y, Vinuela F, Ulhoa A et al. Nonadhesive liquid embolic agent for cerebral arteriovenous malformations: preliminary histopathological studies in swine rete mirabile. Neurosurgery 1998; 43: 1164–75.
29. Jahan R, Murayama Y, Gobin YP et al. Embolization of arteriovenous malformations with Onyx: clinicopathological experience in 23 patients. Neurosurgery 2001; 48: 984–95.
30. Schirmer CM, Zerris V, Malek AM. Electrocautery-induced ignition of spark showers and self-sustained combustion of onyx ethylene-vinyl alcohol copolymer. Neurosurgery 2006; 59: ONS413–8.
31. Yakes WF, Rossi P, Odink H. How I do it. Arteriovenous malformation management. Cardiovasc Intervent Radiol 1996; 19: 65–71.

32. Yakes WF, Krauth L, Ecklund J et al. Ethanol endovascular management of brain arteriovenous malformations: initial results. Neurosurgery 1997; 40: 1145–52.

33. Sorimachi T, Koike T, Takeuchi S et al. Embolization of cerebral arteriovenous malformations achieved with polyvinyl alcohol particles: angiographic reappearance and complications. AJNR Am J Neuroradiol 1999; 20: 1323–28.

34. Mathis JA, Barr JD, Horton JA et al. The efficacy of particulate embolization combined with stereotactic radiosurgery for treatment of large arteriovenous malformations of the brain. AJNR Am J Neuroradiol 1995; 16: 299–306.

35. N-butyl cyanoacrylate embolization of cerebral arteriovenous malformations: results of a prospective, randomized, multi-center trial. AJNR Am J Neuroradiol 2002; 23: 748–55.

36. Wolpert SM, Serbinenko FA. Balloon catheterization and occlusion of major cerebral vessels. J Neurosurg 1974; 41: 1974. AJNR Am J Neuroradiol 2000; 21: 1359–60.

37. Debrun G, Lacour P, Vinuela F et al. Treatment of 54 traumatic carotid-cavernous fistulas. J Neurosurg 1981; 55: 678–92.

38. Debrun G, Fox A, Drake C et al. Giant unclippable aneurysms: treatment with detachable balloons. AJNR Am J Neuroradiol 1981; 2: 167–73.

39. Hieshima GB, Grinnell VS, Mehringer CM. A detachable balloon for therapeutic transcatheter occlusions. Radiology 1981; 138: 227–8.

40. Masaryk TJ, Perl J, Wallace RC, Magdinec M, Chyatte D. Detachable balloon embolization: concomitant use of a second safety balloon. AJNR Am J Neuroradiol 1999; 20: 1103–06.

41. Guglielmi G, Vinuela F, Sepetka I, Macellari V. Electrothrombosis of saccular aneurysms via endovascular approach. Part 1: Electrochemical basis, technique, and experimental results. J Neurosurg 1991; 75: 1–7.

42. Halbach VV, Dowd CF, Higashida RT, Balousek PA, Urwin RW. Preliminary experience with an electrolytically detachable fibered coil. AJNR Am J Neuroradiol 1998; 19: 773–7.

43. Raymond J, Guilbert F, Weill A et al. Long-term angiographic recurrences after selective endovascular treatment of aneurysms with detachable coils. Stroke 2003; 34: 1398–403.

44. Murayama Y, Tateshima S, Gonzalez NR, Vinuela F. Matrix and bioabsorbable polymeric coils accelerate healing of intracranial aneurysms: long-term experimental study. Stroke 2003; 34: 2031–7.

45. Bavinzski G, Talazoglu V, Killer M et al. Gross and microscopic histopathological findings in aneurysms of the human brain treated with Guglielmi detachable coils. J Neurosurg 1999; 91: 284–93.

46. Berenstein A, Song JK, Niimi Y et al. Treatment of cerebral aneurysms with hydrogel-coated platinum coils (HydroCoil): early single-center experience. AJNR Am J Neuroradiol 2006; 27: 1834–40.

47. Cloft HJ. HydroCoil for Endovascular Aneurysm Occlusion (HEAL) study: 3–6 month angiographic follow-up results. AJNR Am J Neuroradiol 2007; 28: 152–4.

48. Cloft HJ. HydroCoil for Endovascular Aneurysm Occlusion (HEAL) study: periprocedural results. AJNR Am J Neuroradiol 2006; 27: 289–92.

49. Deshaies EM, Adamo MA, Boulos AS. A prospective single-center analysis of the safety and efficacy of the hydrocoil embolization system for the treatment of intracranial aneurysms. J Neurosurg 2007; 106: 226–33.

50. Ding YH, Dai D, Lewis DA et al. Angiographic and histologic analysis of experimental aneurysms embolized with platinum coils, Matrix, and HydroCoil. AJNR Am J Neuroradiol 2005; 26: 1757–63.

51. Sterioff S. Etymology of the word stent. Mayo Clin Proc 1997; 72: 377–9.

52. Shiner B. Industrial applications: the all-round performer. Nat Photon 2008; 2: 24–5.

53. Fiorella D, Albuquerque FC, Han P, McDougall CG. Preliminary experience using the Neuroform stent for the treatment of cerebral aneurysms. Neurosurgery 2004; 54: 6–16.

54. Smith TP, Alexander MJ, Enterline DS. Delayed stenosis following placement of a polyethylene terephthalate endograft in the cervical carotid artery. Report of three cases. J Neurosurg 2003; 98: 421–5.

55. Kastrup A, Nagele T, Groschel K et al. Incidence of new brain lesions after carotid stenting with and without cerebral protection. Stroke 2006; 37: 2312–6.

56. Chen CI, Iguchi Y, Garami Z et al. Analysis of emboli during carotid stenting with distal protection device. Cerebrovasc Dis 2006; 21: 223–8.

57. Muller-Hulsbeck S, Stolzmann P, Liess C et al. Vessel wall damage caused by cerebral protection devices: ex vivo evaluation in porcine carotid arteries. Radiology 2005; 235: 454–60.

58. Vos JA, van den Berg JC, Ernst SM et al. Carotid angioplasty and stent placement: comparison of transcranial Doppler US data and clinical outcome with and without filtering cerebral protection devices in 509 patients. Radiology 2005; 234: 493–9.

59. Henry M, Amor M, Henry I et al. Carotid stenting with cerebral protection: first clinical experience using the PercuSurge Guard-Wire system. J Endovasc Surg 1999; 6: 321–31.

60. Stone GW, Rogers C, Hermiller J et al. Randomized comparison of distal protection with a filter-based catheter and a balloon occlusion and aspiration system during percutaneous intervention of diseased saphenous vein aorto-coronary bypass grafts. Circulation 2003; 108: 548–53.

61. Parodi JC, Schonholz C, Parodi FE, Sicard G, Ferreira LM. Initial 200 cases of carotid artery stenting using a reversal-of-flow cerebral protection device.J Cardiovasc Surg (Torino) 2007; 48: 117–24.

62. Asakura F, Kawaguchi K, Sakaida H et al. Diffusion-weighted MR imaging in carotid angioplasty and stenting with protection by the reversed carotid arterial flow. AJNR Am J Neuroradiol 2006; 27: 753–8.

63. Imai K, Mori T, Izumoto H et al. Clot Removal Therapy by Aspiration and Extraction for Acute Embolic Carotid Occlusion. AJNR Am J Neuroradiol 2006; 27: 1521–27.

64. Flint AC, Duckwiler GR, Budzik RF et al. Mechanical thrombectomy of intracranial internal carotid occlusion: pooled results of the MERCI and Multi MERCI Part I trials. Stroke 2007; 38: 1274–80.

65. Gordan R. The alarming history of medicine: amusing anecdotes from Hippocrates to heart transplants. New York: St Martin's Press, 1993.

66. Smith CM. Origin and uses of primum non nocere: above all, do no harm! J Clin Pharmacol 2005; 45: 371–77.

67. Tytle TL, Prati RC Jr, McCormack ST. The 'gooseneck' concept in microvascular retrieval. AJNR Am J Neuroradiol 1995; 16: 1469–71.

68. Fiorella D, Albuquerque FC, Deshmukh VR, McDougall CG. Monorail snare technique for the recovery of stretched platinum coils: technical case report. Neurosurgery 2005; 57: E210.

69. Henkes H, Lowens S, Preiss H et al. A new device for endovascular coil retrieval from intracranial vessels: alligator retrieval device. AJNR Am J Neuroradiol 2006; 27: 327–9.

70. Versnick EJ, Do HM, Albers GW et al. Mechanical thrombectomy for acute stroke. AJNR Am J Neuroradiol 2005; 26: 875–9.

71. Nakagawa Y, Matsuo S, Yokoi H et al. Stenting after thrombectomy with the AngioJet catheter for acute myocardial infarction. Cathet Cardiovasc Diagn 1998; 43: 327–30.

72. Nobuyoshi M, Nakagawa Y. AngioJet thrombectomy catheter for the thrombus-laden lesions. Cathet Cardiovasc Diagn 1998; 45: 394–5.

73. Mayer TE, Hamann GF, Schulte-Altedorneburg G, Bruckmann H. Treatment of vertebrobasilar occlusion by using a coronary waterjet thrombectomy device: a pilot study. AJNR Am J Neuroradiol 2005; 26: 1389–94.

74. Bellon RJ, Putman CM, Budzik RF et al. Rheolytic thrombectomy of the occluded internal carotid artery in the setting of acute ischemic stroke. AJNR Am J Neuroradiol 2001; 22: 526–30.

75. Curtin KR, Shaibani A, Resnick SA et al. Rheolytic catheter thrombectomy, balloon angioplasty, and direct recombinant tissue

plasminogen activator thrombolysis of dural sinus thrombosis with preexisting hemorrhagic infarctions. AJNR Am J Neuroradiol 2004; 25: 1807–11.

76. Dowd CF, Malek AM, Phatouros CC, Hemphill JC III. Application of a rheolytic thrombectomy device in the treatment of dural sinus thrombosis: a new technique. AJNR Am J Neuroradiol 1999; 20: 568–70.

77. Kirsch J, Rasmussen PA, Masaryk TJ et al. Adjunctive rheolytic thrombectomy for central venous sinus thrombosis: technical case report. Neurosurgery 2007; 60: E577-8.

5

The role of endovascular therapies in acute ischemic stroke

Thomas J Masaryk, Shaye Moskowitz and Irene Katzan

According to the Oxford English Dictionary a sudden inexplicable cerebrovascular accident was first likened to a 'stroke of God's hand' in 1599.[1] The relationship of cerebral infarction to an act of God exists in other cultures: the Greek verb *plesso* means 'stroke, hit, or beat' and its derivative *plegia* is the root of the term 'hemiplegia'.

Stroke is the third most common cause of death and the leading cause of adult disability in the USA. It afflicts approximately 700,000 Americans each year.[2] Classically, stroke is defined as a sudden focal, non-convulsive neurological deficit lasting 24 hours or more and caused by disruption of the cerebral circulation. It is a syndrome with multiple potential etiologies: embolism, thrombosis, and hemorrhage. Cerebral infarction, which comprises 80–85% of all strokes, is the result of an irreversible derangement in cellular metabolism that rapidly occurs after interruption of blood flow to a portion of the brain.[3]

Up to the 1980s the approach to patients with acute ischemic stroke was often nihilistic, and to some extent it remains so.[4] It is estimated that following acute vascular occlusion, one loses 1.9 million neurons per minute.[5] However, in the late 1970s experimental evidence began to accumulate that this is not an immediate or an 'all-or-none' phenomenon, and that patients may have additional neural dysfunction far in excess of the initial region of infarction.[6] This border-zone region – ischemic and dysfunctional yet (at least temporarily) potentially viable – became known as 'the ischemic penumbra'.[7,8] It was this knowledge, coupled with the ability of CT to expeditiously exclude hemorrhagic etiologies and cases of completed infarction that prompted early clinical trials for acute stroke treatment to preserve this potentially viable tissue.

Intravenous thrombolytic therapy

The 1990s witnessed a renewed devotion to the treatment of acute ischemic stroke with several randomized prospective trials conducted to assess the outcome of patients treated with thrombolytic agents.[9] The pivotal study was the National Institutes of Neurological Disorders and Stroke (NINDS) randomized, prospective trial of recombinant tissue plasminogen activator (rt-PA) for acute ischemic stroke.[10] Confirmed using other thrombolytic agents,[11] results from this trial demonstrated that with medical intervention within 3 hours of ictus:

- the number of patients with favorable outcomes for each of the primary measurements was higher in the rt-PA group;
- there was a 12% absolute (32% relative) increase in the number of patients with minimal or no disability;
- there was an 11% absolute (55% relative) increase in the number of patients with a National Institutes of Health Stroke Score (NIHSS) of 0 or 1; and
- there was no significant difference in mortality, although symptomatic intracerebral hemorrhage was significantly more common in the rt-PA group (6.4% compared to 0.6% in the placebo group).

There were several key features of this trial, including:

- the routine use of a numeric score assessing the severity of stroke at the time of presentation and at follow-up;
- the rapidity at which treatment was given (within 3 hours from the onset of symptoms); and
- the use of limited, unenhanced computed tomography.

Generalizability of the safety risks in general clinical practice has been demonstrated.[12]

Two clinical, reliable, numeric scoring systems were established. The NIHSS is a 42-point scale used to quantify the severity of stroke deficit (Table 5.1).[13] Although the score is skewed toward the hemisphere involved in language,[14] the scale has been found in multiple stroke treatment trials to be reproducible, and it provides a good sense of the gravity of the clinical problem at hand:[15–17]

- NIHSS 4–10 represents moderate severity of stroke with potential for good outcome
- NIHSS 11–20 represents severe deficit with greater likelihood of severe disability or death
- NIHSS >20 represents impending catastrophe.

Table 5.1 National Institutes of Health Stroke Scale* (NIHSS)

Administer in order shown. Record initial performance (do not go back).

1a. Level of consciousness

0 Alert; keenly responsive
1 Not alert, but arousable by minor stimulation to obey, answer or respond
2 Not alert, requires repeated stimulation to attend, or is obtunded and requires strong painful stimulation to make movements (not stereotyped)
3 Comatose: responds only with reflex motor (posturing) or autonomic effects, or totally unresponsive, flaccid and areflexic]

1b. Level of consciousness questions
Patient is asked the month and his or her age.

0 Answers both questions correctly (no credit for being close)
1 Answers one question correctly or cannot answer because of: ET tube, orotracheal trauma, severe dysarthria, language barrier, or other problem not secondary to aphasia
2 Answers neither question correctly, or is: aphasic, stuporous, or does not comprehend the questions

1c. Level of consciousness commands
Patient is asked to open and close the eyes, and then to grip and release the non-paretic hand. Substitute another one-step command if both hands cannot be used. Credit is given for an unequivocal attempt even if it cannot be completed because of weakness. If there is no response to commands, demonstrate (pantomime) the task. Record only first attempt.

0 Performs both tasks correctly
1 Performs one task correctly
2 Performs neither task correctly

2. Best gaze
Test only horizontal eye movement. Use motion to attract attention of aphasic patients.

0 Normal
1 Partial gaze palsy (gaze abnormal in one or both eyes, but forced deviation or total gaze paresis are not present) or patient has an isolated cranial nerve III, IV or VI paresis
2 Forced deviation or total gaze paresis not overcome by oculocephalic (doll's eyes) maneuvers, do not do caloric testing

3. Visual
Visual fields (upper and lower quadrants) are tested by confrontation. May be scored as normal if patient looks at side of finger movement. Use ocular threat where consciousness or comprehension limits testing. The test with double-sided simultaneous stimulation:

0 No visual loss
1 Partial hemianopia (clear cut asymmetry), or extinction to double-sided simultaneous stimulation
2 Complete hemianopia
3 Bilateral hemianopia (blind, including cortical blindness)

4. Facial palsy

Ask patient (or pantomime to patient) to show their teeth, or raise eyebrows and close eyes. Use painful stimulus and grade grimace response in poorly responsive or non-comprehending patients.

0 Normal symmetrical movement
1 Minor paralysis (flattened nasolabial fold, asymmetry on smiling)
2 Partial paralysis (total or near-total paralysis of lower face)
3 Complete paralysis of one or both sides (absent facial movement in upper and lower face)

(Continued)

Table 5.1 *Continued*

5. Motor arm (5a, left; 5b, right)
Instruct patient to hold the arms outstretched, palms down (at 90° if sitting or 45° if supine). If consciousness or comprehension-impaired, cue patient by actively lifting arms into position while verbally instructing patient to maintain position.

0 No drift (holds arm at 90° or 45° for full 10 seconds)
1 Drift (holds limbs at 90° or 45° position, but drifts before full 10 seconds but does not hit bed or other support)
2 Some effort against gravity (cannot get to or hold initial position, drifts down to bed)
3 No effort against gravity, limb falls
4 No movement
9 Amputation or joint fusion: explain

6. Motor leg (6a, left; 6b, right)
Instruct patient (while patient is supine) to maintain the non-paretic leg at 30°. If consciousness-or comprehension-impaired, cue patient by actively lifting leg into position and verbally instruct patient to maintain position. Then repeat in paretic leg.

0 No drift (holds leg at 30° full 5 seconds)
1 Drift (leg falls before 5 seconds, but does not hit bed)
2 Some effort against gravity (leg falls to bed by 5 seconds)
3 No effort against gravity (leg falls to bed immediately)
4 No movement
9 Amputation or joint fusion: explain

7. Limb ataxia
(Looking for unilateral cerebral lesion.) Finger–nose–finger and heel–knee–shin tests are performed on both sides. Ataxia is scored only if clearly out of proportion to weakness. Ataxia is absent in the patient who cannot comprehend or is paralyzed.

0 Absent
1 Present in one limb
2 Present in two limbs
9 Amputation or joint fusion: explain

8. Sensory
Test with pin. When consciousness- or comprehension-impaired, score sensation as normal unless a deficit is clearly recognized (e.g. clear-cut asymmetry of grimace or withdrawal). Only hemisensory losses attributed to stroke are counted as abnormal.

0 Normal, no sensory loss
1 Mild to moderate sensory loss (pin-prick feels dull or less sharp on the affected side, or loss of superficial pain to pin-prick but patient aware of being touched)
2 Severe to total (patient unaware of being touched in the face, arm, and leg)

9. Best language
In addition to judging comprehension of commands in the preceding neurologic examination, the patient is asked to describe a standard picture, to name common items, and to read and interpret the standard text in the box below. The intubated patient should be asked to write.

> You know how.
> Down to earth.
> I got home from work.
> Near the table in the dining room.
> They heard him speak on the radio last night.

0 Normal, no aphasia
1 Mild to moderate aphasia (some loss of fluency, word-finding errors, naming errors, or paraphasias or impairment of communication by either comprehension or expression disability)
2 Severe aphasia (great need for inference, questioning and guessing by listener; limited range of information can be exchanged)
3 Mute or global aphasia (no usable speech or auditory comprehension) or patient in coma (item 1a = 3)

(Continued)

Table 5.1 *Continued*

10. Dysarthria

Patient may be graded on the basis of information already gleaned during evaluation. If patient is thought to be normal, have the patient read (or repeat) the standard text shown in this box.

> Mama
> Tip-top
> Fifty–fifty
> Thanks
> Huckleberry
> Baseball player
> Caterpillar

0 Normal speech
1 Mild to moderate impairment (slurs some words, can be understood with some difficulty)
2 Severe impairment (unintelligible slurred speech in the absence of, or out of proportion to, any dysphasia, or is mute or anarthric)
9 Intubated or other physical barrier

11. Extinction and inattention (formerly neglect)

Sufficient information to identify neglect may have already be gleaned during evaluation. If the patient has severe visual loss preventing visual double-sided simultaneous stimulation, and the cutaneous stimuli are normal, the score is normal. Scored as abnormal only if present.

0 Normal, no sensory loss
1 Visual, tactile, auditory, spatial, or personal inattention or extinction to double-sided simultaneous stimulation in one of the sensory modalities
2 Profound hemi-inattention or hemi-inattention to more than one modality. Does not recognize own hand or orients to only one side of space

A. Distal motor function (not part of NIHSS) (a, left arm; b, right arm)

Patient's hand is held up at the forearm by the examiner, and patient is asked to extend the fingers as much as possible. If the patient cannot do so, the examiner does it. Do not repeat the command.

0 Normal (no finger flexion after 5 seconds)
1 At least some extension after 5 seconds (any finger movement is scored)
2 No voluntary extension after 5 seconds

Revised January 24, 1991. Based on the Cincinnati stroke scale.[i] Contact the Public Health Service, National Institutes of Health, National Institute of Neurologic Disorders and Stroke, Bethesda, Maryland, USA for copies of a grading form (which has more details on some aspects of grading) and for training information.[ii]
i. Brott T, Adams HP, Ollinger CP et al. Measurements of acute cerebral infarction: a clinical examination scale. Stroke 1991; 20: 864–70.
ii. Lyden P, Brott T, Tilley B et al. Improved reliability of the NIH Stroke Scale using videotraining. Stroke 1994; 25: 2220–6.

Table 5.2 Modified Rankin scale

0 No symptoms at all
1 No significant disability despite symptoms; able to carry out all usual duties and activities
2 Slight disability; unable to carry out all previous activities but able to look after own affairs without assistance
3 Moderate disability requiring some help, but able to walk without assistance
4 Moderate severe disability; unable to walk without assistance and unable to attend to own bodily needs without assistance
5 Severe disability; bedridden, incontinent, and requiring constant nursing care and attention

patients and where personnel are motivated to maintain a certain level of preparedness.[20–22] Implicit within the last statement is the ability of the center to marshal the appropriate personnel and communicate clearly and efficiently the clinical situation:[23–25] the meter is running at 1.9 million neurons per minute. Hence, there must be coordinated efforts with emergency medical services, immediate availability of physicians and surgeons knowledgeable in the diagnosis and management of acute stroke, CT technologists, nurses, and anesthesiologists accessible via emergency pager 24 hours a day and able to be on site within minutes.[26]

Finally, in an effort to meet the time commitment of 3 hours, the NINDS trial adhered to the most basic form of neuroimaging for quickly excluding hemorrhage, neoplasm, and the possibility of fully completed infarction. The combination of clinical history, NIHSS, and simple CT scan creates a heuristic setting in which the diagnosis of ischemic stroke is possible. The interpretation of the unenhanced CT scan is crucial not only in excluding hemorrhage prior to administration of thrombolytic agents, but also in identifying subtle clues to areas of completed infarction.[27–30] Within the parameters of the NINDS trial, predictors of outcome included:

- age[31]
- presenting NIHSS[15,31]
- time to treat[9,31]
- serum glucose level[32–34]
- pre-existing medical regimen (specifically the positive impact of statins and the potentially negative effect of aspirin).[35,36]

Intra-arterial thrombolysis

With the experience gained in the NINDS trial, and careful analysis of contemporary clinical studies, came an appreciation of the full spectrum of ischemic stroke, and also of the limitations of the 3-hour time window and of intravenous thrombolytic infusion therapy.

In angiography-based pilot trials of intravenous rt-PA, the rate of re-canalization of major arterial occlusions was low, with partial or complete re-canalization of only 10% of occluded internal carotid arteries and 25% of occluded proximal middle cerebral arteries.[37,38] The majority of cases in these trials had only partial re-canalization (TIMI-2), with a minority having complete reperfusion (TIMI-3). By comparison, TIMI-3 perfusion flow occurs in 50–55% of subjects with acute myocardial infarction treated with thrombolytic agents and in 75% of subjects treated with primary angioplasty and stenting.[39,40]

The large majority (75–80%) of acute stroke subjects with NIHSS scores ≥10 have occlusions of a major extracranial or

Another routine scale emphasized by the NINDS rt-PA study was the modified Rankin score, used to gauge clinical outcome and disability at 90 days (Table 5.2).

The second, but perhaps most important, feature of the NINDS trial was the fact that all patients were treated in under 3 hours from the onset of symptoms. Other acute stroke trials have confirmed the crucial role played by expediency, with clinical benefit falling off rapidly by 3 hours. (Figure 5.1).[9,11] Indeed, as in many areas of emergency medicine, the ability to distill the delivery of care to rote efficiency is crucial. (Table 5.3).[18,19] This has further led to the recognition that this level of efficiency is likely to be obtained only at well-equipped centers that routinely see stroke

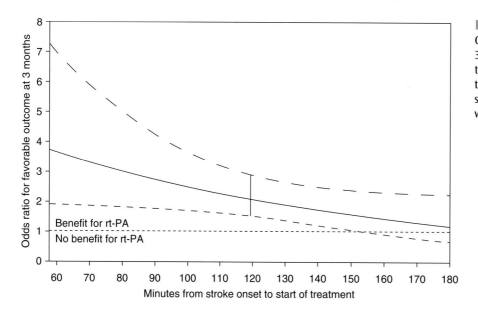

Figure 5.1
Odds ratio for favorable outcome 3 months post-stroke versus time to treatment with intravenous thrombolysis for acute ischemic stroke. rt-PA, alteplase. Reprinted with permission.

Table 5.3 Acute stroke checklist

Time of onset
Age of patient
- Able to consent
- Pregnant

Right- or left-handed
- NIHSS
- Able to consent

Vital signs
- Blood pressure
- Heart rate and rhythm
- Anticoagulation status

Contraindications to thrombolysis
- Recent surgery
- Systolic blood pressure >180 mm Hg
- Coagulopathy
- >3 hours post-ictus
- Known intraparenchymal central nervous system neoplasm

Imaging available
- Blood
- Parenchymal changes in over one-third of the vascular territory
- Vascular occlusion
- Perfusion mismatch

Contact information
- Parent or spouse or medical power of attorney
- Living will
- Immediate activation of emergency endovascular technologist, nurse and physician

NIHSS, National Institutes of Health Stroke Scale.

intracranial trunk artery even after initiation of intravenous rt-PA.[41,42] The overall prognosis for these subjects after rt-PA therapy in the NINDS rt-PA trial was poor (albeit better than for those treated with placebo). Given the apparent failure of intravenous thrombolysis to re-canalize major arterial occlusions in earlier angiography-based trials, the overall outcome in this NINDS rt-PA trial subgroup is not surprising.[43]

Furthermore, these same subjects with a high NIHSS who often failed to re-canalize with intravenous rt-PA were also at increased risk of symptomatic intracranial hemorrhage – risk as high as 17% for an NIHSS >20.[44]

Given the time imperative, the risk of hemorrhage, and the continued high morbidity and mortality of severe strokes treated with intravenous thrombolytic agents, a logical next step was emergency intra-arterial therapy. Trial design poses significant logistical and ethical hurdles in acute stroke, particularly in patients eligible for an accepted intravenous treatment.[45–47] Consequently, data from randomized, controlled trials of intra-arterial thrombolytics (Prolyse in Acute Cerebral Thromboembolism, or PROACT) is limited to the use of recombinant pro-urokinase (proUK) in patients within 6 hours of angiographically documented middle cerebral artery occlusion.[17,48–51] The follow-up study, PROACT II, was conducted at 54 North American centers where 180 patients with middle cerebral artery occlusion within 6 hours of onset of symptoms were randomized to intra-arterial proUK plus heparin or heparin only. A total of 40% of the thrombolysis patients versus 25% of control patients had a modified Rankin score of 2 or less at 90 days ($p = 0.04$), indicating mild to no disability. Mortality was similar between groups, although the early symptomatic hemorrhage rate was higher in the proUK group (10% vs. 2%). While not surprising that the re-canalization rate was higher with lytics than without (66% versus 18%), it is worth noting that the infusion was carried out over 2 hours.[49] Additionally, the median time to start of intra-arterial therapy in the PROACT II was 5.3 hours, and only three subjects had therapy started within 3 hours. Re-canalization, when it occurred, often happened more than 7 hours after stroke onset. Thus, using current intra-arterial strategies and systems, the time from symptom onset to re-canalization is often greater than 7 hours. Two published reports of intra-arterial thrombolytic therapy indicate that treatment begun within 3–4 hours of symptom onset is associated with higher rates of re-canalization and better outcome.[52,53] Additional variables that appeared to affect success of therapy in PROACT were similar to those of the NINDS: age, presenting NIHSS, CT signs of completed stroke, and location of thrombus.[17,51]

Beyond intra-arterial thrombolysis: adjunctive mechanical thrombectomy and stenting

Imaging

The FDA approval of intravenous rt-PA for stroke led to a focus on acute ischemic stroke as a true medical emergency, as well as a careful and continuous reexamination of how acute stroke evaluation and management can be improved.[22,54] Since the publication of the NINDS trial, imaging has evolved that can rapidly identify the vascular anatomy and the location of the occlusion; it can also estimate the degree of completed infarction and potential salvageable surrounding brain parenchyma.[55–66]

Subsequent stroke treatment trials have attempted to use advances in neuroimaging to improve patient selection by identifying specific etiologies responsible for the variety of clinical presentations of ischemic stroke (i.e. cardioembolic stroke, stroke due to small vessel or lacunar disease, stroke of determined etiology such as large vessel disease or dissection, and ischemic stroke of unknown etiology), as well as the patients who may potentially benefit from treatment (i.e. even those beyond the 3-hour window). The primary imaging modalitites include CT angiography and perfusion imaging (Figure 5.2) and magnetic resonance (MR) angiography and diffusion and perfusion imaging (Figure 5.3). Certainly each modality has strengths and weaknesses. Multi-row detector CT scanners (with 16 rows or more) allow ready access to acutely ill patients, can rapidly identify acute hemorrhage, and produce excellent quality angiographic images from the aortic arch to vertex, but provide limited perfusion information (see Figure 5.2). Conversely MR studies are exquisitely sensitive to early changes of hemispheric ischemia with full-coverage perfusion studies, but they must be performed in the somewhat hostile environment of a high magnetic field with limited patient visibility, and they provide somewhat limited angiographic imaging. In the context of how data impact time to treatment (see Figure 5.1), it is our practice to use CT as the modality of choice in cases less than 6 hours from onset of symptoms (see Figure 5.2). Beyond that time, and in cases where there may be fewer negative outcome predictors (particularly age and NIHSS), we often resort to MR studies to assist clinical decision making (see Figure 5.3).

It is worth noting that the sensitivity of diffusion-weighted imaging with b values ≥ 1000 that enables it to detect areas of infarction in patients who might otherwise have been clinically labeled as having transient ischemic attacks is remarkably high ($> 40\%$).[67–69] The propensity for early recurrent infarction in such cases has led to an appreciation of the need to identify and manage such patients more aggressively (Table 5.4).[67–79]

Pharmacological adjuncts

Pharmacologic adjuncts to intravenous therapy have been proposed (in a fashion analogous to treatment for acute myocardial infarction) in an effort to improve both the odds as well as the speed of cerebral artery re-canalization.[80–84] However, analogies to coronary intervention must be tempered by concern for further exacerbating the risk of intracranial hemorrhage.[65,82,85–97]

Glycoprotein IIb–IIIa inhibition certainly has a role in acute intervention involving thrombolytics, implantable stents, and acute coronary syndromes.[84,98–103] These agents are potent anti-platelet agents; they include abciximab, eptifibatide, and tirofiban. Controlled trials of these agents for stroke have been without great success, but they were limited to use of these anti-platelet agents alone.[97] While anecdotal reports of their use in combination with other agents have been more encouraging, their precise role in stroke therapy remains to be defined.[82,91]

Additional pharmacologic manipulation has been directed at minimizing complications from ischemia, both by reducing secondary morbidity and by affording neuroprotection.[35] In both the NINDS rt-PA and PROACT studies, hypertension was aggressively managed in an effort to minimize hemorrhagic complications (Table 5.5). These efforts primarily involved the use of beta-blockers and nitroprusside. Hydroxymethylglutaryl CoA reductase inhibitors (statins) appear to have a neuroprotective effect in ischemia, over and above the intended impact on serum cholesterol.[35,104–106] This positive impact has been appreciated only since the publication of the larger stroke studies. Significant efforts have been made to identify additional pharmacologic agents that can be used as an adjunct to thrombolysis for stoke, including glutamate receptor inhibitors, estrogen, erythropoietin, and anti-oxidants. However, these agents have not proven effective for wide clinical use.

Mechanical devices

On the basis of the limited ability of intravenous thrombolytic therapy to recanalize acute large vessel occlusions, and the logistical and pharmacological delays imposed by intra-arterial therapy, a variety of physical maneuvers have been proposed to expedite re-canalization. These include:

- ultrasound[107–110]
- foreign body retrieval devices (Figures 5.4, 5.5, 5.6)[111–114]
- aspiration systems[115]
- emergent stenting (Figures 5.7, 5.8)[116–118]

The largest experience to date has been with the Merci retriever device (see Figure 5.4). This device is approved by the Food and Drugs Administration (FDA), and it is currently available for use by any interventionalist treating a patient with an acute stroke who is ineligible for intravenous rt-PA or a patient who has failed thrombolytic therapy. The Merci device is a system consisting of a balloon-tip guiding catheter and retriever. The inflated balloon of the guide catheter placed in the proximal vasculature interrupts or reverses flow. The retriever itself is a flexible, tapered core nitinol wire with a helical shaped tip used to ensnare and retrieve the thrombus.

The clinical basis for FDA 510(K) clearance was the Mechanical Embolus Removal in Cerebral Ischemia (MERCI) Trial,[111] which was a prospective, single-arm multicenter trial conducted at 25 US centers in two parts. Part I enrolled 55 subjects and part II enrolled an additional 96 subjects, for a total of 151 subjects. Primary outcomes, which were reported on the basis of an intention-to-treat analysis, were the rate of vessel re-canalization and rate of observed device related complications. Complications were defined as vessel perforation, arterial dissection, or embolization of a previously uninvolved territory. The primary efficacy endpoint of vascular re-canalization (TIMI grades 2 or 3) was compared to the data published on the spontaneous

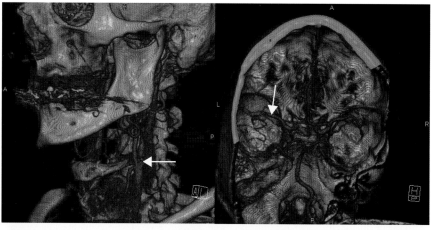

(a)

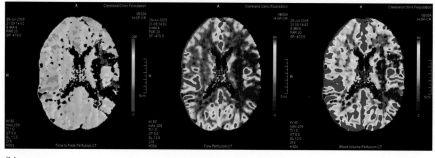

(b)

Figure 5.2

(a) CT angiogram in an acute stroke involving the dominant hemisphere of a 47-year-old man. There is a severe stenosis involving the left internal carotid artery (LICA) origin (left arrow) with a thrombotic saddle embolus in the ipsilateral M1–M2 junction (right arrow). (b) CT perfusion study demonstrating a delayed time-to-peak map (left), limited perfusion map (center), and cerebral blood volume (right), which demonstrates relative preservation of the cortex in the left middle cerebral artery (MCA) territory. (c) Near-complete occlusion of the LICA, which a microcatheter easily passed. When the MCA is injected, the saddle embolus is obvious. Recognizing the need to lyse the thrombus as well as the likely necessity of opening the carotid, 5mg rt-PA was administered as well as half the loading dose of abciximab. (d) While the pharmacologic treatment works (above), the carotid is stented (left, solid arrow). LICA injection post-stent demonstrates early lysis of the thrombus.

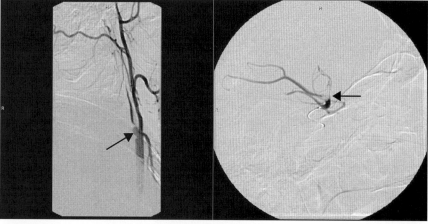

(c)

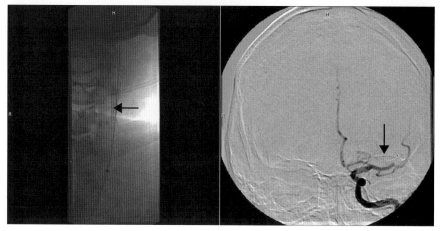

(d)

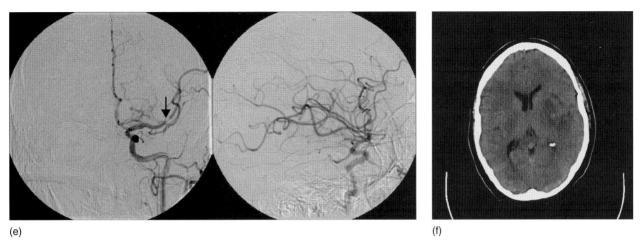

(e)   (f)

Figure 5.2 (*Continued*)
(e) View with an additional 5 mg of rt-PA and additional abciximab has been titrated to 70% inhibition. (f) Follow-up CT. The patient walked out of the hospital on discharge and on return at 8 weeks to clinic he was neurologically normal. Note that this use of rt-PA and abciximab is not FDA-approved.

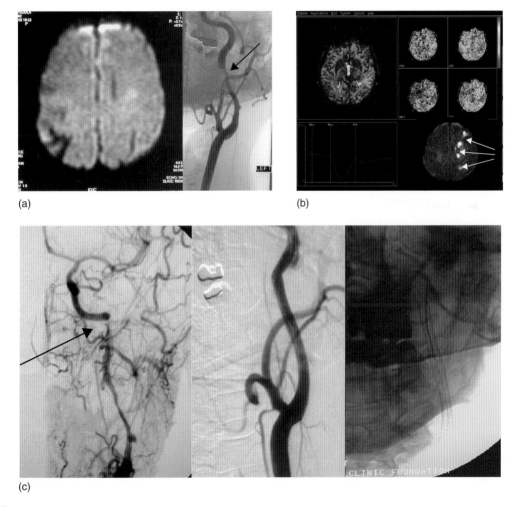

(a)   (b)

(c)

Figure 5.3
(a) Initial MR diffusion scan and angiogram of a 40-year-old woman with transient speech disturbance and hemiparesis caused by left internal carotid artery dissection (arrow). Two days post-admission, symptoms returned while she was being anticoagulated.
(b) The patient was transferred from the outside hospital 72 hours from the time of deterioration. MR diffusion study demonstrates a typical watershed pattern of infarction in the white matter with sparing of the cortex (lower right, arrows). The perfusion study demonstrates markedly delayed time to peak map, diminished cerebral perfusion and compensatory increased cerebral blood volume in the affected left hemisphere. (c) 80 hours after the return of her fixed deficit, repeat angiography demonstrates extension of the dissection (arrow), which was successfully stented (center and right.) The patient slowly improved and was normal at 8 weeks follow-up.

Table 5.4 'ABCD2' patient profile to identify patients at high early risk of stroke after a transient ischemic attack

Age 60 years or older
Blood pressure ≥140/90 mm Hg
Clinical signs and symptoms of hemiparesis or speech disturbance
Duration of symptoms 60 minutes or more
Diabetes

i. Rothwell PM, Giles MF, Flossmann E et al. A simple score (ABCD) to identify individuals at high early risk of stroke after transient ischaemic attack. Lancet 2005; 366: 29–36.
ii. Johnston SC, Rothwell PM, Nguyen-Huynh MN et al. Validation and refinement of scores to predict very early stroke risk after transient ischaemic attack. Lancet 2007; 369: 283–92.

Table 5.5 Management of hypertension after administration of rt-PA for acute cerebrovascular accident

Blood pressure	Intervention
Systolic 180–230 mmHg and/or Diastolic 110–120 mmHg	Labetalol 10 mg intravenously over 1–2 minutes, repeat or double dose every 10–20 minutes up to 150 mg
Systolic >230 mmHg and/or Diastolic 121–140 mmHg	As above, but if labetalol is contraindicated or ineffective, use nitroprusside
Diastolic >140 mmHg	Start nitroprusside 0.5–10 µg per kilogram per minute

recanalization rate in the control arm of the PROACT II study. Under the protocol up to six passes with retriever devices were allowed.

A total of 1809 patients were screened to recruit the 151 subjects. Subjects had to have completed the first pass with the device within 8 hours of onset of symptoms and had to have a baseline NIHSS score of ≥10 in part I or ≥8 in part II. Vessels eligible for treatment with the retriever device included the internal cerebral artery (ICA), the ICA terminal bifurcation, the M1 section of the middle cerebral artery (MCA), the M2 section of the MCA (allowed in Part II), the basilar artery, or the vertebral artery. Ten of the 151 subjects enrolled did not have the device deployed for a variety of reasons, many of which were technical and related to catheter access.

In comparison to PROACT, patients enrolled in the MERCI trial with MCA occlusion presented with slightly higher NIHSS and also a slightly higher rate of modified Rankin score of >2 (mild or no disability) at 90 days. Re-canalization rates for vertebral or basilar artery occlusion were also higher.

This study was followed by the Multi-Merci trial, which was likewise a prospective, single-arm trial of patients with large vessel stroke (vertebral, basilar, ICA, ICA-terminus, M1 or M2 occlusion) treated within 8 hours of symptom onset. Primary outcome was vascular re-canalization (TIMI 2 or TIMI 3) and safety. Physicians used a newer generation device (L5) first and subsequent passes could be made with the L5 or with the first-generation devices (X5 or X6). Adjuvant therapy with intra-arterial rt-PA was allowed after retriever use, with a maximum dose of 24mg.

Preliminary Multi-Merci data indicated that the baseline NIHSS score was similar to that of the MERCI Trial. However, there was significant decrease in the mortality rate, with similar rate of symptomatic hemorrhage when compared with subjects

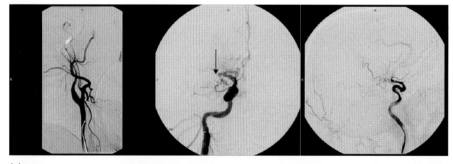

(a)

Figure 5.4

(a) Carotid, AP and lateral RCCA angiographic views demonstating a filling defect (convex margin, arrow) in the right M1 segment. (b) AP and lateral RICA injections after successful thrombectomy using the Merci retriever. A small residual filling defect can been seen in the M1 segment.

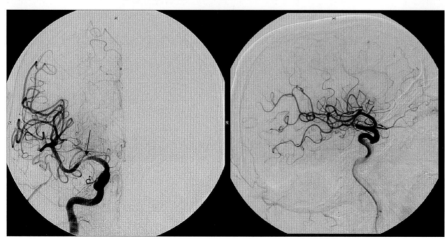

(b)

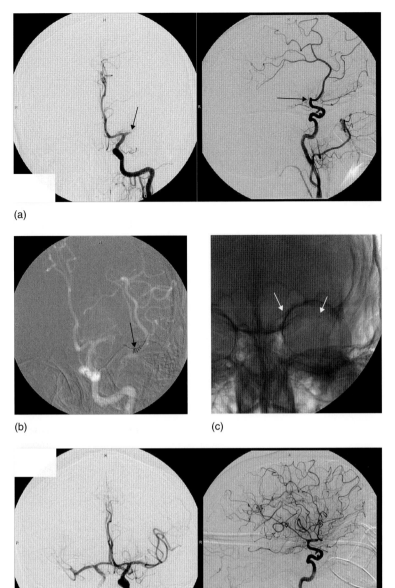

(a)

(b)   (c)

(d)

Figure 5.5
(a) Carotid, anterior–posterior (AP) and lateral right common carotid artery (RCCA) angiographic views demonstating a filling defect (convex margin, arrow) in the left M1 segment. (b) AP view demonstrating Merci retriever at the defect using simultaneous guide and distal micro-catheter roadmap. (c) Following unsuccessful attempts to re-canalize using the Merci device, a stent was placed across the occlusion (tines highlighted by arrows on this unsubtracted view. (d) AP and lateral angiogram after stent placement. Note that this is not an FDA-approved use of intra-cranial stents.

treated in the MERCI trial. On the basis of the preliminary Multi Merci data, the use of intravenous rt-PA before mechanical thrombectomy appears safe, with a symptomatic hemorrhage rate of 7.8%. Mechanical thrombectomy with both first- and second-generation Merci devices is effective to open intracranial vessels, with a re-canalization rate of 48%. This is significantly better than the spontaneous rate of 18% seen in the PROACT II control group. Enthusiasm for the device should be tempered by a comparison with the treatment group for intra-arterial rt-PA in PROACT II, for whom re-canalization occurred in 66%.

These trials also emphasize the observation that clinical outcome is tied to successful re-vascularization. The collective MERCI data demonstrated that clinical improvement was seen with successful re-canalization, whether a device was used or not. Ninety-day outcomes for modified Rankin scores of 0–2 was 39% for those patients in whom recanalization occurred, compared with only 3% for those in whom it did not. Similar patterns were seen for mortality and NIHSS scores. These data support the use

of the Merci device during acute ischemic stroke in patients who are either ineligible for intravenous thrombolytic therapy or in whom intravenous thrombolytic therapy has failed.

Ultrasound-enhanced thrombolysis is another potential combination therapy. The Combined Lysis of Thrombus in Brain ischemia with Transcranial Ultrasound and Systemic Tpa (CLOTBUST) II trial was a prospective randomized clinical trial of 126 patients with MCA occlusions. The patients were randomized to receive intravenous rt-PA alone or rt-PA plus low intensity ultrasound using a 2MHz transcranial Doppler probe placed on the affected artery.[109] Complete re-canalization or dramatic clinical recovery within 2 hours of rt-PA bolus occurred in 49% of the ultrasound plus rt-PA group and in 30% of the rt-PA only group ($p=0.03$). Several trials are currently evaluating the use of microbubble and ultrasound in combination with intravenous thrombolysis in patients with MCA occlusion. Additional studies utilizing locally applied, intra-arterial ultrasound devices have also suggested improved re-canalization rates, although the exact mechanism of therapeutic augmentation is not well understood.[119]

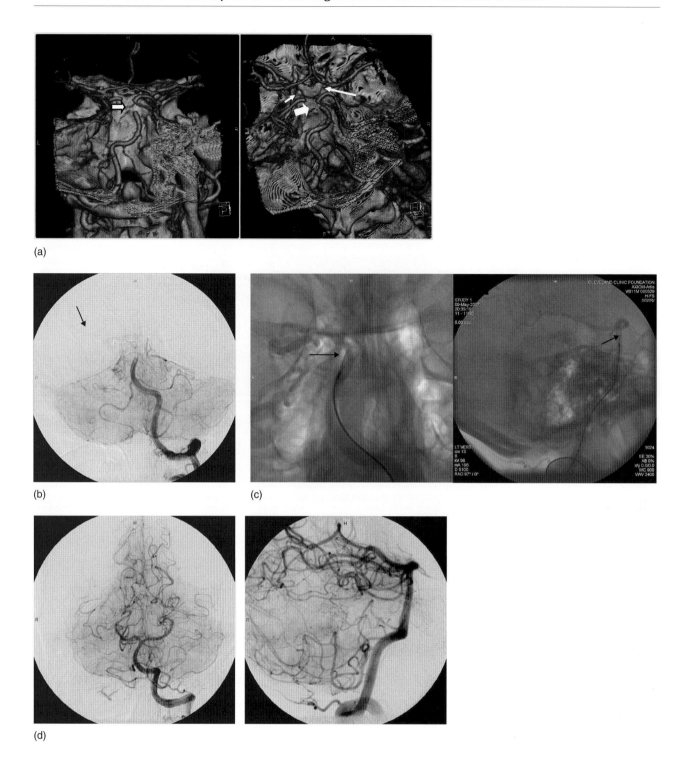

Figure 5.6

(a) CT angiography demonstrates a filling defect secondary to a saddle embolus at the basilar summit (block arrow). Notice the lack of filling of the posterior communicating artery (long arrows). (b) Confirmatory conventional angiogram demonstrating convex margin of the filling defect (arrow). (c) Anterior–posterior (AP) and lateral unsubtracted views of the micro-catheter in the distal basilar artery, from which extends the tines of the alligator retriever (arrows). (d) AP and lateral posterior circulation angiograms post-thrombectomy. Note that this is not an FDA-approved use of the alligator retrieval device.

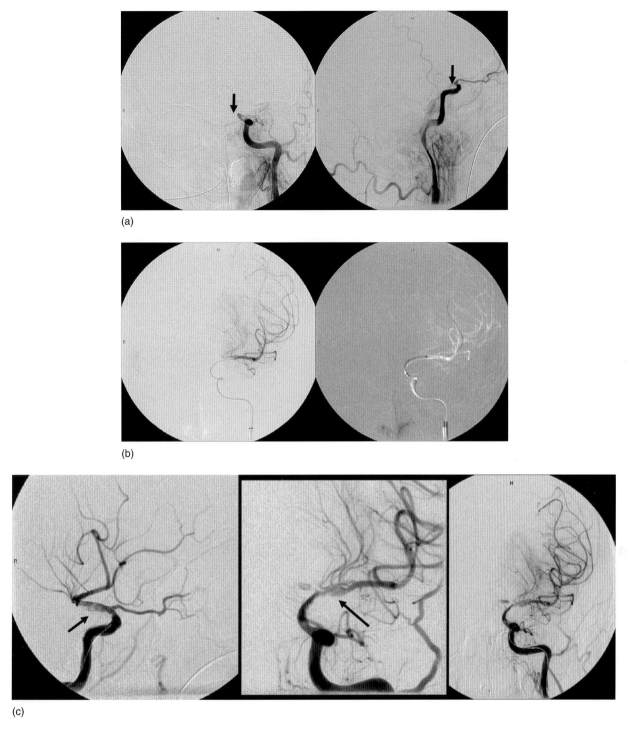

(a)

(b)

(c)

Figure 5.7

(a) Anterior–posterior (AP) and lateral angiogram in a patient with an acute carotid terminus occlusion, probably due to saddle thrombo-embolism (block arrow). (b) Micro-catheter view confirming distal middle cerebral artery patency (left) before stent placement (right). (c) Oblique, AP and lateral left common carotid artery angiographic views post-stent. Stenting across soft thrombus almost universally produces immediate re-canalization, with soft clot bulging at the interstices of the stent creating a 'quilt-like' pattern. Following stent placement and re-canalization, lysis can occur in a more controlled fashion. Note that this is not an FDA-approved use of intra-cranial stents.

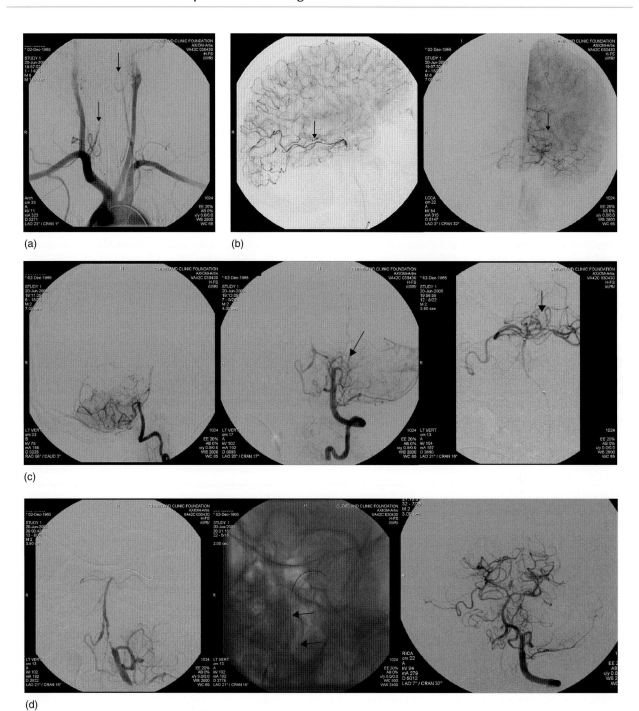

Figure 5.8

(a) Aortic arch angiogram demonstrates delayed filling of both vertebral arteries. (b) Anterior–posterior (AP) and lateral delayed views from a left internal carotid artery angiogram demonstrate watershed collateral circulation and delayed filling to the posterior cerebral artery territory. (c) Lateral and AP left vertebral artery (LVA) angiograms demonstrate poor intracranial filling with a distal LVA stenosis. The right vertebral artery is filling retrogradely. A distal micro-catheter view (right) demonstrates that the distal posterior circulation remains patent. Proximal posterior circulation occlusions are often secondary to thrombosis *in situ,* while thromboemboli are often carried to the basilar summit. (d) Post-angioplasty (left), unsubtracted view, post-Wingspan stent (center), and post-procedure angiogram (right).

Strategy

Optimal therapy for acute ischemic stroke is, at best, a work in progress. Co-ordination of timely patient access, universal imaging protocols, effective pharmacologic regimens, and endovascular devices requires a constant re-calibration of risks versus benefits, particularly in the absence of FDA-endorsed therapies. Guidance on implementing stroke care is available from treatment guidelines and clinical trial protocols,[51] Joint Commission stroke center certification, and Accreditation Council for Graduate Medical Education certification of endovascular training programs.[21,22,120–122]

Certainly one logical strategy to minimize time to treatment while attempting to intervene for patients with large vessel occlusion (who are unlikely to benefit from intravenous treatment alone) is being studied in the Emergency Management of Stroke (EMS) trial and the Interventional Management of Stroke (IMS) trial.[41,123] In these trials patients with suspected large vessel occlusions (NIHSS >10) received intravenous thrombolytics at the earliest possible moment (at two-thirds of the NINDS dose or 0.6mg per kilogram rt-PA over 30 minutes) while the resources are marshaled to initiate intra-arterial treatment. Early results have trended towards improved outcomes with combined treatment when compared with intravenous thrombolysis alone.[123] More recent iterations (such as IMS III) have included mechanical adjuncts to intra-arterial thrombolytics.

Another strategy that is being used in the clinical trials of desmoteplase is to extend the therapeutic time window through improved patient selection with neuroimaging. Patients with 'brain at risk', who may still benefit from re-perfusion beyond the 3-hour window, are identified using diffusion–perfusion mismatch on MR, or cerebral blood volume–cerebral blood flow mismatch on CT.[55,61,64–66] Although preliminary results have established safe dosing guidelines, phase III demonstration of efficacy remains to be demonstrated.

Despite extensive public and professional educational efforts, the acceptance of intravenous rt-PA – the only FDA-approved therapy for acute ischemic stroke – has been slow.[124] Interestingly, US data indicate that off-protocol use of intra-arterial rt-PA is increasing.[125] The 2000–2001 National Hospital Discharge Survey database indicates that there were 1,259,740 admissions for ischemic stroke in the years 2000 and 2001 in the USA, and intra-arterial thrombolysis was performed in 10,370 (0.8%) admissions compared with virtually none 10 years earlier. Outside the prescribed logic of a trial protocol, faced with calls from remote emergency rooms with limited neurological or radiological expertise, the willingness to initiate intravenous therapy for acute ischemic stroke should be encouraged. If in fact the clinical scenario suggests a high NIHSS secondary to large vessel occlusion, or if the patient is beyond the therapeutic window for intravenous thrombolysis, the question then becomes how quickly can the patient reach a facility with additional capability and what the next step should be. This will in part be limited by clinical exclusions, contraindications, availability of informed consent regarding off-label therapies, and time to endovascular access. A relative consideration in the first 6 hours (the PROACT therapeutic window) may be the availability and need for additional imaging to delineate better the area of completed infarction and penumbra.

As suggested by the early IMS results,[123] as well as by multimodal treatment of coronary disease,[39,40] the rapid re-canalization of large vessel occlusion by mechanical means appears to be the path to the future.[126] In cases of tandem disease or occlusions, attention should always be initially directed distally. In cases of carotid thromboembolic disease, flow must be re-established distally before a proximal stenosis or occlusion is opened.[127] For example, a distal embolism should be lysed or retrieved before a proximal bifurcation stenosis is stented. In cases of purely intracranial emboli without proximal vascular disease, a removable mechanical device, such as the Merci system, would not necessitate antiplatelet therapies and their additional risks of hemorrhage.[97] As suggested by Fiorella et al., newer non-implanted devices that readily facilitate re-canalization and adjunctive thrombolysis (while avoiding post-procedure anticoagulation) are likely to be the technique of the future. If however, there is a proximal stenosis or dissection (see Figures 5.2, 5.8) the use of permanent implantable stents will necessitate the use of antiplatelet agents to prevent acute, in-stent thrombosis. In such dire cases, in which the use of antiplatelet agents is pre-ordained, we have followed the experience outside the cerebral circulation and incorporated their administration (calibrated by point-of-service testing to minimize the risk of hemorrhage; see Chapter 3) with any initial attempts at intra-arterial thrombolysis. This may then be followed by proximal stenting during the preliminary period, in which lytic therapy is given the opportunity to work.

References

1. Rolack LA. Neurology trivia. In: Loren A, Rolak, ed. Neurology Secrets. Philadelphia, PA: Mosby Saunders, 2004.
2. Thom T, Haase N, Rosamond W et al. Heart disease and stroke statistics – 2006 update: a report from the American Heart Association Statistics Committee and Stroke Statistics Subcommittee. Circulation 2006; 113: e85–151.
3. Wardlaw JM, Zoppo G, Yamaguchi T, Berge E. Thrombolysis for acute ischaemic stroke. Cochrane Database Syst Rev 2003; 3: CD000213.
4. Biller J, Love BB. Nihilism and stroke therapy. Stroke 1991; 22: 1105–7.
5. Saver JL. Time is brain – quantified. Stroke 2006; 37: 263–6.
6. Hossmann KA. Viability thresholds and the penumbra of focal ischemia. Ann Neurol 1994; 36: 557–65.
7. Astrup J, Symon L, Branston NM, Lassen NA. Cortical evoked potential and extracellular K+ and H+ at critical levels of brain ischemia. Stroke 1977; 8: 51–7.
8. Astrup J, Siesjo BK, Symon L. Thresholds in cerebral ischemia: the ischemic penumbra. Stroke 1981; 12: 723–5.
9. Hacke W, Donnan G, Fieschi C et al. Association of outcome with early stroke treatment: pooled analysis of ATLANTIS, ECASS, and NINDS rt-PA stroke trials. Lancet 2004; 363: 768–74.
10. Tissue plasminogen activator for acute ischemic stroke. The National Institute of Neurological Disorders and Stroke rt-PA Stroke Study Group. N Engl J Med 1995; 333: 1581–7.
11. Yamaguchi T, Mori E, Minematsu K et al. Alteplase at 0.6 mg/kg for acute ischemic stroke within 3 hours of onset: Japan Alteplase Clinical Trial (J-ACT). Stroke 2006; 37: 1810–5.
12. Hill MD, Buchan AM. Thrombolysis for acute ischemic stroke: results of the Canadian Alteplase for Stroke Effectiveness Study. CMAJ 2005; 172: 1307–12.
13. Lyden P, Lu M, Jackson C et al. Underlying structure of the National Institutes of Health Stroke Scale: results of a factor analysis. NINDS tPA Stroke Trial Investigators. Stroke 1999; 30: 2347–54.
14. Woo D, Broderick JP, Kothari RU et al. Does the National Institutes of Health Stroke Scale favor left hemisphere strokes? NINDS t-PA Stroke Study Group. Stroke 1999; 30: 2355–9.
15. Adams HP Jr, Davis PH, Leira EC et al. Baseline NIH Stroke Scale score strongly predicts outcome after stroke: A report of the Trial of Org 10172 in Acute Stroke Treatment (TOAST). Neurology 1999; 53: 126–31.
16. Ueda T, Sakaki S, Kumon Y, Ohta S. Multivariable analysis of predictive factors related to outcome at 6 months after intra-arterial thrombolysis for acute ischemic stroke. Stroke 1999; 30: 2360–5.

17. Wechsler LR, Roberts R, Furlan AJ et al. Factors influencing outcome and treatment effect in PROACT II. Stroke 2003; 34: 1224–9.

18. Hales BM, Pronovost PJ. The checklist – a tool for error management and performance improvement. J Crit Care 2006; 21: 231–5.

19. Gawande A. The checklist: if something so simple can transform intensive care, what else can it do? New Yorker 2007; 86–101.

20. Johnston SC, Nguyen-Huynh MN, Schwarz ME et al. National Stroke Association guidelines for the management of transient ischemic attacks. Ann Neurol 2006; 60: 301–13.

21. Broderick J, Connolly S, Feldmann E et al. Guidelines for the management of spontaneous intracerebral hemorrhage in adults: 2007 update: a guideline from the American Heart Association/American Stroke Association Stroke Council, High Blood Pressure Research Council, and the Quality of Care and Outcomes in Research Interdisciplinary Working Group. Circulation 2007; 116: e391–413.

22. Adams HP Jr, del ZG, Alberts MJ et al. Guidelines for the early management of adults with ischemic stroke: a guideline from the American Heart Association/American Stroke Association Stroke Council, Clinical Cardiology Council, Cardiovascular Radiology and Intervention Council, and the Atherosclerotic Peripheral Vascular Disease and Quality of Care Outcomes in Research Interdisciplinary Working Groups: the American Academy of Neurology affirms the value of this guideline as an educational tool for neurologists. Stroke 2007; 38: 1655–711.

23. Beach C, Croskerry P, Shapiro M. Profiles in patient safety: emergency care transitions. Acad Emerg Med 2003; 10: 364–7.

24. Croskerry P. Cognitive forcing strategies in clinical decisionmaking. Ann Emerg Med 2003; 41: 110–20.

25. Cosby KS, Croskerry P. Profiles in patient safety: authority gradients in medical error. Acad Emerg Med 2004; 11: 1341–5.

26. Acker JE III, Pancioli AM, Crocco TJ et al. Implementation strategies for emergency medical services within stroke systems of care: a policy statement from the American Heart Association/American Stroke Association Expert Panel on Emergency Medical Services Systems and the Stroke Council. Stroke 2007; 38: 3097–115.

27. Pexman JH, Barber PA, Hill MD et al. Use of the Alberta Stroke Program Early CT Score (ASPECTS) for assessing CT scans in patients with acute stroke. AJNR Am J Neuroradiol 2001; 22: 1534–42.

28. Mak HK, Yau KK, Khong PL et al. Hypodensity of >1/3 middle cerebral artery territory versus Alberta Stroke Programme Early CT Score (ASPECTS): comparison of two methods of quantitative evaluation of early CT changes in hyperacute ischemic stroke in the community setting. Stroke 2003; 34: 1194–6.

29. Coutts SB, Demchuk AM, Barber PA et al. Interobserver variation of ASPECTS in real time. Stroke 2004; 35: e103–5.

30. Demchuk AM, Hill MD, Barber PA et al. Importance of early ischemic computed tomography changes using ASPECTS in NINDS rtPA Stroke Study. Stroke 2005; 36: 2110–5.

31. Generalized efficacy of t-PA for acute stroke. Subgroup analysis of the NINDS t-PA Stroke Trial. Stroke 1997; 28: 2119–25.

32. Leigh R, Zaidat OO, Suri MF et al. Predictors of hyperacute clinical worsening in ischemic stroke patients receiving thrombolytic therapy. Stroke 2004; 35: 1903–7.

33. Ribo M, Molina C, Montaner J et al. Acute hyperglycemia state is associated with lower tPA-induced recanalization rates in stroke patients. Stroke 2005; 36: 1705–9.

34. Varez-Sabin J, Molina CA, Ribo M et al. Impact of admission hyperglycemia on stroke outcome after thrombolysis: risk stratification in relation to time to reperfusion. Stroke 2004; 35: 2493–8.

35. Marti-Fabregas J, Gomis M, Arboix A et al. Favorable outcome of ischemic stroke in patients pretreated with statins. Stroke 2004; 35: 1117–21.

36. Wilterdink JL, Bendixen B, Adams HP Jr et al. Effect of prior aspirin use on stroke severity in the trial of Org 10172 in acute stroke treatment (TOAST). Stroke 2001; 32: 2836–40.

37. Wolpert SM, Bruckmann H, Greenlee R et al. Neuroradiologic evaluation of patients with acute stroke treated with recombinant tissue plasminogen activator. The rt-PA Acute Stroke Study Group. AJNR Am J Neuroradiol 1993; 14: 3–13.

38. Mori E, Yoneda Y, Tabuchi M et al. Intravenous recombinant tissue plasminogen activator in acute carotid artery territory stroke. Neurology 1992; 42: 976–82.

39. Keeley EC, Boura JA, Grines CL. Primary angioplasty versus intravenous thrombolytic therapy for acute myocardial infarction: a quantitative review of 23 randomised trials. Lancet 2003; 361: 13–20.

40. Cucherat M, Bonnefoy E, Tremeau G. Primary angioplasty versus intravenous thrombolysis for acute myocardial infarction. Cochrane Database Syst Rev 2003; 3: CD001560.

41. Lewandowski CA, Frankel M, Tomsick TA et al. Combined intravenous and intra-arterial r-TPA versus intra-arterial therapy of acute ischemic stroke: Emergency Management of Stroke (EMS) Bridging Trial. Stroke 1999; 30: 2598–605.

42. Ernst R, Pancioli A, Tomsick T et al. Combined intravenous and intra-arterial recombinant tissue plasminogen activator in acute ischemic stroke. Stroke 2000; 31: 2552–7.

43. Mattle HP, Arnold M, Georgiadis D et al. Comparison of intraarterial and intravenous thrombolysis for ischemic stroke with hyperdense middle cerebral artery sign. Stroke 2008; 39: 379–83.

44. Intracerebral hemorrhage after intravenous t-PA therapy for ischemic stroke. The NINDS t-PA Stroke Study Group. Stroke 1997; 28: 2109–18.

45. del Zoppo GJ. Thrombolysis in acute stroke. Neurologia 1995; 10: 37–47.

46. Furlan AJ, Kanoti G. When is thrombolysis justified in patients with acute ischemic stroke? A bioethical perspective [see comments]. Stroke 1997; 28: 214–8.

47. Ciccone A, Valvassori L, Gasparotti R et al. Debunking 7 myths that hamper the realization of randomized controlled trials on intra-arterial thrombolysis for acute ischemic stroke. Stroke 2007; 38: 2191–5.

48. del Zoppo GJ, Higashida RT, Furlan AJ et al. PROACT: a phase II randomized trial of recombinant pro-urokinase by direct arterial delivery in acute middle cerebral artery stroke. PROACT Investigators. Prolyse in Acute Cerebral Thromboembolism. Stroke 1998; 29: 4–11.

49. Furlan A, Higashida R, Wechsler L et al. Intra-arterial prourokinase for acute ischemic stroke. The PROACT II study: a randomized controlled trial. Prolyse in Acute Cerebral Thromboembolism. JAMA 1999; 282: 2003–11.

50. Kase CS, Furlan AJ, Wechsler LR et al. Cerebral hemorrhage after intra-arterial thrombolysis for ischemic stroke: the PROACT II trial. Neurology 2001; 57: 1603–10.

51. Roberts HC, Dillon WP, Furlan AJ et al. Computed tomographic findings in patients undergoing intra-arterial thrombolysis for acute ischemic stroke due to middle cerebral artery occlusion: results from the PROACT II trial. Stroke 2002; 33: 1557–65.

52. Suarez JI, Sunshine JL, Tarr R et al. Predictors of clinical improvement, angiographic recanalization, and intracranial hemorrhage after intra-arterial thrombolysis for acute ischemic stroke. Stroke 1990; 30: 2094–100.

53. Bendszus M, Urbach H, Ries F, Solymosi L. Outcome after local intra-arterial fibrinolysis compared with the natural course of patients with a dense middle cerebral artery on early CT. Neuroradiology 1998; 40: 54–8.

54. Higashida RT, Furlan AJ, Roberts H et al. Trial design and reporting standards for intra-arterial cerebral thrombolysis for acute ischemic stroke. Stroke 2003; 34: e109–37.

55. Sunshine JL, Bambakidis N, Tarr RW et al. Benefits of perfusion MR imaging relative to diffusion MR imaging in the diagnosis and treatment of hyperacute stroke. AJNR Am J Neuroradiol 2001; 22: 915–21.

56. Prosser J, Butcher K, Allport L et al. Clinical-diffusion mismatch predicts the putative penumbra with high specificity. Stroke 2005; 36: 1700–4.

57. Koga M, Reutens DC, Wright P et al. The existence and evolution of diffusion-perfusion mismatched tissue in white and gray matter after acute stroke. Stroke 2005; 36: 2132–7.

58. Molina CA, Saver JL. Extending reperfusion therapy for acute ischemic stroke: emerging pharmacological, mechanical, and imaging strategies. Stroke 2005; 36: 2311–20.

59. Butcher K, Parsons M, Allport L et al. Rapid assessment of perfusion diffusion mismatch. Stroke 2008; 39: 75–81.

60. Koenig M, Kraus M, Theek C et al. Quantitative assessment of the ischemic brain by means of perfusion-related parameters derived from perfusion CT. Stroke 2001; 32: 431–7.

61. Murphy BD, Fox AJ, Lee DH et al. Identification of penumbra and infarct in acute ischemic stroke using computed tomography perfusion-derived blood flow and blood volume measurements. Stroke 2006; 37: 1771–7.

62. Parsons MW, Pepper EM, Bateman GA, Wang Y, Levi CR. Identification of the penumbra and infarct core on hyperacute noncontrast and perfusion CT. Neurology 2007; 68: 730–6.

63. Tan JC, Dillon WP, Liu S et al. Systematic comparison of perfusion-CT and CT-angiography in acute stroke patients. Ann Neurol 2007; 61: 533–43.

64. Wintermark M, Flanders AE, Velthuis B et al. Perfusion-CT assessment of infarct core and penumbra: receiver operating characteristic curve analysis in 130 patients suspected of acute hemispheric stroke. Stroke 2006; 37: 979–85.

65. Hacke W, Albers G, Al-Rawi Y et al. The Desmoteplase in Acute Ischemic Stroke Trial (DIAS): a phase II MRI-based 9-hour window acute stroke thrombolysis trial with intravenous desmoteplase. Stroke 2005; 36: 66–73.

66. Furlan AJ, Eyding D, Albers GW et al. Dose Escalation of Desmoteplase for Acute Ischemic Stroke (DEDAS): evidence of safety and efficacy 3 to 9 hours after stroke onset. Stroke 2006; 37: 1227–31.

67. Ay H, Koroshetz WJ, Benner T et al. Transient ischemic attack with infarction: a unique syndrome? Ann Neurol 2005; 57: 679–86.

68. Purroy F, Montaner J, Rovira A et al. Higher risk of further vascular events among transient ischemic attack patients with diffusion-weighted imaging acute ischemic lesions. Stroke 2004; 35: 2313–9.

69. Kidwell CS, Alger JR, Di SF et al. Diffusion MRI in patients with transient ischemic attacks. Stroke 1999; 30: 1174–80.

70. Daffertshofer M, Mielke O, Pullwitt A, Felsenstein M, Hennerici M. Transient ischemic attacks are more than "ministrokes". Stroke 2004; 35: 2453–8.

71. Eliasziw M, Kennedy J, Hill MD et al. Early risk of stroke after a transient ischemic attack in patients with internal carotid artery disease. CMAJ 2004; 170: 1105–9.

72. Hill MD, Yiannakoulias N, Jeerakathil T et al. The high risk of stroke immediately after transient ischemic attack: a population-based study. Neurology 2004; 62: 2015–20.

73. Howard G, Toole JF, Frye-Pierson J, Hinshelwood LC. Factors influencing the survival of 451 transient ischemic attack patients. Stroke 1987; 18: 552–7.

74. Johnston SC, Gress DR, Browner WS, Sidney S. Short-term prognosis after emergency department diagnosis of TIA. JAMA 2000; 284: 2901–6.

75. Johnston SC, Rothwell PM, Nguyen-Huynh MN et al. Validation and refinement of scores to predict very early stroke risk after transient ischaemic attack. Lancet 2007; 369: 283–92.

76. Kleindorfer D, Panagos P, Pancioli A et al. Incidence and short-term prognosis of transient ischemic attack in a population-based study. Stroke 2005; 36: 720–3.

77. Lisabeth LD, Ireland JK, Risser JM et al. Stroke risk after transient ischemic attack in a population-based setting. Stroke 2004; 35: 1842–6.

78. Lovett JK, Dennis MS, Sandercock PA et al. Very early risk of stroke after a first transient ischemic attack. Stroke 2003; 34: e138–40.

79. Rothwell PM, Giles MF, Flossmann E et al. A simple score (ABCD) to identify individuals at high early risk of stroke after transient ischaemic attack. Lancet 2005; 366: 29–36.

80. Broderick JP, Hacke W. Treatment of acute ischemic stroke: Part II: neuroprotection and medical management. Circulation 2002; 106: 1736–40.

81. Broderick JP, Hacke W. Treatment of acute ischemic stroke: Part I: recanalization strategies. Circulation 2002; 106: 1563–9.

82. Mangiafico S, Cellerini M, Nencini P, Gensini G, Inzitari D. Intravenous glycoprotein IIb/IIIa Inhibitor (Tirofiban) followed by intra-arterial urokinase and mechanical thrombolysis in stroke. AJNR Am J Neuroradiol 2005; 26: 2595–601.

83. Zhang L, Zhang ZG, Zhang C, Zhang RL, Chopp M. Intravenous administration of a GPIIb/IIIa receptor antagonist extends the therapeutic window of intra-arterial tenecteplase-tissue plasminogen activator in a rat stroke model. Stroke 2004; 35: 2890–5.

84. Combining thrombolysis with the platelet glycoprotein IIb/IIIa inhibitor lamifiban: results of the Platelet Aggregation Receptor Antagonist Dose Investigation and Reperfusion Gain in Myocardial Infarction (PARADIGM) trial. J Am Coll Cardiol 1998; 32: 2003–10.

85. Emergency administration of abciximab for treatment of patients with acute ischemic stroke: results of a randomized phase 2 trial. Stroke 2005; 36: 880–90.

86. Abciximab in acute ischemic stroke: a randomized, double-blind, placebo-controlled, dose-escalation study. The Abciximab in Ischemic Stroke Investigators. Stroke 2000; 31: 601–9.

87. Alteplase for thrombolysis in acute ischemic stroke. Med Lett Drugs Ther 1996; 38: 99–100.

88. Clark WM, Wissman S, Albers GW et al. Recombinant tissue-type plasminogen activator (Alteplase) for ischemic stroke 3 to 5 hours after symptom onset. The ATLANTIS Study: a randomized controlled trial. Alteplase Thrombolysis for Acute Noninterventional Therapy in Ischemic Stroke. JAMA 1999; 282: 2019–26.

89. Clark WM, Albers GW, Madden KP, Hamilton S. The rtPA (alteplase) 0- to 6-hour acute stroke trial, part A (A0276g) : results of a double-blind, placebo-controlled, multicenter study. Thromblytic therapy in acute ischemic stroke study investigators. Stroke 2000; 31: 811–6.

90. Dundar Y, Hill R, Dickson R, Walley T. Comparative efficacy of thrombolytics in acute myocardial infarction: a systematic review. QJM 2003; 96: 103–13.

91. Eckert B, Koch C, Thomalla G et al. Aggressive therapy with intravenous abciximab and intra-arterial rtPA and additional PTA/stenting improves clinical outcome in acute vertebrobasilar occlusion: combined local fibrinolysis and intravenous abciximab in acute vertebrobasilar stroke treatment (FAST): results of a multicenter study. Stroke 2005; 36: 1160–5.

92. Liberatore GT, Samson A, Bladin C, Schleuning WD, Medcalf RL. Vampire bat salivary plasminogen activator (desmoteplase): a unique fibrinolytic enzyme that does not promote neurodegeneration. Stroke 2003; 34: 537–43.

93. Mangiafico S, Cellerini M, Nencini P, Gensini G, Inzitari D. Intravenous tirofiban with intra-arterial urokinase and mechanical thrombolysis in stroke: preliminary experience in 11 cases. Stroke 2005; 36: 2154–8.

94. Ovbiagele B. HMG-CoA reductase inhibitors improve acute ischemic stroke outcome. Stroke 2005; 36: 2344.

95. Sherman DG, Atkinson RP, Chippendale T et al. Intravenous ancrod for treatment of acute ischemic stroke: the STAT study: a randomized controlled trial. Stroke Treatment with Ancrod Trial. JAMA 2000; 283: 2395–403.

96. Zhang L, Zhang ZG, Zhang C, Zhang RL, Chopp M. Intravenous administration of a GPIIb/IIIa receptor antagonist extends the therapeutic window of intra-arterial tenecteplase-tissue plasminogen activator in a rat stroke model. Stroke 2004; 35: 2890–5.

97. Adams HP Jr, Effron MB, Torner J et al. Emergency administration of abciximab for treatment of patients with acute ischemic stroke: results of an international phase III trial: Abciximab in Emergency Treatment of Stroke Trial (AbESTT-II). Stroke 2008; 39: 87–99.

98. Rebeiz AG, Johanson P, Green CL et al. Comparison of ST-segment resolution with combined fibrinolytic and glycoprotein IIb/IIIa inhibitor therapy versus fibrinolytic alone (data from four clinical trials). Am J Cardiol 2005; 95: 611–4.

99. Di MC, Bolognese L, Maillard L et al. Combined Abciximab REteplase Stent Study in acute myocardial infarction (CARESS in AMI). Am Heart J 2004; 148: 378–85.

100. Giugliano RP, Roe MT, Harrington RA et al. Combination reperfusion therapy with eptifibatide and reduced-dose tenecteplase for ST-elevation myocardial infarction: results of the integrilin and tenecteplase in acute myocardial infarction (INTEGRITI) Phase II Angiographic Trial. J Am Coll Cardiol 2003; 41: 1251–60.

101. Lincoff AM, Califf RM, Van de WF et al. Mortality at 1 year with combination platelet glycoprotein IIb/IIIa inhibition and reduced-dose fibrinolytic therapy vs conventional fibrinolytic therapy for acute myocardial infarction: GUSTO V randomized trial. JAMA 2002; 288: 2130–5.

102. Brener SJ, Zeymer U, Adgey AA et al. Eptifibatide and low-dose tissue plasminogen activator in acute myocardial infarction: the integrilin and low-dose thrombolysis in acute myocardial infarction (INTRO AMI) trial. J Am Coll Cardiol 2002; 39: 377–86.

103. Cannon CP. Bridging the gap with new strategies in acute ST elevation myocardial infarction: bolus thrombolysis, glycoprotein IIb/IIIa inhibitors, combination therapy, percutaneous coronary intervention, and "facilitated" PCI. J Thromb Thrombolysis 2000; 9: 235–41.

104. Tseng MY, Hutchinson PJ, Czosnyka M et al. Effects of acute pravastatin treatment on intensity of rescue therapy, length of inpatient stay, and 6-month outcome in patients after aneurysmal subarachnoid hemorrhage. Stroke 2007; 38: 1545–50.

105. McGirt MJ, Blessing R, Alexander MJ et al. Risk of cerebral vasospasm after subarachnoid hemorrhage reduced by statin therapy: A multivariate analysis of an institutional experience. J Neurosurg 2006; 105: 671–4.

106. Kennedy J, Quan H, Buchan AM, Ghali WA, Feasby TE. Statins are associated with better outcomes after carotid endarterectomy in symptomatic patients. Stroke 2005; 36: 2072–6.

107. Pfaffenberger S, vcic-Kuhar B, Kollmann C et al. Can a commercial diagnostic ultrasound device accelerate thrombolysis? An in vitro skull model. Stroke 2005; 36: 124–8.

108. Daffertshofer M, Gass A, Ringleb P et al. Transcranial low-frequency ultrasound-mediated thrombolysis in brain ischemia: increased risk of hemorrhage with combined ultrasound and tissue plasminogen activator: results of a phase II clinical trial. Stroke 2005; 36: 1441–6.

109. Alexandrov AV, Wojner AW, Grotta JC. CLOTBUST: design of a randomized trial of ultrasound-enhanced thrombolysis for acute ischemic stroke. J Neuroimaging 2004; 14: 108–12.

110. Alexandrov AV, Molina CA, Grotta JC et al. Ultrasound-enhanced systemic thrombolysis for acute ischemic stroke. N Engl J Med 2004; 351: 2170–8.

111. Smith WS, Sung G, Starkman S et al. Safety and efficacy of mechanical embolectomy in acute ischemic stroke: results of the MERCI trial. Stroke 2005; 36: 1432–8.

112. Merci retriever. Clin Privil White Pap 2004; 225: 1–8.

113. Gobin YP, Starkman S, Duckwiler GR et al. MERCI 1: a phase 1 study of Mechanical Embolus Removal in Cerebral Ischemia. Stroke 2004; 35: 2848–54.

114. Flint AC, Duckwiler GR, Budzik RF, Liebeskind DS, Smith WS. Mechanical thrombectomy of intracranial internal carotid occlusion: pooled results of the MERCI and Multi MERCI Part I trials. Stroke 2007; 38: 1274–80.

115. Lutsep HL, Clark WM, Nesbit GM, Kuether TA, Barnwell SL. Intraarterial suction thrombectomy in acute stroke. AJNR Am J Neuroradiol 2002; 23: 783–6.

116. Fitzsimmons BF, Becske T, Nelson PK. Rapid stent-supported revascularization in acute ischemic stroke. AJNR Am J Neuroradiol 2006; 27: 1132–4.

117. Gupta R, Jovin TG, Tayal A, Horowitz MB. Urgent stenting of the M2 (superior) division of the middle cerebral artery after systemic thrombolysis in acute stroke. AJNR Am J Neuroradiol 2006; 27: 521–3.

118. Jovin TG, Gupta R, Uchino K et al. Emergent stenting of extracranial internal carotid artery occlusion in acute stroke has a high revascularization rate. Stroke 2005; 36: 2426–30.

119. Mahon BR, Nesbit GM, Barnwell SL et al. North American clinical experience with the EKOS MicroLysUS infusion catheter for the treatment of embolic stroke. AJNR Am J Neuroradiol 2003; 24: 534–8.

120. Smaha LA. The American Heart Association. Get With The Guidelines program. Am Heart J 2004; 148: S46–8.

121. Stradling D, Yu W, Langdorf ML et al. Stroke care delivery before vs after JCAHO stroke center certification. Neurology 2007; 68: 469–70.

122. Higashida RT, Hopkins LN, Berenstein A, Halbach VV, Kerber C. Program requirements for residency/fellowship education in neuroendovascular surgery/interventional neuroradiology: a special report on graduate medical education. AJNR Am J Neuroradiol 2000; 21: 1153–9.

123. The Interventional Management of Stroke (IMS) II Study. Stroke 2007; 38: 2127–35.

124. Leira EC, Pary JK, Davis PH, Grimsman KJ, Adams HP Jr. Slow progressive acceptance of intravenous thrombolysis for patients with stroke by rural primary care physicians. Arch Neurol 2007; 64: 518–21.

125. Qureshi AI, Suri MF, Nasar A et al. Changes in cost and outcome among US patients with stroke hospitalized in 1990 to 1991 and those hospitalized in 2000 to 2001. Stroke 2007; 38: 2180–4.

126. Furlan AJ, Fisher M. Devices, drugs, and the Food and Drug Administration: increasing implications for ischemic stroke. Stroke 2005; 36: 398–9.

127. Nesbit GM, Clark WM, O'Neill OR, Barnwell SL. Intracranial intraarterial thrombolysis facilitated by microcatheter navigation through an occluded cervical internal carotid artery. J Neurosurg 1996; 84: 387–92.

128. Johnston SC. Clinical practice. Transient ischemic attack. N Engl J Med 2002; 347: 1687–92.

6

Subacute and elective revascularization of the cerebral vasculature

Thomas J Masaryk, Irene Katzan and David Fiorella

Hippocrates was the first to describe transient ischemic attacks (TIA's), noting that 'unaccustomed attacks of numbness and anesthesia are signs of impending apoplexy.'[1,2] And while Sir Thomas Willis appreciated the significance of the communicating arteries in preserving cerebral collateral flow,[3] it was not until the 1950s that C Miller Fisher associated TIAs with carotid bifurcation disease and stroke.[4] The first successful carotid endarterectomy (CEA) was performed shortly thereafter.[5,6] By the early 1980s CEA was the most frequently performed vascular surgical procedure. Nevertheless, the subsequent failure of the external carotid–internal carotid bypass operation to prevent stroke[7] and the absence of randomized clinical endarterectomy trial data provoked challenges about the procedure's safety and efficacy.[8] In early 1990s, six randomized clinical trials established the efficacy of CEA plus aspirin compared with aspirin alone in preventing stroke in patients with atherosclerotic carotid bifurcation stenosis. (Figures 6.1, 6.2).[9–16] Similarly, long-term outcome studies have better defined the natural history of intracranial atherosclerotic disease treated medically (Figure 6.3).

Minimally invasive, percutaneous techniques to re-establish arterial blood flow paralleled the development of vascular surgery (although in a delayed fashion, reflecting the evolution and ultimate digitization of real-time angiography). In 1964, Charles Dotter and Melvin Judkins reported the first transluminal angioplasty using a series of catheters of ever-increasing diameter.[17] Subsequently Andreas Grundzig reported and popularized balloon angioplasty for (initially) the coronary circulation and (ultimately) the peripheral circulation.[18] Almost 10 years later, Palmaz was the first to report the implantation of vascular stents to preserve luminal diameter following angioplasty.[19]

One of the benefits of large, well-controlled randomized surgical trials is the establishment of accepted primary and secondary outcome benchmarks as well as the natural history of the underlying disease. Enthusiasm for the adaptation of the endovascular innovations of angioplasty to the cerebral circulation was initially tempered by a healthy respect for potential thromboembolic complications, intracranial hemorrhage, and the excellent results achievable by capable surgeons as documented using these benchmarks. Nevertheless, in the context of what is now known regarding the natural history of the disease[9–16,20,21] and further refinements in percutaneous techniques, selective application of angioplasty and stenting has become established as a tool in the armamentarium against stroke.[22–25] In the USA in 2005, carotid revascularization volumes include 103,000 CEA,[26] and there are ever-increasing numbers of carotid artery stenting procedures. Indications may include selective instances of extra- and intracranial atherosclerosis, dissection, post-surgical re-stenosis, arteritis, erosion and stenosis by neoplasm, and penetrating trauma.

Atherosclerotic cerebrovascular disease

Atherosclerosis accounts for up to one-third of all strokes. Approximately 50% of strokes occur in the territory of the carotid arteries, and while extracranial carotid disease is more frequent in Caucasians, intracranial disease is more frequent in non-whites (Figure 6.4).[27–29] Carotid disease that is amenable to revascularization accounts for 5–12% of new strokes.[30–32] Carotid atherosclerosis is typically unifocal, and 90% of lesions are located within 2cm of the origin of the internal carotid artery (ICA) (see Figure 6.4).[4,33] The degree of carotid stenosis is associated with stroke risk in symptomatic patients. Carotid atherosclerosis can produce retinal and cortical symptoms by either progressive carotid stenosis leading to hypoperfusion (less commonly) or by intracranial arterial embolization (more commonly). The risk of progression of carotid stenosis is 9.3% per year, and risk factors for progression include:[34]

- ipsilateral or contralateral ICA stenosis greater than >50%;
- ipsilateral external carotid artery (ECA) stenosis >50%; and
- systolic blood pressure >160 mmHg.[34]

Nearly 80% of strokes due to carotid atherosclerosis occur without warning, emphasizing the need for careful screening and follow-up.[30–32] In patients who do present with a sentinel TIA, the risk of secondary stroke in temporal proximity to the initial symptoms is high.[35,36]

Medical therapy

A demographic profile can gauge the risk of stroke based on age, systolic blood pressure, antihypertensive therapy, diabetes,

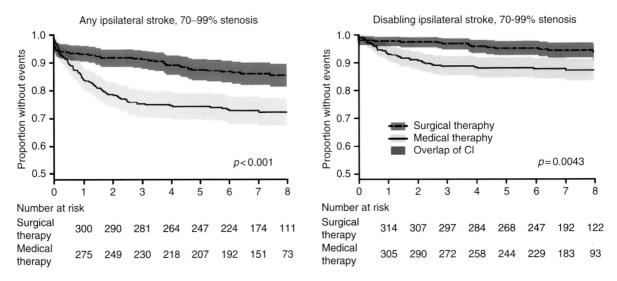

Figure 6.1

NASCET Kaplan–Meier survival curves for stroke in symptomatic patients with severe carotid stenoses treated by surgery (red) or best medical therapy (blue). (Reprinted with permission from Barnett et al.[10])

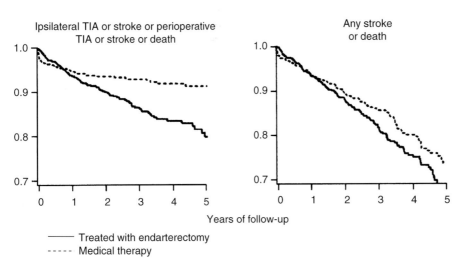

Figure 6.2

Survival curves for asymptomatic patients with severe carotid stenoses treated with endarterectomy and medical therapy. TIA, transient ischemic attack. Reprinted with permission from: Endarterectomy for Asymptomatic Carotid Artery Stenosis. JAMA 1995; 273: 1421–28.

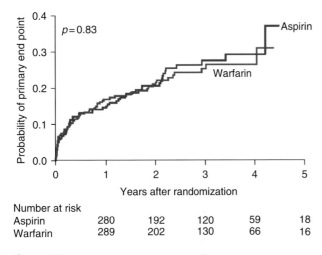

Figure 6.3

Cumulative incidence of ischemic stroke, intracranial hemorrhage and death in patients with intracranial stenoses treated with either aspirin or warfarin. (Reprinted with permission from Chimowitz MI et al.[20])

cigarette smoking, and history of coronary artery disease (CAD), congestive heart failure, or atrial fibrillation.[35,37] Clinical findings must be correlated with brain and vascular imaging to determine whether or not suspected atherosclerotic cerebrovascular disease is symptomatic. Imaging is critical to assess the anatomy and structural pathology of the brain (e.g. mass, old or new stroke, presence of hemorrhage) and the cervical vessels (e.g. stenosis, plaque morphology, dissection), and to guide treatment. In asymptomatic patients there are no guidelines to support routine carotid imaging, except for some candidates for coronary artery bypass grafting (CABG.) Prior to CABG, carotid duplex studies are recommended in asymptomatic patients who are older than 65 years or who have left main coronary artery stenosis; peripheral arterial disease; a history of smoking, TIA, or stroke; or a carotid bruit.[12]

Hypertension is major risk factor for all forms of cerebrovascular disease by virtue of its direct atherogenic effects on the systemic and cerebral circulations, and by association with CAD and atrial fibrillation.[38] Control of blood pressure is key to modification of atherogenic risk factors: there is a linear relationship between increasing blood pressure and stroke risk.

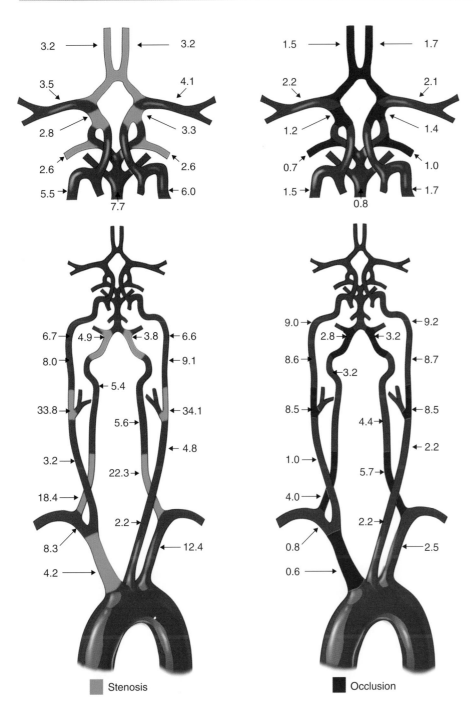

Figure 6.4
Percentage distribution of atherosclerotic stenoses (green) and occlusion (blue). (Adapted from the work of Fields et al. and Hass et al., JAMA 1968; 203: 955–60, 961–68.)

Even small reductions in systolic pressure (10 mmHg) and diastolic pressure (3–6 mmHg) result in a 30–42% decline in the risk of stroke.[39,40] Systolic hypertension is an especially important risk factor in the elderly.[41]

Recent trials of angiotensin converting enzyme (ACE) inhibitors and angiotensin receptor blockers (ARBs) suggest that these agents may have benefits for stroke reduction that extend beyond their antihypertensive effects. The Heart Outcomes and Prevention Evaluation (HOPE) trial studied 9297 patients with high cardiovascular risk, including 1013 patients with previous TIA or stroke.[42] Patients were randomized to ramipril 10 mg daily or placebo, and ramipril was associated with a 32% reduction in stroke over 5 years. Although ramipril was associated with a significant antihypertensive effect (2–3 mmHg decline in systolic and diastolic blood pressure) these benefits were felt to be insufficient to explain the dramatic decline in stroke. In the Losartan Intervention for Endpoint (LIFE) trial, losartan and atenolol achieved similar degrees of blood pressure reduction, but losartan was associated with a 13% reduction in cardiovascular events and a 25% reduction in stroke.[43] Potential added benefits of ACE inhibitors and ARBs include inhibition of angiotensin II-mediated vasoconstriction and vascular smooth cell hyperplasia, improved endothelial function, and enhanced fibrinolysis.

Smoking increases the risk of ischemic and hemorrhagic stroke (particularly subarachnoid hemorrhage), and the risk is directly proportional to the number of cigarettes smoked.[44,45] The risk is higher in female smokers who use oral contraceptives. Passive exposure to cigarette smoke nearly doubles the risk of stroke in spouses of smokers.[46] The risk of stroke decreases to that of non-smokers within 5 years of smoking cessation.[47]

The relationship between dyslipidemia and stroke has not been demonstrated consistently. However, there is a relationship between total cholesterol, low-density lipoprotein cholesterol, and the extent of extracranial carotid artery atherosclerosis and wall thickness.[48] Furthermore, efforts to manage hypercholesterolemia with statins may have the added benefit of a protective effect in the event of actual ischemic insult.[49–54]

Gemfibrozil reduced stroke rates by 24% in the Veterans Affairs High Density Lipoprotein Cholesterol Intervention Trial (VA-HIT) study.[55] Niacin reduced stroke by 22% in the Coronary Drug Project.[56] Pravastatin, simvastatin, and atorvastatin are approved by the Food and Drug Administration (FDA) in the USA for stroke prevention in patients with CAD,[49,51,57] although the benefits may be mediated by anti-inflammatory, plaque stabilization, and neuroprotective effects (rather than by direct cholesterol reduction). The Stroke Prevention with Aggressive Reduction of Cholesterol Levels (SPARCL) trial studied atorvastatin 20mg for secondary prevention of stroke in 4731 patients without CAD and documented a 16% relative risk reduction for recurrent stroke.[54,58]

Statins may be effective for secondary prevention in patients undergoing CEA.[59] The National Cholesterol Education Program (NCEP) guidelines and the American Stroke Association (ASA) recommend statins in patients with prior TIA or stroke or carotid stenosis >50%.[50,60]

Diabetes is a major independent risk factor for stroke.[61,62] The combination of diabetes and hypertension increases the risk of stroke six-fold compared with normal patients, and the risk is two-fold higher than in normotensive diabetics. Abdominal obesity contributes more than body mass index to the presence of insulin resistance, hypertension, and dyslipidemia, and secondarily to the risk for stroke;[63] however, there are no reports correlating weight loss with reduced stroke risk.

Additional risk factors include the use of oral contraceptives (especially in women over 35 years), elevated fibrinogen, and elevated C-reactive protein.[64–67] These factors exacerbate the primary risk factors of hypertension, smoking, and diabetes listed above.

Risk factor modification with medical therapy is recommended to limit progression of atherosclerosis and to decrease clinical events, irrespective of carotid artery revascularization.[68,69] Therapy should also include an antiplatelet agent. For asymptomatic patients with one or more cardiovascular risk factors, antiplatelet therapy is indicated. For symptomatic patients (with a recent TIA or minor cerebrovascular accident), the recommendations for antiplatelet therapy are based on large stroke prevention studies[70–81] that included patients with a variety of stroke etiologies.

The relative risk reduction conferred by aspirin therapy is 16% for fatal stroke and 28% for nonfatal stroke.[82] Randomized trials indicate that aspirin is superior to CEA for symptomatic patients with carotid stenosis <50%[9,10,13,14] and for asymptomatic patients with carotid stenosis <60%.[83,84] Early studies suggested benefit with low-dose aspirin.[70–72] The risk of myocardial infarction, stroke, and death within 1–3 months of CEA was lower for patients taking low-dose aspirin (81mg or 325mg daily) than for those taking high-dose aspirin (650mg or 1300mg daily).[73]

Ticlopidine has been shown to be useful for secondary prevention after stroke in the Canadian–American Ticlopidine Study (CATS); it resulted in a 23% reduction in cardiovascular events.[76] The Ticlopidine Aspirin Stroke Study (TASS) looked at patients after TIA or major stroke;[77] ticlopidine caused significantly fewer cerebrovascular events and less bleeding, but neutropenia complicated therapy in 0.9% of patients. Clopidogrel has largely replaced ticlopidine because of a superior safety profile and its once-daily dosing. For preventing stroke in secondary prevention trials, clopidogrel was similar to aspirin in the Clopidogrel versus Aspirin in Patients at Risk of Ischemic Events (CAPRIE) trial.[78] The combination of clopidogrel plus aspirin was similar to aspirin alone in the Clopidogrel for High Atherothrombotic Risk and Ischemic Stabilization, Management, and Avoidance (CHARISMA) trial.[80] In the Atherothrombosis with Clopidogrel in High-Risk Patients With Recent Transient Ischemic Attack or Ischemic Stroke (MATCH) trial, the combination of aspirin plus clopidogrel increased the risk of systemic and intracerebral hemorrhage, but it did not decrease the risk of stroke compared with clopidogrel alone.[74] Hence, aspirin and clopidogrel appear to have similar efficacy, but the combination may increase the risk of serious bleeding and is not superior to either drug alone.[82] Nevertheless, In cases of recurrent symptoms despite antiplatelet therapy, dual therapy with may be warranted.

Warfarin is recommended for primary and secondary prevention of stroke in patients with atrial fibrillation. However, in patients with non-cardioembolic stroke there were no differences between warfarin and aspirin in stroke, death, or major bleeding.[81] Moreover, the Warfarin Aspirin Symptomatic Intracranial Disease (WASID) trial failed to show an advantage for warfarin compared with aspirin, and there was additional morbidity.[85]

In summary, antiplatelet therapy is favored over warfarin in patients with cerebral atherosclerotic disease who are not at risk of cardioembolic stroke

Revascularization of carotid atherostenosis

Work-up and indications

Indications for carotid stenting must always be framed in the context of the more established alternative, endarterectomy. Guidelines from the American Heart Association (AHA) recommend CEA in symptomatic patients with a stenosis of 50–99%, when the risk of periprocedure stroke or death is less than 6%.[69] Pooled analysis of 6092 patients with 35,000 patient–years follow-up (using uniform definitions of stenosis severity and outcome) revealed a 1.1% mortality and a 7.1% incidence of stroke or death at 30 days after CEA.[86] After 5 years, CEA was associated with a 48% relative risk reduction in ipsilateral stroke in patients with a stenosis of 70–99%, a 28% relative risk reduction in ipsilateral stroke in patients with a stenosis of 50–69%, and no benefit in patients with stenosis of less than 50%.

For asymptomatic patients, AHA guidelines recommend CEA for patients with a stenosis of 60–99%, when the risk of perioperative stroke or death is less than 3%. Pooled analysis of asymptomatic carotid endarterectomy trials include 5,223 patients with 17,037 patient years follow-up, averaging 3.3 years per patient.[87] At 30 days, the risk of stroke or death after CEA was 2.9%. In comparison with aspirin alone, CEA was associated with a 31% relative risk reduction in stroke or perioperative death during the study period, but the absolute risk reduction was only 1% per year. Interestingly, all of the risk was in men (51% relative risk reduction) rather than in women (4% relative risk reduction), and in younger patients. Also, outcome after CEA in asymptomatic patients was not associated with stenosis severity.

Implicit in these guidelines is the accurate assement of carotid stenosis as measured the in the North American Symptomatic Carotid Endarterectomy Trial (NASCET) and the Asymptomatic Carotid Atherosclerosis Study (ACAS). This method utilizes the diameter of the proximal ICA above the carotid bulb as the reference diameter relative to the diameter of the stenosis, as seen in the projection in which it appears most severe.[88] All patients being considered for carotid artery stenting (CAS) must meet these angiographic criteria. Nevertheless, carotid duplex studies, magnetic resonance angiography (MRA), and CT angiography (CTA) are often recommended for the initial evaluation of patients with carotid artery disease.

The mainstay of carotid duplex evaluation is the determination of flow velocity using spectral Doppler analysis. Meta-analyses[89,90] and a multidisciplinary consensus conference[91] suggest that peak systolic velocity is the single most accurate duplex parameter for determination of stenosis severity. Compared with angiography, carotid duplex has a sensitivity of between 77% and 98% and a specificity of between 53% and 82% for identifying or excluding an ICA stenosis >70%.[89] Women have higher flow velocities than men.[92] In patients with a severe carotid stenosis or occlusion, compensatory increases in contralateral blood flow may result in spuriously high velocities in the patent ICA. In this situation, the ratio of peak systolic flow velocities in the proximal ICA and the distal common carotid artery (the ICA–CCA peak systolic velocity ratio) is a better determinant of stenosis severity.[93,94] The accuracy of diagnostic criteria may vary substantially between laboratories,[95–97] optimal diagnostic criteria may change over time,[98] and there is significant intraobserver variability.[89,95,99] Hence ultrasound laboratories must have strict quality-assurance programs to establish optimal internal diagnostic criteria. When carotid duplex results are unclear, diagnostic accuracy may increase to >90% when it is used in conjunction with CTA and/or MRA.[100]

MRA allows imaging of aortic arch, cervical carotid and intracranial lesions that are not accessible by carotid duplex studies.[101] Newer reconstruction algorithms[101] as well as newer contrast agents have increased speed and study consistency.[102,103] When compared with conventional angiography, first-pass contrast enhanced three-dimensional MRA maximum-intensity projections correlate with angiography stenosis in 90% of cases, and correlation is best for severe stenoses.[102] Additional benefits include the ability to image the aortic arch and the circle of Willis as well as highly sensitive diffusion techniques for acute ischemic brain injury (within minutes, up to 14 days).[104,105] Limitations include the inability to perform MRA because of claustrophobia, pacemakers, implantable defibrillators, and obesity.

The combination of these ultrasound and MRA techniques provides better concordance with digital subtraction angiography than either test alone (combined 96% sensitivity and 80% specificity), but is not cost-effective for routine use.[106] MRA following stent placement is safe and has been attempted; however, magnetic susceptibility artifact and Faraday shielding significantly degrade the image about the implant.[104,105,107–111]

CTA with multi-row spiral scanners (with more than 16 rows) allows axial carotid imaging at speeds capable capturing a three-dimensional arterial snapshot from the aortic arch to the vertex of the cerebrum. Like MRA, CTA is useful when carotid duplex studies are ambiguous, permitting as it does visualization of aortic arch or high bifurcation pathology, reliable differentiation of total and subtotal occlusion, assessment of ostial and tandem stenoses, and evaluation of carotid disease in patients with arrhythmias, valvular heart disease, or cardiomyopathy. When compared with carotid duplex, CTA is more specific for high-grade lesions,

and in one study it altered surgical planning in 11% of cases.[112] Comparing CTA with enhanced MRA, one study showed that CTA was less reliable.[101] With CTA, the sensitivity and specificity for detecting carotid stenosis of more than 70% was 85–95% and 93–98%, respectively.[113,114] CTA sensitivity and accuracy can be increased by examining axial source images[113] and volume-rendered projections,[115] and by the use of faster, high-resolution multi-slice scanners.[116]

Carotid and cerebral angiography has the same complications as other arterial catheterization techniques: access site injury, blood loss requiring transfusion, contrast nephropathy, anaphylactoid reactions, and stroke. In symptomatic patients undergoing cerebral angiography, the risk of stroke is 0.5–5.7%, and the risk of TIA is 0.6–6.8%.[117] In asymptomatic patients in the ACAS trial, stroke occurred in 1.2% of patients after angiography.[118] More recent studies reported stroke and TIA rates of less than 1%, suggesting that the risk may be lower.[119] Possible explanations include faster digital equipment, technique, operator experience, and the use of antiplatelet agents.

In the USA, Medicare and Medicaid reimbursement for carotid stenting is limited to the use of facilities and to physicians that meet minimum standards and use FDA-approved stents and emboli protection devices (EPDs) for high-risk patients with symptomatic stenosis >70%. The minimum standards include credentialing of all operators as well as a continuous quality assessment program. The term 'high risk' applies to conditions outlined in Table 6.1. Additional high-risk patients (symptomatic stenosis >50%, asymptomatic stenosis >80%) may also be eligible if enrolled in a category B Investigational Device Exemption (IDE) trial or post-approval studies that are under FDA sponsorship and FDA Institutional Review Board supervision.

Stenting carotid atherosclerotic stenosis: risks and benefits

The risk of stroke in patients with carotid stenosis is primarily dependent on symptom status and stenosis severity,[10] and it is

---

Table 6.1 High-risk conditions for carotid endarterectomy

Previous radiation therapy to the neck

Previous CEA with recurrent re-stenosis

High cervical internal carotid artery stenosis or below-the-clavicle common carotid artery stenosis

Severe tandem lesions

Contralateral carotid artery occlusion

Contralateral laryngeal nerve palsy

Age >80 years

Severe pulmonary disease.

Significant cardiac co-morbidity
- Congestive heart failure (New York Heart Association Class III or IV) and/or known severe left ventricular dysfunction;
- Open heart surgery needed within 6 weeks
- Recent myocardial infarction (more than 24 hours and less than 4 weeks ago)
- Unstable angina (Canadian Cardiovascular Society Class III or IV)

CEA, carotid endarterectomy.

secondarily influenced by the presence of silent infarction, contralateral disease, extent of collaterals, atherosclerotic risk factors, plaque morphology, and other clinical features.[120,121]

Patients with asymptomatic carotid bruits are more commonly seen than patients with symptomatic carotid stenosis. A carotid bruit is identified in 4–5% of patients aged between 45 and 80 years (it is higher in patients with known atherosclerosis), and it may be appreciated in most patients with carotid stenosis ≥75%.[122,123] Carotid stenoses ≥50% have been identified in 7% of men and 5% of women older than 65 years. However, a bruit may be absent if there is slow flow through a severe stenosis, so cervical bruits are neither specific nor sensitive for identifying severe carotid stenosis.

In asymptomatic patients, the annual stroke risk is less than 1% for carotid stenoses <60% and 1–2.4% for carotid stenoses >60%.[84,118] In the Asymptomatic Carotid Surgery Trial (ACST), there was no relationship between the risk of stroke and increasing stenosis severity from 60% to 99% for asymptomatic patients.[84] Patients referred for CABG have a particularly high incidence of asymptomatic carotid stenosis with a prevalence of 17–22% for carotid stenosis >50% and 6–12% for carotid stenosis >80%. The risk of perioperative stroke after CABG is 2% for carotid stenosis <50%, 10% for carotid stenosis of 50–80%, and as high as 19% for carotid stenosis >80%.[12]

The prevalence of silent cerebral infarction in patients with asymptomatic carotid stenosis is estimated to be 15–20%,[118] and appears to be associated with a higher risk of subsequent stroke. In patients with ICA occlusion, the annual stroke risk is influenced by the number of intracranial collateral pathways.[124]

The risk of stroke is substantial in symptomatic patients;[10,15] and it is highest immediately after the initial ischemic event. In NASCET, the risk of stroke in the first year was 11% for carotid stenosis of 70–79% and 35% for carotid stenosis ≥90%.[9,10,35] Patients with carotid stenosis of 70–99% had a 2-year ipsilateral stroke risk of 26%. Somewhat perversely, patients with near-occlusion have a lower stroke risk.[125,126]

Other factors that influence the risk of stroke include the clinical manifestations, contralateral disease, intracranial disease, intracranial collaterals, and plaque morphology.[120,127] In the NASCET, the 3-year risk of ipsilateral stroke was 10% after retinal TIAs and 20.3% after hemispheric TIAs.[128] The presence of concomitant intracranial disease raised the 3-year risk of stroke from 25% to 46% in patients with carotid stenosis of 85–99%.[129] In NASCET patients with carotid stenosis of 70–99%, the presence of contralateral carotid occlusion increased stroke risk by more than two-fold,[130] whereas the presence of collaterals decreased the stroke risk by more than two-fold.[131] Stroke risk in symptomatic patients may also be influenced by plaque morphology, including the presence of hypoechoic or echolucent plaque[132,133] and plaque ulceration,[127,134] irrespective of the degree of stenosis.

Beyond stroke risk, many patients with carotid stenosis are elderly and may have additional co-morbidities. Given the risk of revascularization, patients must live several years to reap the full benefit of either CEA or CAS (see the Kaplan–Meier survival curves in Figures 6.1, 6.2) Indeed, in the European Long-term Carotid Artery Stenting Registry (ELOCAS), which included 2172 CAS patients from four centers, despite a high rate of procedural success at 1, 3, and 5 years of follow-up, stroke or death occurred in 4.1%, 10.1%, and 15.1%, respectively.[135] Similarly, the early experience in the Carotid Revascularization Endarterectomy versus Stent Trial (CREST) cautioned against stenting in octogenarians.[136] The fact that CEA is associated with more risk in patients with co-morbidities does not mandate that patients

undergo CAS. A list of contraindications to carotid stenting is included in Table 6.2

Carotid artery stenting: technique

Beyond indications and informed estimation of risk versus benefit, there are additional lessons to be learned from the experience of CEA. Centers were selected to participate in CEA trials based on volume and vetting of low complication rates, raising concern that the results might not be applicable to community practice.[137] In fact, operative mortality is higher in Medicare audits[138,139] and in high-risk patients who would have been excluded from the randomized trials.[139] Bond et al. have also confirmed lower complication rates for high-volume operators and high-volume centers.[140,141] This raises the often prickly issue of credentialing for CAS (Table 6.3).[117] Additionally, the standard medical therapy for the randomized CEA trials was aspirin, and many physicians believe that 'best medical therapy' with statins, ACE inhibitors, and stricter control of risk factors may be superior to aspirin alone.[142] Finally, standard practice after CEA does not include routine evaluation by a neurologist. In a large meta-analysis of nearly 16,000 symptomatic patients with CEA, the 30-day risk of stroke and death was 7.7% if a neurologist evaluated the patient, and 2.3% if a vascular surgeon performed the evaluation.[143] These data support the need for independent neurological evaluation pre- and post-CAS.

A summary of pre-CAS evaluation and preparation is included in Table 6.4. With rare exceptions great care must be taken to optimize fully the patient's medical regimen prior to the procedure. In particular it has become our practice to insure that the patient is therapeutic (>70% inhibition of platelet function) relative to aspirin and clopidogrel prior to CAS and that the patient is receiving statins.[50,53]

Initial intraprocedure management consists of mild sedation and analgesia, anticoagulation, hemodynamic monitoring (ECG and arterial pressure monitoring) and support, and intermittent neurological assessment. Once arterial access has been achieved, unfractionated heparin is given to maintain the activated clotting time between 250 and 300 seconds. There are no published data on low-molecular-weight heparin. The use of bivalirudin was

---

Table 6.2 Contraindications to carotid artery stenting

Clinical
- Life expectancy < 5 years
- Strict contraindication to antiplatelet agents
- Renal dysfunction precluding contrast administration

Neurological
- Sustained major functional or cognitive impairment
- Major stroke within 4 weeks

Anatomical
- Inability to achieve safe vascular access
- Severe tortuosity of aortic arch
- Severe tortuosity of common carotid artery or the internal carotid artery
- Extensive plaque calcification
- Intra-luminal thrombus
- Total occlusion
- Intracranial aneurysm, arterial–venous malformation or primary intra-axial neoplasm requiring treatment

Table 6.3 Requirements for performance of carotid artery stenting[117]

Cognitive requirements

I. A fund of knowledge regarding stroke syndromes and TIA etiologies, evaluation of traumatic and/or atherosclerotic neurovascular lesions, and inflammatory conditions of the central nervous system

II. Formal training that imparts an adequate depth of cognitive knowledge of the brain and its associated pathophysiological vascular processes, including management of complications of endovascular procedures

III. Diagnostic and therapeutic acumen, including the ability to recognize and manage procedural complications

IV. Ability to recognize clinical intra- or post-procedural neurological symptoms, as well as pertinent angiographic findings and the proper cognitive and technical skills to offer the most appropriate therapy. This might also entail optimal hemodynamic management necessitating sufficient neurointensive skills

Technical requirements

I. Technical requirements for performance of carotid stenting, including adequate procedural skill achieved by repetitive training in an approved clinical setting by a qualified instructor. This includes the ability to correctly interpret a cervicocerebral angiogram, which serves as the prerequisite and foundation for the technical performance of cervicocerebral angiography. Minimum numbers of procedures to achieve competence: 100 diagnostic cervicocerebral angiograms

Clinical management requirements

I. In addition to procedural technical experience requirements, a minimum of 6 months of formal cognitive neuroscience training in a program in radiology, neuroradiology, neurosurgery, neurology, and/or vascular neurology approved by the Accreditation Council for Graduate Medical Education is required

II. Formal training and competency in the National Institutes of Health Stroke Scale

III. Maintenance of proficiency by lifelong continuing medical education and continuing performance of cases with adequate success and outcomes with minimal complications

Table 6.4 pre-carotid artery stent protocol

History and physical examination

- NIHSS
- Rankin score

Vascular imaging of vascular anatomy (carotid duplex scans, CTA, or MRA)

- Preferably to include aortic arch
- Brain imaging in symptomatic cases

Basic laboratory tests including renal function, coagulation profile (including aspirin and clopidogrel platelet function testing), and blood counts

Medication

- Aspirin 81–325 mg per day for at least 4 days
- Clopidogrel: 600mg loading dose, then 75mg per day (orally)
- Statins
- ACE inhibitors (If indicated)

NIHSS, National Institutes of Health Stroke Scale; CTA, computed tomography angiography; MRA, magnetic resonance angiography; ACE, angiotensin converting enzyme

permitted in some CAS trials, but data in large numbers of patients are not available.[144] Potential advantages with bivalirudin include lower bleeding risk, rapid offset that permits early sheath removal, and no need for monitoring of the activated clotting time. The use of glycoprotein IIb–IIIa inhibitors has not been established as routine with CAS.[145,146]

Experience accessing the brachiocephalic vessels is also integral to successful CAS planning.[147,148] It is important to recognize the type of aortic arch, the configuration of the great vessels, and the anatomic variants, because these features influence the complexity of the procedure and, by extension, the choice of catheters. (see Chapter 2). Although most procedures are performed utilizing femoral access to the CCA, a brachial or radial approach may in rare instances be necessary.

Following preliminary angiography to assess the precise location of the target lesion, a 6F interventional sheath or an 8F guiding catheter (internal diameter 0.087–0.090 inches, 2.2–2.3 mm) may be exchanged to provide a conduit from the femoral access site to the target lesion. For CCA lesions at the brachiocephalic origins, the conduit may only extend to the aortic arch. Alternatively in the more common case of a lesion at the bifurcation, the guide or sheath is placed in the CCA

proximal to the bifurcation, usually by exchange over a relatively stiff 0.035-inch (0.9 mm) exchange length (300cm) guidewire with the tip located in a distal branch of the ECA artery under roadmap guidance. The guide is connected to a pressurized heparin flush solution (4,000 IU/liter), which is fixed to a rotating hemostatic valve.

As with angioplasty performed elsewhere in the body, the stenosis is first crossed with a guidewire under roadmap guidance. Given the eloquent nature of the end-organ, this and any future manipulation of the atherosclerotic plaque must be kept to a minimum and performed with great care to avoid embolic events. Several systems or EPDs have been developed to minimize this risk. There are two categories of EPDs: proximal EPDs and distal EPDs.

Proximal EPDs rely on transient occlusion of the CCA proximal to the target lesion (with a balloon) and the ECA (with a smaller balloon), resulting in stagnant or reversed flow in the ICA.[107,149,150] An advantage of such a system is that embolic protection is established even before the lesion is crossed with a guidewire. After stent placement and angioplasty, aspiration of blood from the carotid bifurcation removes any debris; this is followed by re-establishment of antegrade flow with balloon deflation.

Distal EPDs are deployed after crossing the stenosis.[104,125,151–161] Generally these systems consists of a 0.014-inch (0.36 mm) guidewire-mounted occlusive balloon or filter, over which angioplasty and stenting are performed. Disadvantages of this design include the necessity of traversing the atherostenosis prior to full deployment of the balloon or filter, as well as the fact that the diameter of the filter sheath is substantially larger than the guidewire alone. In the case of balloon occlusion, once it has been inflated, debris is aspirated from the occluded carotid artery after manipulation and prior to deflation and re-establishment of antegrade flow. With filter devices, collected debris within the filter is captured and removed when the filter is reconstrained with a sheath (Figures 6.5, 6.6).

Controlled studies of proximal and distal EPDs for CAS have not been performed, and to date distal EPDs have advantages as well as limitations.[107,149,152–154,156,157,159–162] Certainly even in skilled hands these devices do not guarantee that an embolic event will not occur as the result of failed deployment, vascular trauma, or incomplete capture of debris.[156,163,164] Furthermore, certain situations such as severe tortuosity of the ICA or precarious positioning of the guide catheter extending from the arch may predispose to such failures and are relative contraindications to the use of EPDs.[153]

If a patient does develop focal neurological symptoms or signs during the procedure, removal of the protection device (or deflation of the occlusion balloon) may result in resolution. Alternatively if, after this maneuver, the patient remains symptomatic, it is important to assess for evidence of distal emboli. Distal ICA or proximal middle cerebral artery occlusions are associated with a high degree of morbidity and should entertain consideration of mechanical means of thrombectomy (see Chapter 5). Alternatively if there is no evidence of occlusion, and particularly if symptoms are accompanied by acute headache, hypertension, and bradycardia, an emergent head CT scan (conventional or cone bean with flat-panel digital systems) should be obtained to exclude hemorrhage.

After placement of the EPD, the stenosis is usually underdilated with a small diameter angioplasty balloons (2–4 mm in diameter and 20 mm in length) to allow passage of the stent delivery system. With placement of the stent, the carotid stenosis is again dilated using an undersized balloon (typically 5 mm in diameter and 15–30 mm in length) to expand the stent more fully (Figure 6.7). Because over-aggressive balloon inflation increases the risk of embolic complications there is no need for an angiographically perfect result. Additionally, in previously unoperated

carotid bifurcations, stimulation of the carotid sinus may lead to significant hemodynamic instability with profound bradycardia and hypotension, despite pre-medication with anticholinergics (atropine or glycopyrrolate). Vasopressors such as phenylephrine (10–100 mg per minute intravenously) and dopamine (5–15 µg per kilogram per minute intravenously) should be pre-drawn and available in case hypotension does not respond to fluid administration and anticholinergics. Sustained bradycardia is unusual, but a temporary transvenous pacemaker should be readily available. Hypertension should be treated if the systolic blood pressure is >180 mmHg, to decrease the risk of intracranial hemorrhage. A more complete list of complications of CAS is presented in Table 6.5.

With respect to stent selection, balloon expandable stents are generally used for ostial lesions of the brachiocephalic origins (as they allow for relatively precise placement), while cervical stenoses are addressed by self-expanding (nitinol) stents (primarily because they resist deformation during neck movement or compression). Many companies manufacture stents with rapid-exchange delivery systems; some also have tapered designs for the transition from the common to the internal carotid artery (see Chapter 4).

Carotid artery stenting: results

Initial experience in the USA included a variety of stents and variable pre-medication and anticaogulation regimens, and the procedures were performed without the routine use of emboli protection. In an effort to address these limitations, one study reported the results of CAS after pooling data from 26 observational studies between 1990 and 2002, which included nearly 3,500 CAS procedures.[165] This analysis suggested that stroke or death at 30 days was observed in 5.5% of patients who were treated without EPD and 1.8% of patients who were treated with EPD. Furthermore, CAS without EPD was associated with more cases of major (1.1% vs. 0.3%) and minor (3.7% vs. 0.5%) strokes. Nevertheless, it should be noted that operator experience, devices, and medical regimens also evolved over this same period.

Subsequently, the Global Carotid Artery Stent Registry[166] surveyed 12,392 CAS procedures in 11,243 patients from 53 sites from 1997 to 2002.[166] The technical success rate was 98.9%; while at 30 days TIA was noted in 3.1% of patients, minor stroke in

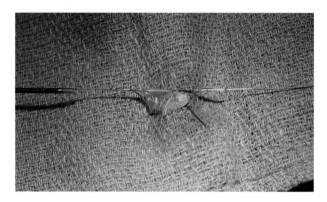

Figure 6.5
FilterWire (Boston Scientific, Natick, Massachusetts) post-carotid angioplasty, demonstrating atherosclerotic debris (arrow).

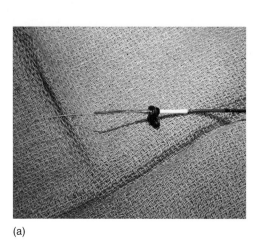

(a)

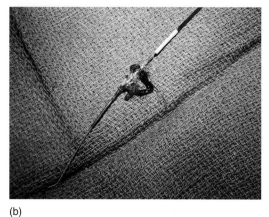

(b)

Figure 6.6
Accunet (Abbott Vascular, Abbott Park, Illinois) closed (above) and open (below), demonstrating a captured thrombotic embolus.

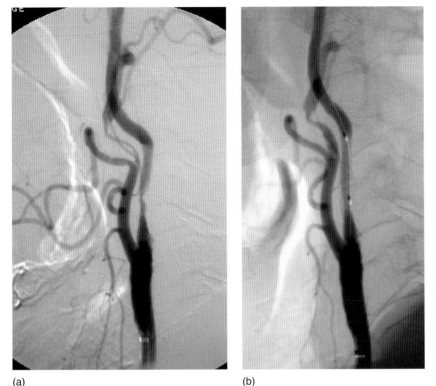
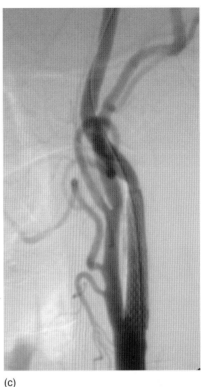

(a)   (b)   (c)

Figure 6.7
(a) Severe carotid stenosis with guide catheter in place. (a) Relatively straight distal internal carotid is optimal for the use of an emboli protection device. (b) Angioplasty balloon in place following pre-dilatation with a 3 mm × 20 mm balloon. (c) Angiogram following stent deployment and post-dilatation.

Table 6.5 Complications of carotid artery stenting

Cardiovascular
- Vasovagal reaction (5–10%)
- Vasodepressor reaction (5–10%)
- Myocardial infarction (1%)

Carotid artery
- Dissection (≤1%)
- Thrombosis (≤1%)
- Perforation (≤1%)
- External carotid artery stenosis or occlusion (5–10%)
- Transient vasospasm (10–15%)
- Re-stenosis (3–5%)

Neurological
- Transient ischemic attack (1–2%)
- Stroke (2–3%)
- Intracranial hemorrhage (≤1%)
- Hyperperfusion syndrome (≤1%)
- Seizures (≤1%)

General
- Access site injury (5%)
- Blood transfusion (2–3%)
- Contrast nephropathy (2%)
- Contrast reactions (1%)
- Death (1%)

2.1%, major stroke in 1.2%, death in 0.6%, and stroke or death in 4.7%. The risk of stroke or death was 6.2% without EPD and 2.8% with EPD. Stroke or death was seen in 4.9% of symptomatic patients and in 2.9% of asymptomatic patients. During the first 3 years of follow-up, re-stenosis rates (by carotid duplex studies)

were roughly 2.5%, and ipsilateral neurological events were observed in approximately 1.5% of patients (Figure 6.8). The Prospective Registry of Carotid Angioplasty and Stenting (Pro-CAS) was started the following year, and showed similarly high rates of technical success.[167] However, in-hospital events included TIA in 6.0% of patients, stroke in 2.5%, and stroke or death in 2.8%. The risk of stroke or death was 2.1% with EPD, 2.2% without EPD, 3.1% in symptomatic patients, and 2.4% in asymptomatic patients.

Early randomized trials of CAS compared with CEA suffered from patient selection bias, rudimentary technology, and operator inexperience; not surprisingly, results were mixed. The first trial enrolled symptomatic low-risk patients with carotid stenosis >70%.[168] After five of seven CAS patients suffered a stroke, the study was terminated. The Wallstent trial was similarly halted prematurely when the 30-day incidence of stroke or death was 12.1% after CAS and 4.5% after CEA.[169] Brooks et al. reported 104 patients with symptomatic stenosis >70% and 85 patients with asymptomatic stenosis >80%; there was no in-hospital stroke or death after CEA or CAS.[170] The Carotid and Vertebral Artery Transluminal Angioplasty Study (CAVATAS) randomized 504 patients, but only 22% of the angioplasty group received stents.[139] Although stroke or death rates at 30 days occurred in 10% of patients in both groups, angioplasty was associated with lower rates of cranial neuropathy, major hematoma, myocardial infarction, and pulmonary embolism, and with a higher rate of restenosis at 1 year. The rate of stroke or death at 3 years was similar.[139]

More recently the Stenting and Angioplasty with Protection in Patients at High Risk for Endarterectomy (SAPPHIRE) study randomized high-risk patients and compared CAS with EPD

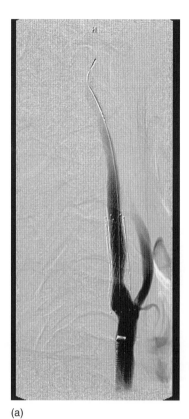
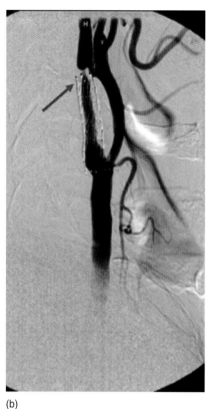

(a)   (b)

Figure 6.8
(a) Post-stent severe re-stenosis at the distal tines of the initial stent.
(b) Postangioplasty and re-stenting of the distal margin of the first stent. Notice the degree of persistent intimal hyperplasia at the proximal margin of the stent.

against CEA; the trial was stopped prematurely because of slow enrollment due to high surgical risk for CEA.[171] Inclusion criteria included symptomatic stenosis >50% or asymptomatic stenosis >80%, plus at least one high-risk criterion (see Table 6.1). Technical success was achieved in 95.6% of CAS patients. The incidence of the composite endpoints (myocardial infarction, stroke, or death within 30 days or ipsilateral stroke or death at 1 year) was 12% after CAS and 20.1% after CEA ($p = 0.048$). However, when myocardial infarction was excluded, the difference in stroke and death between CAS and CEA was not statistically significantly different. In the patients with symptomatic stenosis, the primary endpoints after CAS and CEA were 16.8% vs. 16.5%, while in asymptomatic patients, there were fewer primary endpoints after CAS (9.9%) vs. CEA (21.5%) ($p = 0.02$).

Post-procedure care

Post-procedure monitoring should include assessment of the arterial puncture site as well as routine neurological checks in a unit capable of hemodynamic monitoring. All patients should undergo a formal National Institutes of Health Stroke Scale (NIHSS) assessment within 24 hours of CAS, or sooner if symptomatic. Patients who are neurologically and hemodynamically stable (90% of patients) can usually be discharged the following day with continuation of statins, clopidogrel, and aspirin. Aspirin is typically given indefinitely while clopidogrel is discontinued at 6–8 weeks. Patients who have no deficits but are hemodynamially unstable will require fluids, and possibly pressors, usually for 24–48 hours. Patients with stroke or TIA will require appropriate imaging (usually diffusion-weighted MRI), intensive care, and supportive measures based on the extent of injury.

Carotid duplex surveillance is performed at 6 months and 1 year to check for re-stenosis. Anecdotally, personal experience would lead us to believe that re-stenosis is commoner in patients with accelerated intimal hyperplasia post-endarterectomy and in patients who have previously had radiation therapy to the affected region. Before the era of drug-eluting coronary stents, there were case reports of successful intraluminal brachytherapy coronary systems adapted for carotid in-stent stenosis.[172,173] In the absence of such systems (plagued by both FDA and Nuclear Regulatory Commission (NRC regulations), there are few alternatives. One promising technology may be the use of angioplasty balloons impregnated with paclitaxel.[174]

Revascularization of intracranial atherosclerotic stenoses

As noted previously, intracranial atherosclerotic disease is more frequently identified in non-whites (see Figure 6.4).[27–29] Nevertheless, many patients with asymptomatic intracranial disease are identified during evaluation for suspected carotid artery disease. The presence of asymptomatic intracranial stenosis usually does not influence decision-making about extracranial carotid revascularization.[129,175]

As with carotid atherosclerotic stenosis, symptomatic high-grade (>70%) intracranial atheromatous disease is characterized by a malignant natural history despite optimal medical therapy.[20,21] In the recent Warfarin–Aspirin Symptomatic Intracranial Disease (WASID) study, 25% of patients presenting with 70–99% stenosis experienced a stroke in the ipsilateral vascular territory within 2 years despite treatment with either warfarin or aspirin.[21] However, unlike lesions of the bifurcation, there is no commonly accepted surgical option.[7] Consequently, there have been numerous attempts to apply a variety endovascular techniques and devices to intracranial stenoses, many of them not originally designed for this purpose.

Data continue to demonstrate that angioplasty alone is a safe and often effective treatment.[176–178] The major limitations of angioplasty without stenting include vessel recoil with acute re-stenosis and acute vessel occlusion secondary either to procedural dissection or to recoil with regional platelet aggregation.

Additionally, series have suggested that some patients often require multiple procedures, owing to recurrent stenosis. Mori et al. reported a series of 42 patients undergoing angioplasty for symptomatic intracranial stenoses in which the procedural success rate was 76% (32 of 42 lesions).[178] Two of 42 patients (4.8%) experienced major procedural strokes, and an additional eight lesions could not be treated. Of the 32 patients treated successfully, nine (28%) demonstrated re-stenosis at follow up and were re-treated one or more times. During these secondary treatments, two patients had experienced ipsilateral TIAs and one patient suffered a subarachnoid hemorrhage. A very useful contribution from this work was the characterization of stenoses (according to length, shape, and so on) such that relative risk as well as benefit could be stratified (Table 6.6).[178] In effect, the more focal the stenosis and the less tortuous the vessel, the better the results are likely to be.

Marks et al. analyzed 36 patients with symptomatic ICA disease who underwent angioplasty only. Two procedural deaths and one symptomatic re-perfusion hemorrhage occurred. Eleven of 36 patients had radiographic dissections. Clinical follow-up (average 52.9 months) in the surviving 34 patients showed two strokes occurring in the ipsilateral hemisphere (15.3%). A more recent, multi-center, retrospective experience of 120 patients reported a 5.8% rate of stroke and death within 30 days of the procedure, with an additional 5.2% of patients experiencing a recurrent stroke during long-term (average 42.3 months) follow-up.[176]

Angioplasty with balloon-mounted coronary stents has been associated with high rates of procedural morbidity and mortality.[179–181] In one of the largest available series of patients with symptomatic vertebrobasilar insufficiency undergoing treatment with balloon-expandable stents, nine periprocedural neurological complications (stroke or death) were encountered during the treatment of 39 patients (23.1%).[179] Hence, even those patients who are at the greatest risk of recurrent stroke on best medical therapy (take those with high-grade intracranial stenoses presenting with stroke) are exposed to the equivalent of up to 2 years of stroke risk on medical therapy during attempted placement of these devices.

Table 6.6 Mori classification of intracranial stenoses[178]

Type A
- Short, focal ($\leq$ 5mm)
- Concentric or moderately eccentric
- Non-occlusive

Type B
- Tubular (5–10mm)
- Extremely eccentric, and moderately angulated
- Occluded (< 3 months)

Type C
- Diffuse ($\geq$10mm)
- Severely angulated or tortuous proximal segment
- Chronic occlusion (>3 months)

Intracranial angioplasty and stenting: technique

More recently, a prospective, multi-center study reported on the use of a self-expanding stent and angioplasty balloon system specifically tailored to the intracranial circulation (Wingspan System, Boston Scientific).[24,25] In this system, guide catheter access and anticoagulation regimens are similar for cervical stent procedures. The diameter of the stenotic lesion was measured using biplane angiography, and compared to a reference diameter of the normal vessel (usually proximal to the lesion) using the technique in the WASID study.[20] Subsequently, a 2.3F micro-catheter is passed under roadmap guidance across the target lesion using a 0.014-inch (0.36 mm) guidewire. The micro-catheter is then exchanged over a 0.014-inch (0.36mm), 300 cm exchange wire for a Gateway angioplasty balloon. The balloon diameter is typically under-sized to 80% of the 'normal' parent vessel diameter proximal to the lesion. The balloon length is selected to match the length of the lesion. Angioplasty is performed with a slow graded inflation of the balloon to a pressure of between 6 and 12 atmospheres, typically for a duration of 120 seconds. Following angioplasty, the balloon is removed and conventional angiography is repeated (Figure 6.9).

The Wingspan delivery system is then prepared and manipulated over the exchange wire across the target lesion. The stent is purposely sized to exceed the diameter of the normal parent vessel by 0.5–1mm. The stent length is selected to equal or exceed the length of the angioplasty balloon and diseased segment.

Preliminary results using this technique suggest a far lower complication rate (2%) than seen with previously used balloon mounted stents.[24] Additional evidence of procedural safety was provided in this study by post-procedure diffusion-weighted MRI, which revealed new embolic lesions in only 29% of patients (seven of 24 patients for whom this information is available, all but one of whom were asymptomatic) – a rate that compares very favorably with the 70% rate of diffusion-positive lesions reported after the use of balloon-mounted coronary stents.[182] The dramatic reduction in procedural complications can be attributed to the device design and to the recommended treatment strategy of under-sizing the angioplasty balloon and over-sizing the self-expanding stent to achieve the desired angiographic result (Figures 6.10, 6.11).

Turk et al. reported follow-up (mean 7.3 months) of 93 of 155 intracranial stenoses (equally distributed in the anterior and posterior circulation) treated with Wingspan.[25] In this series, re-stenoses were more commonly seen in patients under the age of 55 years (odds ratio 2.6) and more often seen in the anterior circulation (particularly the supraclinoid internal carotid artery – 88.9% of this subset).[25] Excluding supraclinoid lesions, the re-stenosis rate was only 24.4%. Similarly symptoms were more likely to return in carotid lesions (40%) versus other intracranial sites (3.9%) – a much more favorable comparison to medical therapy. In-stent stenosis generally appears within the first 6 months and typically presents with TIA (delayed stroke more commonly presents as a result of failure of medical therapy.) As with carotid re-stenosis, treatment options are limited to angioplasty[174] or rarely, re-stenting.

Follow-up: transcranial Doppler

Imaging evaluation of symptomatic intracranial stenosis is similar to that of extracranial atherosclerotic disease. In the presence of

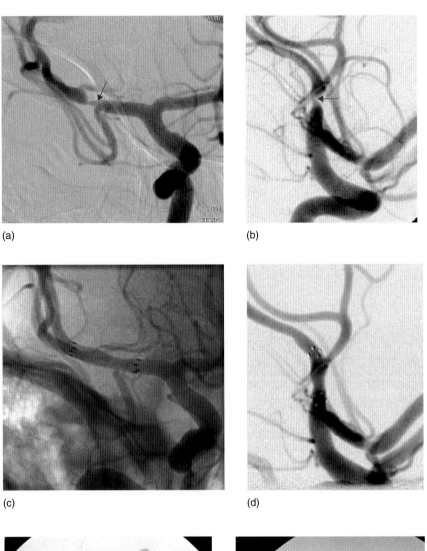

(a)

(b)

Figure 6.9
(a, b) Anterior–posterior and oblique views of a focal stenosis of the distal right middle cerebral artery beyond the origin of the anterior temporal branches. (c, d) Corresponding views after Gateway and Wingspan revascularization.

(c)

(d)

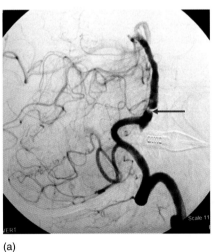

(a)

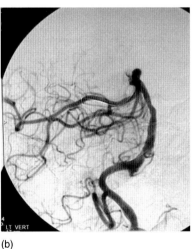

(b)

Figure 6.10
Lateral views. (a) Before and (b) after Gateway and Wingspan revascularization of a severe, focal proximal basilar artery stenosis (Mori type A).

symptoms, preliminary evaluation is likely to include initial imaging of the brain. Given the availability of multi-row spiral CT scanners and MRI, CTA and MRA are both reasonable first steps in the work-up. However, because of the unknowns regarding re-stensosis of treated intracranial lesions, regular follow-up is needed. Both CTA and MRA may be subject to significant post-stent artifact as well, and the expense may limit their utility for routine follow-up in the absence of symptoms. Transcranial Doppler, like carotid duplex studies, measures intracranial blood flow patterns and so indirectly assesses stenoses.[183] Additionally, in cases of immediate post-procedure symptoms, transcranial Doppler may be useful to detect emboli and secondarily to assess the effectiveness of the anticoagulation regimen.[184,185]

Dissection and blunt trauma

Dissection of the carotid artery is uncommon with an average annual incidence of 2.6 per 100,000 (Rochester, Minnesota

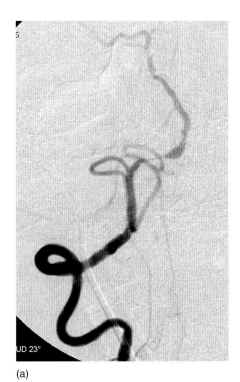

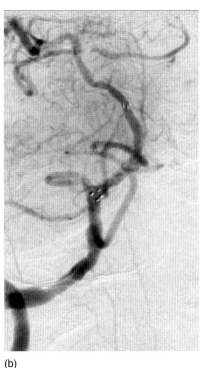

(a)   (b)

Figure 6.11
Oblique views. (a) Before and (b) after Gateway and Wingspan revascularization of a longer segment of atherosclerotic stenosis of the basilar artery (Mori type B).

epidemiologic data from the Mayo Clinic).[186] Nevertheless, it should be emphasized that dissection represents a significant cause of stroke in young adults.[187,188] In some series, up to 80% of patients with carotid dissection will present during the first month with ipsilateral symptoms of cerebral ischemia.[189] Equally concerning is the report by Mokri et al., which documented subsequent development of stroke as late as 6–10 years after the initial insult.[190]

The diagnosis cervical vascular dissection requires a high index of suspicion, as the presenting symptoms are frequently non-specific. Headache is the most common symptom, often with pain in the neck directly over the course of the ipsilateral carotid artery and/or ipsilateral headache. A total of 90% of patients experience symptoms within the first month after the injury.[191] Other clinical manifestations in decreasing order of frequency include: focal cerebral ischemic symptoms, neck pain, bruit, and tinnitus. Less common symptoms are Horner's syndrome, syncope, scalp tenderness, or neck swelling.[192,193]

Most carotid dissections are either a result of blunt trauma or occur spontaneously (and are frequently idiopathic).[190,194] The role of minor trauma in the absence of an arteriopathy has been questioned because of the difference in the clinical course of dissections resulting from severe trauma and spontaneous dissection or those resulting from minor trauma.[193,195] In his review, Mokri analyzed 70 patients with spontaneous dissection and 21 patients with traumatic dissection, with a follow-up period of 64 months for the spontaneous group and 40 months for the traumatic group.[196] In this series traumatic dissections were less common than spontaneous dissections, although traumatic were associated with a worse prognosis. The traumatic group had a higher incidence of focal cerebral ischemic manifestations than the spontaneous group (71% versus 61%), although the difference was not statistically significant. Patients with traumatic dissections demonstrated a higher incidence of aneurysmal degeneration with a lower likelihood that the aneurysms would resolve with conservative treatment. Also, more of

the stenoses in the traumatic group progressed to occlusion.[196] These data suggest that the insult in traumatic dissection is probably more severe than that of the spontaneous group, as might be expected.

The association of intrinsic arteriopathies with dissection, including fibromuscular dysplasia, Marfan syndrome, Ehlers–Danlos syndrome type IV, and cystic medial necrosis, is well known. It is estimated that 15% of intrinsic arteriopathies are related to underlying fibromuscular disease (Figure 6.12)[193,195,197,198] In such cases,[197,198] multiple cervical arteries may be involved at the time of diagnosis, although recurrent dissection is uncommon and rarely involves the same vessel segment in the absence of underlying vasculopathy.[193,195,198–200]

Whatever the etiology, the injury to the vessel results in blood penetrating the intima into the vessel wall, with variable cephalad extension though rarely beyond the petrous segment.[193,197–199] Dissections involving the intracranial vessels have a catastrophic clinical course.[187,201,202]

Imaging manifestations

Classically, the angiographic findings have been described as a tapered narrowing that begins in or about the carotid bulb and ends at the base of the skull.[203] In addition to luminal compromise and vessel thrombosis, irregularity and pseudoaneurysms may occur.[193,204] Houser et al. detailed the temporal evolution of the angiographic findings in dissection in 1984.[197] In their series, the appearance of the dissection varied, depending on its severity and extent and the interval between onset and angiography. The disruption initially manifested itself as an eccentric tapered stenosis in 47% of cases, a tapered stenosis and a dissecting aneurysm in 28%, an occlusion in 18%, and a dissecting aneurysm alone in 7%. Subsequently, stenotic dissections angiographically resolved in 60% of cases, improved in 20%, and progressed in 15%, while dissecting aneurysms diminished in half

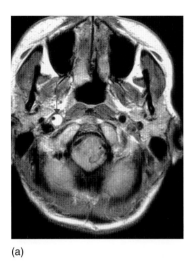
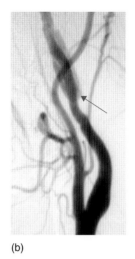
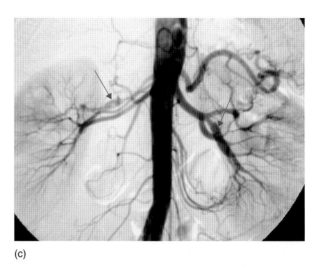

(a)   (b)   (c)

Figure 6.12
(a) Axial T1-weighted MRI with flow saturation demonstrating subintimal thrombus compromising the lumen (arrow) in a right carotid artery dissection. (b) Corresponding angiogram. Beaded distal appearance suggested fibromuscular disease. (c) Aortic angiogram demonstrating renal artery involvement by fibromuscular dysplasia (arrow).

and resolved in one-quarter of cases. An angiographic residuum was evident in 25% of dissections.

MRI and color-flow Doppler ultrasound are efficacious, non-invasive methods of diagnosis and longitudinal evaluation of a patient with a clinical suspicion of dissection,[205] and they are frequently complementary.[188,206] Ultrasound may demonstrate both the true and false lumen. The true lumen is perhaps best identified with color-flow Doppler as antegrade signal in the absence of atherosclerotic change (plaque or calcification), and it may gradually re-canalize (in 68% of cases) after the initial injury.[207] Alternatively, the appearance of the false lumen is quite variable depending on the extent of dissection and the presence of thrombus, but it is typically described as having high-resistance flow, which may be forwards, reversed, or bidirectional.[208] A key limitation in the ultrasound evaluation of dissection is the limited ability to establish reliably the distal extent of the flap.[209]

MR scanners may apply multiple techniques to the diagnosis of carotid dissection. Conventional T1-weighted MRI may directly image subintimal thrombus with its high signal paramagnetic effect in addition to the patent lumen, which is characterized by low signal on the basis of persistent flow (this can be best visualized with the elimination of flow artifacts with special presaturation pulses (see Figure 6.12a)[205,210–212] MRA with or without contrast may also be used to evaluate the brachiocephalic vessels, although because of the method by which these images are produced, subacute intramural thrombus may erroneously produce an image of a dilated (rather than tapered) lumen. Unencumbered by facial and skull bones, MRI is helpful in assessing the distal extent of dissection as well as its temporal resolution with medical management. Levy et al., in a prospective blinded study, compared MRI to three-dimensional time-of-flight MRA to conventional angiography in a series of 19 patients with spontaneous or traumatic dissections (comprising 19 carotid and 5 vertebral vessels).[205] MRI and MRA demonstrated excellent sensitivity and specificity (84% and 99%, respectively, for MRI, and 95% and 99%, respectively, for MRA).[205] MRA is also useful in follow-up of patients with dissections by monitoring the resolution of an intramural hematoma or the development of complications of dissection.[204,210,213,214] Djouhri et al. followed

20 patients with 26 spontaneous dissecting aneurysms with MRA over a mean duration of 41 months; no progression was noted, four dissecting aneurysms decreased in size, and two resolved.[215]

Medical treatment of dissection

The etiology for the ischemic symptoms begins with thrombus formation on the damaged endothelial surface. Subsequently the natural history is one of either complete thrombosis of the arterial lumen or distal embolization leading to stroke in the majority of cases.[189] Therefore, the initial treatment for patients with carotid dissections, of any etiology, has centered on the use of anticoagulation in an attempt to limit this potential for embolization or vessel thrombosis.[204] At this time, no data exist from controlled randomized trials; however, through the use of transcranial Doppler monitoring, therapeutic levels of systemic heparin resulted in reduced frequency of high-intensity transient signals corresponding to a reduced incidence of intracranial emboli.[216] In uncomplicated dissection, the initial therapy remains anticoagulation for a period of 3 months followed by surveillance using either duplex scanning or MRA.[217,218] If there is a persistent abnormality, anticoagulation is usually continued for a period of 3 more months, with repeat imaging. It has been reported that 47–85% of stenosed or occluded arteries will re-canalize over a period of 6 months with anticoagulation.[193,199]

In a minority of patients (7–14%), new ischemic neurologic symptoms will develop despite adequate anticoagulation. These are related either to embolization or to occlusion of the dissected carotid artery, the majority being related to embolization.[193,219,220] In their review of the literature on traumatic carotid dissections, Krajewski and Hertzer noted a much higher complication rate in the patients with traumatic carotid dissections treated conservatively.[221] Their evaluation revealed that 86% of patients treated non-surgically suffered either death or severe neurologic deficit, while only 53% of those undergoing surgical intervention and correction suffered the same fate.

Revascularization strategy for dissection

In the setting of an acute dissection, there are two indications for immediate intervention. The primary indication is fluctuating or deteriorating neurologic symptoms despite adequate anticoagulation. Additionally, there are a number of patients who are poor candidates for anticoagulation who may be offered surgical or endovascular repair, even though some would argue that these patients may be adequately treated with antiplatelet therapy alone. In the setting of the chronic dissection, there are two sequelae – persistent high-grade stenosis and aneurysmal degeneration – which offer relative indications for therapeutic intervention. Normally, those patients with a persistent aneurysm in the setting of chronic dissection may be offered treatment to minimize the risk of thromboembolization and subsequent stroke. However, these pseudoaneurysms rarely enlarge and there are no reports of ruptured extracranial ICA aneurysms secondary to dissection in the literature to date.[222]

Surgical treatment of the dissected carotid artery is associated with a much higher morbidity and mortality than is open surgery for atherosclerotic stenosis of the carotid artery; these higher rates are primarily related to the greater cephalocaudad extent of disease. Additionally, there has been reported a higher incidence of facial and lower cranial nerve palsies. The major morbidity associated with the high cervical exposure necessary for repair is injury to the pharyngeal and superior laryngeal branches of the vagus nerve. This usually leads to dysphasia and dysphonia, which are usually transient. Additionally, the incidence of neurological complications of surgical repair of carotid dissection is also higher (9–10%) than after CEA.[222]

Contemporary experience suggests that endovascular techniques have a significant role in carotid dissection with symptomatic high-grade stenosis or pseudo-aneurysm. Key to the success of these maneuvers is the judicious use of digital roadmapping in order to navigate safely and access the true lumen with a guidewire; failure to do so will undoubtedly lead to inadvertent extension of the false lumen. This maneuver may also be safer with the pre-operative knowledge of the cephalocaudal extent of the lesion on pre-procedure imaging studies. Given these limitations and the underlying pathologic process, the use of EPDs is contraindicated.

These procedures include balloon angioplasty and stent placement in patients with stenotic lesions, and stenting in conjunction with coil embolization of the aneurysm through the struts of the stent in patients with aneurysmal degeneration of the carotid artery. Typically, the self-expanding stents are preferred in this location because of the sustained radial force that they provide. Balloon-expandable stents are occasionally utilized in the higher cervical or intracranial portions of the carotid artery.

Liu et al. reported a series of seven patients over an 8-year period who were treated with angioplasty and stenting of carotid artery dissection.[223] They placed a total of 11 stents [eight Palmaz (balloon-expandable) stents and three Wallstents (self-expanding)] with an initial technical success rate of 100%. A total of 86% of the patients (six of the seven) demonstrated no evidence of re-stenosis at a mean follow-up of 20.2 months (1–67 months). One patient who was treated for pseudo-aneurysm of the carotid artery as a direct result of a dissection occluded at 3 months. This patient was treated with a polytetrafluoroethylene-covered stent. None of the seven patients experienced new or recurrent ischemic neurologic symptoms. The mean follow-up for this study was 42.9 months (13–72 months).[223]

Another retrospective review from Malek et al. included 10 patients over an 18-month period treated with angioplasty and stenting.[224] The etiology of the dissection was spontaneous in five patients, iatrogenic in three, and traumatic in two. They used Wallstents in eight patients, SMART stents in two patients, and GFX balloon-expandable stents in one patient (some patients required multiple stents), with an initial technical success rate of 100% as well. The stenoses improved form a mean stenosis of $74\pm5.5\%$ to $5.5\pm2.8\%$ without any peri-procedural TIAs, cerebrovascular accidents, or deaths, and without the use of any angioprotection devices. The mean follow-up was 16.5 ± 1.9 months, during which time there was one cerebrovascular accident. This complication was in a patient with a contralateral ICA occlusion, and it followed an episode of hypotension 8 months after the initial procedure.[224]

Schievink et al. reported a retrospective review focusing only on the surgical treatment of extracranial ICA aneurysms secondary to dissection.[222] In this study, there were 22 patients with chronic carotid dissections and subsequent aneurysm formation. The etiology of the initial dissection was traumatic in 11 patients and spontaneous in 11 patients. The mean age of the patients was 39 years (21–57 years). Five patients underwent cervical carotid ligation, 13 patients were treated with resection of the aneurysm and reconstruction, and the final four patients were treated with ECA–ICA bypass. In this group of patients, there were two postoperative strokes (9%). Cranial nerve complications were again frequent; they included 12 cases of transient palsies. There were no long-term neurologic sequelae during the mean follow-up of 6.2 years.[222] In the context of contemporary endovascular techniques, such pseudoaneurysms are better treated with covered stents (if the vessel is relatively straight) or with stenting followed by coil embolization in cases involving the skull base or where there is significant tortuosity.

Penetrating trauma

The frequency of firearm-related injuries has increased dramatically in many US urban centers.[225] It is estimated that there are 7.4 non-fatal shootings for each murder, with firearms fatalities rivaling those from motor vehicle trauma in the USA.[226,227]

The leading cause of death in penetrating neck trauma is vascular injury.[228] However, predicting vascular injury in gunshot wounds of the neck is difficult because of erratic trajectories and the variety of ballistic missiles, which can have different characteristics, and because cavitation and bullet fragmentation can produce tissue damage far beyond the immediate path of the primary projectile.[229,230] High-velocity weapons impart kinetic energy in a radial direction, stretching tissue[231] and creating a temporary cavity that can be 30 times larger than the bullet diameter.[232] Bleeding, shock from injury to the major vessels in the neck, and compromise of the airway are the major factors causing death after penetrating neck injury. Clinical evidence of active bleeding, shock, or an expanding hematoma or airway compromise all mandate immediate surgical exploration.[228,233,234]

Classification and clinical course

In the absence of clinical evidence of cervical vascular injury, a grading scheme is used to classify penetrating neck injuries on the basis of the anatomic zone of the injury:[235,236]

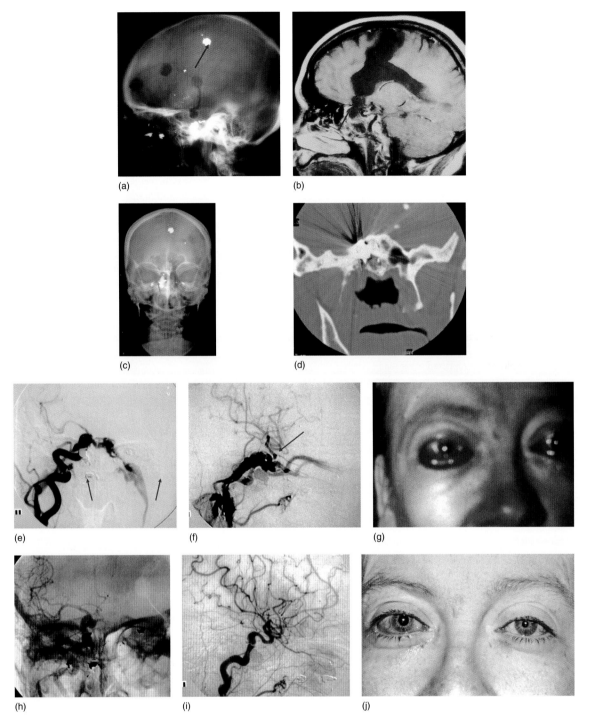

Figure 6.13
(a) Lateral plain film, and (b) MRI of a 55-year-old woman with a self-inflicted high-caliber (short arrow) gunshot wound 20 years previously, transecting the left optic nerve (long arrow). (c) Anterior–posterior (AP) Plain film and the coronal CT (d) demonstrating recent self-inflicted small-caliber rifle wound with the missile embedded in the sphenoid bone (arrow). (e) AP and (f) Lateral right internal carotid artery angiogram demonstrating a high-flow carotid cavernous fistula secondary to as lacerated carotid artery within the cavernous sinus. Extensive venous outflow (arrows) is compromising vision in the remaining right eye (g) Clinical image.
(h) AP unsubtracted and (i) lateral subtracted angiogram following detachable balloon embolization (block arrow) (j) Clinical image 24 hours post-embolization (notice the persistent pupillary defect on the right).

- zone I extends from the root of the neck and involves the area from thoracic inlet to the cricoid cartiledge
- zone II extends from the cricoid region to the angle of the mandible
- zone III extends from the angle of the mandible to the base of the skull.

Although there are no prospective data demonstrating significant advantages of a surgical approach, often the injury zone dictates the treatment strategy. Surgical exploration is often recommended for asymptomatic patients with zone II injuries because such surgery is associated with low morbidity and mortality. Vascular injuries in zone I have the highest mortality rate, owing to concomitant injury to the subclavian and innominate arteries and veins, which results in rapid exsanguination.[228] Physical examination of zones I and III is very difficult, and angiography is often performed in these circumstances.

Endovascular management

In the past, expectant management was often recommended for asymptomatic zone I and III injuries, because these areas are difficult to explore and exploration was associated with greater surgical morbidity and mortality; conversely, endovascular access to these regions is relatively straightforward. This approach is dictated by three factors:

- the hemodynamic status of the patient and presence of hypovolemic shock;

- the neurologic status of the patient and the ability to respond to commands during a test balloon occlusion (Figure 6.13); and
- the extent of non-cerebrovascular injury and the extent to which this may limit post-procedure anticoagulation.

In the event of significant hemodynamic instability, all bets are off: the hemorrhage must be stopped even if by vascular sacrifice (Figure 6.14). Under optimal conditions this would be best accomplished by test balloon occlusion (TBO) for 30 minutes followed by hypotensive challenge to ensure neurologic integrity by virtue of collateral support (e.g. from the circle of Willis). (Of course, this procedure requires an interactive, oriented, and non-medicated patient.) If the patient were to pass the TBO, the injured vessel could merely be sacrificed.

Alternatively if the patient fails TBO, another option would be stenting following by embolization or possibly primary treatment utilizing a covered stent. The presumption in these cases is that the patient can be anticoagulated with antiplatelet agents.

Arteritis

Takayasu arteritis (TA) is a chronic, inflammatory vascular disease that affects the aorta and its primary branches (Figure 6.15). It was initially described by an ophthalmologist, Mikito Takayasu, who reported the case of a 21-year-old woman who had sudden loss of vision accompanied by a wreath of vessels around the optic disc on fundoscopic examination.[237] Although originally described

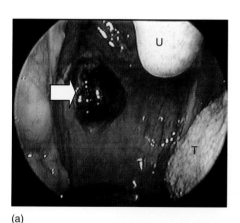

(a)

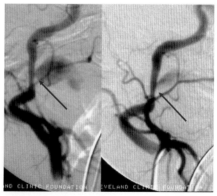

(b)   (c)

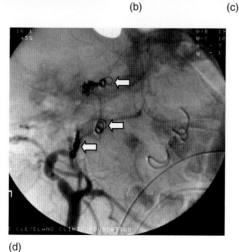

(d)

Figure 6.14
(a) Laryngoscopic image of the oropharynx in a 2-year-old child referred for severe epistaxis demonstrates a puncture wound on the right (block arrow). Uvula (u) and tongue (t). This was believed to have resulted from fall while the child was chewing on a sharpened pencil. (b) The patient was emergently intubated followed by torrential hemorrhage. Rapid vascular access and angiography demonstrated a right internal carotid artery (RICA) pseudoaneurysm, with serial views (c) demonstrating rupture and extravazation. The patient suffered cardiovascular collapse and arrested twice on the angiography table. Despite the lack of complete angiography or test balloon occlusion, (d) the RICA was sacrificed in desperation using detachable and fibered (pushable) coils. The patient sustained no neurological deficit and was discharged to home 4 days later.

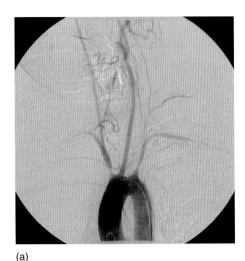

(a)

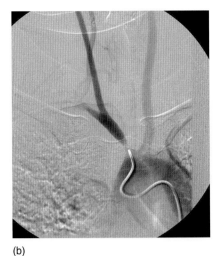

(b)

Figure 6.15
(a) Aortic arch angiogram demonstrating diffuse smooth, long segment stenoses at the brachiocephalic origins consistent with Takayasu's arteritis.
(b) Selective innominate injection.

in Asia and predominantly in women, TA afflicts people in a wide variety of ethnic and racial populations.

Clinical course

Early reports from Asia described a progressive, inflammatory vasculopathy of the brachiocephalic and renal vessels, which occasionally produces significant morbidity and death.[238,239] It has since become appreciated as a multiphasic disease; vascular inflammation may be present in patients who appear clinically quiescent.[240,241] however, monophasic disease is reported in a minority of patients (7–20%).[240,242]

Morbidity associated with TA includes: hypertension (50–75% of patients),[243,244] vascular claudication (>30%),[240,242,244] and aortic valvular insufficiency (25%).[240,242–244] Aortic insufficiency leading to congestive heart failure is the most common cause of death (40–50% of mortalities).[243,245,246] Neurological complications (stroke and TIAs) may result from progressive arterial stenosis or from uncontrolled hypertension; they occur in 20% and 5% of cases, respectively.[239,240,242–245,247,249]

Medical therapy

In most cohorts, patients who have active disease are controlled with corticosteroid therapy. However, even among patients who achieve remission, relapse is common upon steroid withdrawal, which may necessitate alternative immunosuppressive agents.[240,242,247,248]

Revascularization

Early studies examining percutaneous transluminal angioplasty in TA appeared promising. In 1992, Sharma et al. reported an initial success rate of 82% for renal artery PTCA in the treatment of 33 renal artery lesions in 20 patients who had TA.[250] The patency rate at a mean follow-up of 8 months was 79%. Similar findings were reported by Tyagi et al. in a study of

45 patients who had TA, with a preliminary success rate of 89% and a patency rate of 79% at a mean follow-up of 43 months.[251] More recent US data were less optimistic, with initial success rates of 56% and a high rate of complication, including re-stenosis in (up to 80% of cases).[240,242] One factor that has been associated with the procedural failure is the presence of active inflammatory disease at the time of revascularization.[252]

Conclusion

The treatment of all forms of ischemic cerebrovascular disease has changed dramatically in the past 10 years. Endovascular techniques are now often considered a first-line means of treatment for many conditions. Nevertheless, many additional refinements remain to be implemented in an effort to broaden the scope of endovascular treatment to the majority of ischemic stroke patients.

References

1. Rolack LA. Neurology Trivia. In: Rolak LA, ed. Neurology Secrets. 4th ed. Philadelphia, PA: Mosby Saunders; 2004.
2. Robicsek F, Roush TS, Cook JW, Reames MK. From Hippocrates to Palmaz–Schatz, the history of carotid surgery. Eur J Vasc Endovasc Surg 2004; 27: 389–97.
3. Wolpert SM. The circle of Willis. AJNR Am J Neuroradiol 1997; 18: 1033–34.
4. Fisher M. Occlusion of the internal carotid artery. AMA Arch Neurol Psychiatry 1951; 65: 346–77.
5. DeBakey ME. Successful carotid endarterectomy for cerebrovascular insufficiency. Nineteen-year follow-up. JAMA 1975; 233: 1083–85.
6. Eastcott HH, Pickering GW, Rob CG. Reconstruction of internal carotid artery in a patient with intermittent attacks of hemiplegia. Lancet 1954; 267: 994–6.
7. Failure of extracranial–intracranial arterial bypass to reduce the risk of ischemic stroke. Results of an international randomized trial. The EC/IC Bypass Study Group. N Engl J Med 1985; 313: 1191–200.
8. Chambers BR, Norris JW. The case against surgery for asymptomatic carotid stenosis. Stroke 1984; 15: 964–7.
9. Beneficial effect of carotid endarterectomy in symptomatic patients with high-grade carotid stenosis. North American Symptomatic

Carotid Endarterectomy Trial Collaborators. N Engl J Med 1991; 325: 445–53.

10. Barnett HJ, Taylor DW, Eliasziw M et al. Benefit of carotid endarterectomy in patients with symptomatic moderate or severe stenosis. North American Symptomatic Carotid Endarterectomy Trial Collaborators. N Engl J Med 1998; 339: 1415–25.

11. Endarterectomy for asymptomatic carotid artery stenosis. Executive Committee for the Asymptomatic Carotid Atherosclerosis Study. JAMA 1995; 273: 1421–28.

12. Eagle KA, Guyton RA, Davidoff R et al. ACC/AHA 2004 guideline update for coronary artery bypass graft surgery: a report of the American College of Cardiology/American Heart Association Task Force on Practice Guidelines (Committee to Update the 1999 Guidelines for Coronary Artery Bypass Graft Surgery). Circulation 2004; 110: e340–437.

13. MRC European Carotid Surgery Trial: interim results for symptomatic patients with severe (70–99%) or with mild (0–29%) carotid stenosis. European Carotid Surgery Trialists' Collaborative Group. Lancet 1991; 337: 1235–43.

14. Randomised trial of endarterectomy for recently symptomatic carotid stenosis: final results of the MRC European Carotid Surgery Trial (ECST). Lancet 1998; 351: 1379–87.

15. Mayberg MR, Wilson SE, Yatsu F et al. Carotid endarterectomy and prevention of cerebral ischemia in symptomatic carotid stenosis. Veterans Affairs Cooperative Studies Program 309 Trialist Group. JAMA 1991; 266: 3289–94.

16. Hobson RW, Weiss D, Fields W et al. Efficacy of carotid endarterectomy for asymptomatic carotid stenosis. NEJM 1993; 328: 221–7.

17. Friedman SG. Charles Dotter: interventional radiologist. Radiology 1989; 172: 921–4.

18. Gruntzig A. Transluminal dilatation of coronary-artery stenosis. Lancet 1978; 1: 263.

19. Palmaz JC, Sibbitt RR, Tio FO et al. Expandable intraluminal vascular graft: a feasibility study. Surgery 1986; 99: 199–205.

20. Chimowitz MI, Lynn MJ, Howlett-Smith H et al. Comparison of warfarin and aspirin for symptomatic intracranial arterial stenosis. N Engl J Med 2005; 352: 1305–16.

21. Kasner SE, Chimowitz MI, Lynn MJ et al. Predictors of ischemic stroke in the territory of a symptomatic intracranial arterial stenosis. Circulation 2006; 113: 555–63.

22. Roubin GS, Iyer S, Halkin A, Vitek J, Brennan C. Realizing the potential of carotid artery stenting: proposed paradigms for patient selection and procedural technique. Circulation 2006; 113: 2021–30.

23. Bates ER, Babb JD, Casey DE Jr, Vitek J, Brennan C. ACCF/SCAI/ SVMB/SIR/ASITN 2007 clinical expert consensus document on carotid stenting: a report of the American College of Cardiology Foundation Task Force on Clinical Expert Consensus Documents (ACCF/ SCAI/SVMB/SIR/ASITN Clinical Expert Consensus Document Committee on Carotid Stenting). J Am Coll Cardiol 2007; 49: 126–70.

24. Fiorella D, Levy EI, Turk AS et al. US multicenter experience with the wingspan stent system for the treatment of intracranial atheromatous disease: periprocedural results. Stroke 2007; 38: 881–7.

25. Turk AS, Levy EI, Albuquerque FC et al. Influence of patient age and stenosis location on Wingspan in-stent restenosis. AJNR Am J Neuroradiol 2008; 29: 23–7.

26. Rosamond W, Flegal K, Friday G et al. Heart disease and stroke statistics – 2007 update: a report from the American Heart Association Statistics Committee and Stroke Statistics Subcommittee. Circulation 2007; 115: e69–171.

27. Bamford J, Sandercock P, Dennis M, Burn J, Warlow C. Classification and natural history of clinically identifiable subtypes of cerebral infarction. Lancet 1991; 337: 1521–26.

28. Gorelick PB. Distribution of atherosclerotic cerebrovascular lesions. Effects of age, race, and sex. Stroke 1993; 24: 116–19.

29. Sacco RL, Kargman DE, Gu Q, Zamanillo MC. Race-ethnicity and determinants of intracranial atherosclerotic cerebral infarction. The Northern Manhattan Stroke Study. Stroke 1995; 26: 14–20.

30. Bogousslavsky J, Van MG, Regli F. The Lausanne Stroke Registry: analysis of 1, 000 consecutive patients with first stroke. Stroke 1988; 19: 1083–92.

31. Foulkes MA, Wolf PA, Price TR, Mohr JP, Hier DB. The Stroke Data Bank: design, methods, and baseline characteristics. Stroke 1988; 19: 547–54.

32. Inzitari D, Eliasziw M, Gates P et al. The causes and risk of stroke in patients with asymptomatic internal-carotid-artery stenosis. North American Symptomatic Carotid Endarterectomy Trial Collaborators. N Engl J Med 2000; 342: 1693–700.

33. Estol CJ. Dr C. Miller Fisher and the history of carotid artery disease. Stroke 1996; 27: 559–66.

34. Muluk SC, Muluk VS, Sugimoto H et al. Progression of asymptomatic carotid stenosis: a natural history study in 1004 patients. J Vasc Surg 1999; 29: 208–14.

35. Johnston SC, Gress DR, Browner WS, Sidney S. Short-term prognosis after emergency department diagnosis of TIA. JAMA 2000; 284: 2901–06.

36. Kleindorfer D, Panagos P, Pancioli A et al. Incidence and short-term prognosis of transient ischemic attack in a population-based study. Stroke 2005; 36: 720–23.

37. Wolf PA, D'Agostino RB, Belanger AJ, Kannel WB. Probability of stroke: a risk profile from the Framingham Study. Stroke 1991; 22: 312–18.

38. Blood pressure, cholesterol, and stroke in eastern Asia. Eastern Stroke and Coronary Heart Disease Collaborative Research Group. Lancet 1998; 352: 1801–07.

39. Collins R, Peto R, MacMahon S et al. Blood pressure, stroke, and coronary heart disease. Part 2, Short-term reductions in blood pressure: overview of randomised drug trials in their epidemiological context. Lancet 1990; 335: 827–38.

40. Staessen JA, Gasowski J, Wang JG et al. Risks of untreated and treated isolated systolic hypertension in the elderly: meta-analysis of outcome trials. Lancet 2000; 355: 865–72.

41. Vaccarino V, Berger AK, Abramson J et al. Pulse pressure and risk of cardiovascular events in the systolic hypertension in the elderly program. Am J Cardiol 2001; 88: 980–86.

42. Yusuf S, Sleight P, Pogue J et al. Effects of an angiotensin-converting-enzyme inhibitor, ramipril, on cardiovascular events in high-risk patients. The Heart Outcomes Prevention Evaluation Study Investigators. N Engl J Med 2000; 342: 145–53.

43. Lindholm LH, Ibsen H, Dahlof B et al. Cardiovascular morbidity and mortality in patients with diabetes in the Losartan Intervention For Endpoint reduction in hypertension study (LIFE): a randomised trial against atenolol. Lancet 2002; 359: 1004–10.

44. Shinton R, Beevers G. Meta-analysis of relation between cigarette smoking and stroke. BMJ 1989; 298: 789–94.

45. Wolf PA, D'Agostino RB, Kannel WB et al. Cigarette smoking as a risk factor for stroke. The Framingham Study. JAMA 1988; 259: 1025–29.

46. You RX, Thrift AG, McNeil JJ, Davis SM, Donnan GA. Ischemic stroke risk and passive exposure to spouses' cigarette smoking. Melbourne Stroke Risk Factor Study (MERFS) Group. Am J Public Health 1999; 89: 572–5.

47. Kawachi I, Colditz GA, Stampfer MJ et al. Smoking cessation and decreased risk of stroke in women. JAMA 1993; 269: 232–6.

48. Fine-Edelstein JS, Wolf PA, O'Leary DH et al. Precursors of extracranial carotid atherosclerosis in the Framingham Study. Neurology 1994; 44: 1046–50.

49. White HD, Simes RJ, Anderson NE et al. Pravastatin therapy and the risk of stroke. N Engl J Med 2000; 343: 317–26.

50. Statins after ischemic stroke and transient ischemic attack: an advisory statement from the Stroke Council, American Heart Association and American Stroke Association. Stroke 2004; 35: 1023.

51. Collins R, Armitage J, Parish S, Sleight P, Peto R. Effects of cholesterol-lowering with simvastatin on stroke and other major vascular events in 20536 people with cerebrovascular disease or other high-risk conditions. Lancet 2004; 363: 757–67.

52. Amarenco P, Lavallee PC, Labreuche J, Touboul PJ. Stroke prevention, blood cholesterol and statins. Acta Neurol Taiwan 2005; 14: 96–112.

53. Kennedy J, Quan H, Buchan AM et al. Statins are associated with better outcomes after carotid endarterectomy in symptomatic patients. Stroke 2005; 36: 2072–76.

54. Amarenco P, Bogousslavsky J, Callahan A III et al. High-dose atorvastatin after stroke or transient ischemic attack. N Engl J Med 2006; 355: 549–59.

55. Rubins HB, Robins SJ, Collins D et al. Gemfibrozil for the secondary prevention of coronary heart disease in men with low levels of high-density lipoprotein cholesterol. Veterans Affairs High-Density Lipoprotein Cholesterol Intervention Trial Study Group. N Engl J Med 1999; 341: 410–18.

56. Canner PL, Berge KG, Wenger NK et al. Fifteen year mortality in Coronary Drug Project patients: long-term benefit with niacin. J Am Coll Cardiol 1986; 8: 1245–55.

57. Sever PS, Dahlof B, Poulter NR et al. Prevention of coronary and stroke events with atorvastatin in hypertensive patients who have average or lower-than-average cholesterol concentrations, in the Anglo-Scandinavian Cardiac Outcomes Trial–Lipid Lowering Arm (ASCOT-LLA): a multicentre randomised controlled trial. Lancet 2003; 361: 1149–58.

58. Amarenco P, Bogousslavsky J, Callahan AS et al. Design and baseline characteristics of the stroke prevention by aggressive reduction in cholesterol levels (SPARCL) study. Cerebrovasc Dis 2003; 16: 389–395.

59. McGirt MJ, Perler BA, Brooke BS et al. 3-hydroxy-3-methylglutaryl coenzyme A reductase inhibitors reduce the risk of perioperative stroke and mortality after carotid endarterectomy. J Vasc Surg 2005; 42: 829–36.

60. Grundy SM, Cleeman JI, Merz CN et al. Implications of recent clinical trials for the National Cholesterol Education Program Adult Treatment Panel III guidelines. Circulation 2004; 110: 227–39.

61. Ribo M, Molina C, Montaner J et al. Acute hyperglycemia state is associated with lower tPA-induced recanalization rates in stroke patients. Stroke 2005; 36: 1705–09.

62. Leigh R, Zaidat OO, Suri MF et al. Predictors of hyperacute clinical worsening in ischemic stroke patients receiving thrombolytic therapy. Stroke 2004; 35: 1903–07.

63. Rexrode KM, Hennekens CH, Willett WC et al. A prospective study of body mass index, weight change, and risk of stroke in women. JAMA 1997; 277: 1539–45.

64. Further analyses of mortality in oral contraceptive users. Royal College of General Practitioners' Oral Contraception Study. Lancet 1981; 1: 541–6.

65. Wilhelmsen L, Svardsudd K, Korsan-Bengtsen K et al. Fibrinogen as a risk factor for stroke and myocardial infarction. N Engl J Med 1984; 311: 501–5.

66. Rost NS, Wolf PA, Kase CS et al. Plasma concentration of C-reactive protein and risk of ischemic stroke and transient ischemic attack: the Framingham study. Stroke 2001; 32: 2575–9.

67. Boushey CJ, Beresford SA, Omenn GS, Motulsky AG. A quantitative assessment of plasma homocysteine as a risk factor for vascular disease. Probable benefits of increasing folic acid intakes. JAMA 1995; 274: 1049–57.

68. Smith SC Jr, Allen J, Blair SN et al. AHA/ACC guidelines for secondary prevention for patients with coronary and other atherosclerotic vascular disease: 2006 update: endorsed by the National Heart, Lung, and Blood Institute. Circulation 2006; 113: 2363–72.

69. Sacco RL, Adams R, Albers G et al. Guidelines for prevention of stroke in patients with ischemic stroke or transient ischemic attack: a statement for healthcare professionals from the American Heart Association/American Stroke Association Council on Stroke: co-sponsored by the Council on Cardiovascular Radiology and Intervention: the American Academy of Neurology affirms the value of this guideline. Circulation 2006; 113: e409–49.

70. Swedish Aspirin Low-Dose Trial (SALT) of 75 mg aspirin as secondary prophylaxis after cerebrovascular ischaemic events. The SALT Collaborative Group. Lancet 1991; 338: 1345–9.

71. Farrell B, Godwin J, Richards S, Warlow C. The United Kingdom transient ischaemic attack (UK-TIA) aspirin trial: final results. J Neurol Neurosurg Psychiatry 1991; 54: 1044–54.

72. A comparison of two doses of aspirin (30 mg vs. 283 mg a day) in patients after a transient ischemic attack or minor ischemic stroke. The Dutch TIA Trial Study Group. N Engl J Med 1991; 325: 1261–66.

73. Taylor DW, Barnett HJM, Haynes RB et al. Low-dose and high-dose acetylsalicylic acid for patients undergoing carotid endarterectomy: a randomised controlled trial. Lancet 1999; 353: 2179–84.

74. Diener HC, Cunha L, Forbes C et al. European Stroke Prevention Study. 2. Dipyridamole and acetylsalicylic acid in the secondary prevention of stroke. J Neurol Sci 1996; 143: 1–13.

75. Halkes PH, van GJ, Kappelle LJ et al. Aspirin plus dipyridamole versus aspirin alone after cerebral ischaemia of arterial origin (ESPRIT): randomised controlled trial. Lancet 2006; 367: 1665–73.

76. Gent M, Blakely JA, Easton JD et al. The Canadian American Ticlopidine Study (CATS) in thromboembolic stroke. Lancet 1989; 1: 1215–20.

77. Hass WK, Easton JD, Adams HP Jr et al. A randomized trial comparing ticlopidine hydrochloride with aspirin for the prevention of stroke in high-risk patients. Ticlopidine Aspirin Stroke Study Group. N Engl J Med 1989; 321: 501–7.

78. A randomised, blinded, trial of clopidogrel versus aspirin in patients at risk of ischaemic events (CAPRIE). CAPRIE Steering Committee. Lancet 1996; 348: 1329–39.

79. Diener HC, Bogousslavsky J, Brass LM et al. Aspirin and clopidogrel compared with clopidogrel alone after recent ischaemic stroke or transient ischaemic attack in high-risk patients (MATCH): randomised, double-blind, placebo-controlled trial. Lancet 2004; 364: 331–7.

80. Bhatt DL, Fox KA, Hacke W et al. Clopidogrel and aspirin versus aspirin alone for the prevention of atherothrombotic events. N Engl J Med 2006; 354: 1706–17.

81. Mohr JP, Thompson JL, Lazar RM et al. A comparison of warfarin and aspirin for the prevention of recurrent ischemic stroke. N Engl J Med 2001; 345: 1444–51.

82. Albers GW, Amarenco P, Easton JD et al. Antithrombotic and thrombolytic therapy for ischemic stroke: the Seventh ACCP Conference on Antithrombotic and Thrombolytic Therapy. Chest 2004; 126: 483S–512S.

83. Toole JF. ACAS recommendations for carotid endarterectomy. ACAS Executive Committee [letter; comment]. Lancet 1996; 347: 121.

84. Halliday A, Mansfield A, Marro J et al. Prevention of disabling and fatal strokes by successful carotid endarterectomy in patients without recent neurological symptoms: randomised controlled trial. Lancet 2004; 363: 1491–1502.

85. Chimowitz MI, Kokkinos J, Strong J et al. The Warfarin–Aspirin Symptomatic Intracranial Disease Study. Neurology 1995; 45: 1488–93.

86. Rothwell PM, Eliasziw M, Gutnikov SA et al. Analysis of pooled data from the randomised controlled trials of endarterectomy for symptomatic carotid stenosis. Lancet 2003; 361: 107–16.

87. Chambers BR, Donnan GA. Carotid endarterectomy for asymptomatic carotid stenosis. Cochrane Database Syst Rev 2005; 4: CD001923.

88. Fox AJ. How to measure carotid stenosis. Radiology 1993; 186: 316–318.

89. Sabeti S, Schillinger M, Mlekusch W et al. Quantification of internal carotid artery stenosis with duplex US: comparative analysis of different flow velocity criteria. Radiology 2004; 232: 431–9.

90. Blakeley DD, Oddone EZ, Hasselblad V, Simel DL, Matchar DB. Noninvasive carotid artery testing. A meta-analytic review. Ann Intern Med 1995; 122: 360–67.

91. Grant EG, Benson CB, Moneta GL et al. Carotid artery stenosis: gray-scale and Doppler US diagnosis–Society of Radiologists in Ultrasound Consensus Conference. Radiology 2003; 229: 340–46.

92. Comerota AJ, Salles-Cunha SX, Daoud Y, Jones L, Beebe HG. Gender differences in blood velocities across carotid stenoses. J Vasc Surg 2004; 40: 939–44.

93. Busuttil SJ, Franklin DP, Youkey JR, Elmore JR. Carotid duplex overestimation of stenosis due to severe contralateral disease. Am J Surg 1996; 172: 144–7.

94. Fujitani RM, Kafie F. Screening and preoperative imaging of candidates for carotid endarterectomy. Semin Vasc Surg 1999; 12: 261–74.

95. Howard G, Baker WH, Chambless LE et al. An approach for the use of Doppler ultrasound as a screening tool for hemodynamically significant stenosis (despite heterogeneity of Doppler performance). A multicenter experience. Asymptomatic Carotid Atherosclerosis Study Investigators. Stroke 1996; 27: 1951–7.

96. Kuntz KM, Polak JF, Whittemore AD, Skillman JJ, Kent KC. Duplex ultrasound criteria for the identification of carotid stenosis should be laboratory specific. Stroke 1997; 28: 597–602.

97. Alexandrov AV. Ultrasound and angiography in the selection of patients for carotid endarterectomy. Curr Cardiol Rep 2003; 5: 141–7.

98. Elgersma OE, van LM, Buijs PC et al. Changes over time in optimal duplex threshold for the identification of patients eligible for carotid endarterectomy. Stroke 1998; 29: 2352–6.

99. Qureshi AI, Suri MF, Ali Z et al. Role of conventional angiography in evaluation of patients with carotid artery stenosis demonstrated by Doppler ultrasound in general practice. Stroke 2001; 32: 2287–91.

100. Patel MR, Kuntz KM, Klufas RA et al. Preoperative assessment of the carotid bifurcation. Can magnetic resonance angiography and duplex ultrasonography replace contrast arteriography? Stroke 1995; 26: 1753–8.

101. Wutke R, Lang W, Fellner C et al. High-resolution, contrast-enhanced magnetic resonance angiography with elliptical centric k-space ordering of supra-aortic arteries compared with selective X-ray angiography. Stroke 2002; 33: 1522–9.

102. Remonda L, Senn P, Barth A et al. Contrast-enhanced 3D MR angiography of the carotid artery: comparison with conventional digital subtraction angiography. AJNR Am J Neuroradiol 2002; 23: 213–19.

103. Turski PA, Korosec FR, Carroll TJ et al. Contrast-Enhanced magnetic resonance angiography of the carotid bifurcation using the time-resolved imaging of contrast kinetics (TRICKS) technique. Top Magn Reson Imaging 2001; 12: 175–81.

104. Krapf H, Nagele T, Kastrup A et al. Risk factors for periprocedural complications in carotid artery stenting without filter protection A serial diffusion-weighted MRI study. J Neurol 2006; 253: 364–71.

105. Roh HG, Byun HS, Ryoo JW et al. Prospective analysis of cerebral infarction after carotid endarterectomy and carotid artery stent placement by using diffusion-weighted imaging. AJNR Am J Neuroradiol 2005; 26: 376–84.

106. Buskens E, Nederkoorn PJ, Buijs-Van Der WT et al. Imaging of carotid arteries in symptomatic patients: cost-effectiveness of diagnostic strategies. Radiology 2004; 233: 101–12.

107. Asakura F, Kawaguchi K, Sakaida H et al. Diffusion-weighted MR imaging in carotid angioplasty and stenting with protection by the reversed carotid arterial flow. AJNR Am J Neuroradiol 2006; 27: 753–8.

108. Cosottini M, Michelassi MC, Puglioli M et al. Silent cerebral ischemia detected with diffusion-weighted imaging in patients treated with protected and unprotected carotid artery stenting. Stroke 2005; 36: 2389–93.

109. Gonzalez A, Pinero P, Martinez E et al. Silent cerebral ischemic lesions after carotid artery stenting with distal cerebral protection. Neurol Res 2005; 27: S79–83.

110. Kastrup A, Nagele T, Groschel K et al. Incidence of new brain lesions after carotid stenting with and without cerebral protection. Stroke 2006; 37: 2312–16.

111. Teng MM, Tsai F, Liou AJ et al. Three-dimensional contrast-enhanced magnetic resonance angiography of carotid artery after stenting. J Neuroimaging 2004; 14: 336–41.

112. Belsky M, Gaitini D, Goldsher D, Hoffman A, Daitzchman M. Color-coded duplex ultrasound compared to CT angiography for detection and quantification of carotid artery stenosis. Eur J Ultrasound 2000; 12: 49–60.

113. Hollingworth W, Nathens AB, Kanne JP et al. The diagnostic accuracy of computed tomography angiography for traumatic or atherosclerotic lesions of the carotid and vertebral arteries: a systematic review. Eur J Radiol 2003; 48: 88–102.

114. Koelemay MJ, Nederkoorn PJ, Reitsma JB, Majoie CB. Systematic review of computed tomographic angiography for assessment of carotid artery disease. Stroke 2004; 35: 2306–12.

115. Addis KA, Hopper KD, Iyriboz TA et al. CT angiography: in vitro comparison of five reconstruction methods. AJR Am J Roentgenol 2001; 177: 1171–6.

116. Chen CJ, Lee TH, Hsu HL et al. Multi-Slice CT angiography in diagnosing total versus near occlusions of the internal carotid artery: comparison with catheter angiography. Stroke 2004; 35: 83–5.

117. Connors JJ III, Sacks D, Furlan AJ et al. Training, competency, and credentialing standards for diagnostic cervicocerebral angiography, carotid stenting, and cerebrovascular intervention: a joint statement from the American Academy of Neurology, American Association of Neurological Surgeons, American Society of Interventional and Therapeutic Radiology, American Society of Neuroradiology, Congress of Neurological Surgeons, AANS/CNS Cerebrovascular Section, and Society of Interventional Radiology. Radiology 2005; 234: 26–34.

118. Executive Committee for the Asymptomatic Carotid Atherosclerosis Study. Endarterectomy for asymptomatic carotid artery stenosis. JAMA 1995; 273: 1421–8.

119. Fayed AM, White CJ, Ramee SR, Jenkins JS, Collins TJ. Carotid and cerebral angiography performed by cardiologists: cerebrovascular complications. Catheter Cardiovasc Interv 2002; 55: 277–80.

120. Sundt TM, Sandok BA, Whisnant JP. Carotid endarterectomy. Complications and preoperative assessment of risk. Mayo Clin Proc 1975; 50: 301–6.

121. Eliasziw M, Streifler JY, Spence JD et al. Prognosis for patients following a transient ischemic attack with and without a cerebral infarction on brain CT. North American Symptomatic Carotid Endarterectomy Trial (NASCET) Group. Neurology 1995; 45: 428–31.

122. Wolf PA, Kannel WB, Sorlie P, McNamara P. Asymptomatic carotid bruit and risk of stroke. The Framingham study. JAMA 1981; 245: 1442–5.

123. Simons PC, Algra A, Eikelboom BC, Grobbee DE, van der GY. Carotid artery stenosis in patients with peripheral arterial disease: the SMART study. SMART study group. J Vasc Surg 1999; 30: 519–25.

124. Vernieri F, Pasqualetti P, Matteis M et al. Effect of collateral blood flow and cerebral vasomotor reactivity on the outcome of carotid artery occlusion. Stroke 2001; 32: 1552–8.

125. Rothwell PM, Warlow CP. Low risk of ischemic stroke in patients with reduced internal carotid artery lumen diameter distal to severe symptomatic carotid stenosis: cerebral protection due to low poststenotic flow? On behalf of the European Carotid Surgery Trialists' Collaborative Group. Stroke 2000; 31: 622–30.

126. Morgenstern LB, Fox AJ, Sharpe BL et al. The risks and benefits of carotid endarterectomy in patients with near occlusion of the carotid artery. North American Symptomatic Carotid Endarterectomy Trial (NASCET) Group. Neurology 1997; 48: 911–5.

127. Streifler JY, Eliasziw M, Fox AJ et al. Angiographic detection of carotid plaque ulceration. Comparison with surgical observations in a multicenter study. North American Symptomatic Carotid Endarterectomy Trial. Stroke 1994; 25: 1130–32.

128. Benavente O, Eliasziw M, Streifler JY et al. Prognosis after transient monocular blindness associated with carotid-artery stenosis. N Engl J Med 2001; 345: 1084–90.

129. Kappelle LJ, Eliasziw M, Fox AJ et al. Importance of intracranial atherosclerotic disease in patients with symptomatic stenosis of the internal carotid artery. The North American Symptomatic Carotid Endarterectomy Trail. Stroke 1999; 30: 282–6.

130. Gasecki AP, Eliasziw M, Ferguson GG, Hachinski V, Barnett HJ. Long-term prognosis and effect of endarterectomy in patients with symptomatic severe carotid stenosis and contralateral carotid stenosis or occlusion: results from NASCET. North American Symptomatic Carotid Endarterectomy Trial (NASCET) Group. J Neurosurg 1995; 83: 778–82.

131. Henderson RD, Eliasziw M, Fox AJ, Rothwell PM, Barnett HJ. Angiographically defined collateral circulation and risk of stroke in patients with severe carotid artery stenosis. North American Symptomatic Carotid Endarterectomy Trial (NASCET) Group. Stroke 2000; 31: 128–32.

132. Polak JF, Shemanski L, O'Leary DH et al. Hypoechoic plaque at US of the carotid artery: an independent risk factor for incident

stroke in adults aged 65 years or older. Cardiovascular Health Study. Radiology 1998; 208: 649–54.

133. Mathiesen EB, Bonaa KH, Joakimsen O. Echolucent plaques are associated with high risk of ischemic cerebrovascular events in carotid stenosis: the Tromsø study. Circulation 2001; 103: 2171–5.

134. Sitzer M, Muller W, Siebler M et al. Plaque ulceration and lumen thrombus are the main sources of cerebral microemboli in high-grade internal carotid artery stenosis. Stroke 1995; 26: 1231–3.

135. Bosiers M, Peeters P, Deloose K et al. Does carotid artery stenting work on the long run: 5-year results in high-volume centers (ELOCAS Registry). J Cardiovasc Surg (Torino) 2005; 46: 241–7.

136. Hobson RW, Howard VJ, Roubin GS et al. Carotid artery stenting is associated with increased complications in octogenarians: 30-day stroke and death rates in the CREST lead-in phase. J Vasc Surg 2004; 40: 1106–11.

137. Barnett HJ, Eliasziw M, Meldrum HE, Taylor DW. Do the facts and figures warrant a 10-fold increase in the performance of carotid endarterectomy on asymptomatic patients? [see comments]. Neurology 1996; 46: 603–8.

138. Hsia DC, Moscoe LM, Krushat WM. Epidemiology of carotid endarterectomy among Medicare beneficiaries: 1985–1996 update. Stroke 1998; 29: 346–50.

139. Endovascular versus surgical treatment in patients with carotid stenosis in the Carotid and Vertebral Artery Transluminal Angioplasty Study (CAVATAS): a randomised trial. Lancet 2001; 357: 1729–37.

140. Bond R, Rerkasem K, Rothwell PM. Systematic review of the risks of carotid endarterectomy in relation to the clinical indication for and timing of surgery. Stroke 2003; 34: 1–12.

141. Bond R, Rerkasem K, Shearman CP, Rothwell PM. Time trends in the published risks of stroke and death due to endarterectomy for symptomatic carotid stenosis. Cerebrovasc Dis 2004; 18: 37–46.

142. Chaturvedi S, Bruno A, Feasby T et al. Carotid endarterectomy–an evidence-based review: report of the Therapeutics and Technology Assessment Subcommittee of the American Academy of Neurology. Neurology 2005; 65: 794–801.

143. Rothwell PM, Slattery J, Warlow CP. A systematic review of the risks of stroke and death due to endarterectomy for symptomatic carotid stenosis. Stroke 1996; 27: 260–65.

144. Bush RL, Lin PH, Mureebe L et al. Routine bivalirudin use in percutaneous carotid interventions. J Endovasc Ther 2005; 12: 521–2.

145. Kapadia SR, Bajzer CT, Ziada KM et al. Initial experience of platelet glycoprotein IIb/IIIa inhibition with abciximab during carotid stenting: a safe and effective adjunctive therapy. Stroke 2001; 32: 2328–32.

146. Wholey MH, Wholey MH, Eles G et al. Evaluation of glycoprotein IIb/IIIa inhibitors in carotid angioplasty and stenting. J Endovasc Ther 2003; 10: 33–41.

147. Layton KF, Kallmes DF, Cloft HJ, Lindell EP, Cox VS. Bovine aortic arch variant in humans: clarification of a common misnomer. AJNR Am J Neuroradiol 2006; 27: 1541–2.

148. Akers DL, Markowitz IA, Kerstein MD. The value of aortic arch study in the evaluation of cerebrovascular insufficiency. Am J Surg 1987; 154: 230–32.

149. Parodi JC, Schonholz C, Parodi FE, Sicard G, Ferreira LM. Initial 200 cases of carotid artery stenting using a reversal-of-flow cerebral protection device. J Cardiovasc Surg (Torino) 2007; 48: 117–24.

150. Adami CA, Scuro A, Spinamano L et al. Use of the Parodi anti-embolism system in carotid stenting: Italian trial results. J Endovasc Ther 2002; 9: 147–54.

151. Henry M, Amor M, Henry I et al. Carotid stenting with cerebral protection: first clinical experience using the PercuSurge GuardWire system. J Endovasc Surg 1999; 6: 321–31.

152. Chen CI, Iguchi Y, Garami Z et al. Analysis of emboli during carotid stenting with distal protection device. Cerebrovasc Dis 2006; 21: 223–8.

153. Eckert B, Zeumer H. Editorial comment: Carotid artery stenting with or without protection devices? Strong opinions, poor evidence! Stroke 2003; 34: 1941–3.

154. Eskandari MK. Cerebral embolic protection. Semin Vasc Surg 2005; 18: 95–100.

155. Hill MD, Morrish W, Soulez G et al. Multicenter evaluation of a self-expanding carotid stent system with distal protection in the treatment of carotid stenosis. AJNR Am J Neuroradiol 2006; 27: 759–5.

156. Muller-Hulsbeck S, Stolzmann P, Liess C et al. Vessel wall damage caused by cerebral protection devices: ex vivo evaluation in porcine carotid arteries. Radiology 2005; 235: 454–60.

157. Ohki T, Veith FJ. Critical analysis of distal protection devices. Semin Vasc Surg 2003; 16: 317–25.

158. Sprouse LR, Peeters P, Bosiers M. The capture of visible debris by distal cerebral protection filters during carotid artery stenting: Is it predictable? J Vasc Surg 2005; 41: 950–55.

159. Stone GW, Rogers C, Hermiller J et al. Randomized comparison of distal protection with a filter-based catheter and a balloon occlusion and aspiration system during percutaneous intervention of diseased saphenous vein aorto-coronary bypass grafts. Circulation 2003; 108: 548–53.

160. Vos JA, van den B, erg JC, Ernst SM et al. Carotid angioplasty and stent placement: comparison of transcranial Doppler US data and clinical outcome with and without filtering cerebral protection devices in 509 patients. Radiology 2005; 234: 493–9.

161. White CJ, Iyer SS, Hopkins LN, Katzen BT, Russell ME. Carotid stenting with distal protection in high surgical risk patients: the BEACH trial 30 day results. Catheter Cardiovasc Interv 2006; 67: 503–12.

162. Iyer V, de DG, Deloose K et al. The type of embolic protection does not influence the outcome in carotid artery stenting. J Vasc Surg 2007; 46: 251–6.

163. Casserly IP, bou-Chebl A, Fathi RB et al. Slow-flow phenomenon during carotid artery intervention with embolic protection devices: predictors and clinical outcome. J Am Coll Cardiol 2005; 46: 1466–72.

164. Poppert H, Wolf O, Resch M et al. Differences in number, size and location of intracranial microembolic lesions after surgical versus endovascular treatment without protection device of carotid artery stenosis. J Neurol 2004; 251: 1198–203.

165. Kastrup A, Groschel K, Krapf H et al. Early outcome of carotid angioplasty and stenting with and without cerebral protection devices: a systematic review of the literature. Stroke 2003; 34: 813–19.

166. Wholey MH, Al-Mubarek N, Wholey MH. Updated review of the global carotid artery stent registry. Catheter Cardiovasc Interv 2003; 60: 259–66.

167. Theiss W, Hermanek P, Mathias K et al. Pro-CAS: a prospective registry of carotid angioplasty and stenting. Stroke 2004; 35: 2134–39.

168. Naylor AR, Bolia A, Abbott RJ et al. Randomized study of carotid angioplasty and stenting versus carotid endarterectomy: A stopped trial. J Vasc Surg 1998; 28: 326–34.

169. Alberts M. Results of a multicenter prospective randomized trial of carotid artery stenting vs. carotid endarterectomy (abstract) Stroke 2001; 32: 325.

170. Brooks WH, McClure RR, Jones MR, Coleman TC, Breathitt L. Carotid angioplasty and stenting versus carotid endarterectomy: randomized trial in a community hospital. J Am Coll Cardiol 2001; 38: 1589–95.

171. Yadav JS, Wholey MH, Kuntz RE et al. Protected carotid-artery stenting versus endarterectomy in high-risk patients. N Engl J Med 2004; 351: 1493–501.

172. Seemann JH, Leppien A, Feyer P, Felix R. Peripheral vascular disease: carotid and vertebral brachytherapy for in-stent restenosis. Catheter Cardiovasc Interv 2005; 65: 412–15.

173. Chan AW, Roffi M, Mukherjee D et al. Carotid brachytherapy for in-stent restenosis. Catheter Cardiovasc Interv 2003; 58: 86–92.

174. Scheller B, Hehrlein C, Bocksch W et al. Treatment of coronary in-stent restenosis with a paclitaxel-coated balloon catheter. N Engl J Med 2006; 355: 2113–24.

175. Rouleau PA, Huston J III, Gilbertson J et al. Carotid artery tandem lesions: frequency of angiographic detection and consequences for endarterectomy. AJNR Am J Neuroradiol 1999; 20: 621–5.

176. Marks MP, Wojak JC, Al-Ali F et al. Angioplasty for symptomatic intracranial stenosis: clinical outcome. Stroke 2006; 37: 1016–20.

177. Marks MP, Marcellus ML, Do HM et al. Intracranial angioplasty without stenting for symptomatic atherosclerotic stenosis: long-term follow-up. AJNR Am J Neuroradiol 2005; 26: 525–30.

178. Mori T, Fukuoka M, Kazita K, Mori K. Follow-up study after intracranial percutaneous transluminal cerebral balloon angioplasty. AJNR Am J Neuroradiol 1998; 19: 1525–33.

179. Chow MM, Masaryk TJ, Woo HH, Mayberg MR, Rasmussen PA. Stent-assisted angioplasty of intracranial vertebrobasilar atherosclerosis: midterm analysis of clinical and radiologic predictors of neurological morbidity and mortality. AJNR Am J Neuroradiol 2005; 26: 869–74.

180. Levy EI, Horowitz MB, Koebbe CJ et al. Transluminal stent-assisted angiplasty of the intracranial vertebrobasilar system for medically refractory, posterior circulation ischemia: early results. Neurosurgery 2001; 48: 1215–21.

181. Yu W, Smith WS, Singh V et al. Long-term outcome of endovascular stenting for symptomatic basilar artery stenosis. Neurology 2005; 64: 1055–57.

182. Tsumoto T, Terada T, Tsuura M et al. Diffusion-weighted imaging abnormalities after percutaneous transluminal angioplasty and stenting for intracranial atherosclerotic disease. AJNR Am J Neuroradiol 2005; 26: 385–9.

183. Navarro JC, Mikulik R, Garami Z, Alexandrov AV. The accuracy of transcranial Doppler in the diagnosis of stenosis or occlusion of the terminal internal carotid artery. J Neuroimaging 2004; 14: 314–18.

184. Jordan WD, Voellinger DC, Plyuscheva NP, Fisher WS, McDowell HA. Microemboli detected by transcranial Doppler monitoring in patients during carotid angioplasty versus carotid endarterectomy. Cardiovasc Surg 1999; 7: 33–8.

185. Spence JD, Tamayo A, Lownie SP, Ng WP, Ferguson GG. Absence of microemboli on transcranial Doppler identifies low-risk patients with asymptomatic carotid stenosis. Stroke 2005; 36: 2373–8.

186. Schievink WI, Mokri B, Whisnant JP. Internal carotid artery dissection in a community. Rochester, Minnesota, 1987–1992. Stroke 1993; 24: 1678–80.

187. O'Sullivan R, Robertson W, Nugent R, Berry K, Turnbull I. Supraclinoid carotid artery dissection following unusual trauma. AJNR Am J Neuroradiol 1990; 11: 1150–2.

188. Mullges W, Ringelstein EB, Leibold M. Non-invasive diagnosis of internal carotid artery dissections. J Neurol Neurosurg Psychiatry 1992; 55: 98–104.

189. Sturzenegger M. Spontaneous internal carotid artery dissection: early diagnosis and management in 44 patients. J Neurol 1995; 242: 231–8.

190. Mokri B, Piepgras DG, Houser OW. Traumatic dissections of the extracranial internal carotid artery. J Neurosurg 1988; 68: 189–97.

191. Biousse V, nglejan-Chatillon J, Massiou H, Bousser MG. Head pain in non-traumatic carotid artery dissection: a series of 65 patients. Cephalalgia 1994; 14: 33–6.

192. Hart R, Easton J. Dissections and trauma of cervico-cerebral arteries. In: Barnett H, Mohr J, Stein B, Yatsu F, eds. Stroke: Pathophysiology, Diagnosis and Management. New York: Churchill Livingstone, 1986; 775–8.

193. Mokri B, Sundt TMJ, Houser OW, Piepgras DG. Spontaneous dissection of the cervical internal carotid artery. Ann Neurol 1986; 19: 126–38.

194. Malek AM, Higashida RT, Phatouros CC et al. Endovascular management of extracranial carotid artery dissection achieved using stent angioplasty. AJNR Am J Neuroradiol 2000; 21: 1280–92.

195. Schievink WI, Mokri B, O'Fallon WM. Recurrent spontaneous cervical-artery dissection. N Engl J Med 1994; 330: 393–7.

196. Mokri B. Traumatic and spontaneous extracranial internal carotid artery dissections. J Neurol 1990; 237: 356–61.

197. Houser OW, Mokri B, Sundt TMJ, Baker HLJ, Reese DF. Spontaneous cervical cephalic arterial dissection and its residuum: angiographic spectrum. AJNR Am J Neuroradiol 1984; 5: 27–34.

198. O'Dwyer JA, Moscow N, Trevor R, Ehrenfeld WK, Newton TH. Spontaneous dissection of the carotid artery. Radiology 1980; 137: 379–85.

199. Pozzati E, Giuliani G, Acciarri N, Nuzzo G. Long-term follow-up of occlusive cervical carotid dissection. Stroke 1990; 21: 528–31.

200. Schievink WI, Mokri B, O'Fallon WM. Recurrent spontaneous cervical-artery dissection. N Engl J Med 1994; 330: 393–7.

201. Kitani R, Itouji T, Noda Y, Kimura M, Uchida S. Dissecting aneurysms of the anterior circle of Willis arteries. J Neurosurg 1987; 67: 296–300.

202. Morgan K, Besser M, Johnston I, Chaseling R. Intracranial carotid artery injury in closed head trauma. J Neurosurg 1987; 66: 192–7.

203. Ehrenfeld WK, Wylie EJ. Spontaneous dissection of the internal carotid artery. Arch Surg 1976; 111: 1294–301.

204. Fisher C, Ojemann R, Robertson G. Spontaneous dissection of cervico-cerebral arteries. Can J Neurol Sci 1978; 5: 9–19.

205. Levy C, Laissy J, Raveau V. Carotid and vertebral artery dissections: three-dimensional time-of-flight MR angiography and MR imaging versus conventional angiography. Radiology 1994; 190: 97–103.

206. Rothrock JF, Lim V, Press G, Gosink B. Serial magnetic resonance and carotid duplex examinations in the management of carotid dissection. Neurology 1989; 39: 686–92.

207. Steinke W, Rautenberg W, Schwartz A, Hennerici M. Noninvasive monitoring of internal carotid artery dissection. Stroke 1994; 25: 998–1005.

208. Sidhu PS, Jonker ND, Khaw KT et al. Spontaneous dissections of the internal carotid artery: appearances on colour Doppler ultrasound. Br J Radiol 1997; 70: 50–7.

209. de Bray JM, Lhoste P, Dubas F, Emile J, Saumet JL. Ultrasonic features of extracranial carotid dissections: 47 cases studied by angiography. J Ultrasound Med 1994; 13: 659–64.

210. Gelbert F, Assouline E, Hodes J. MRI in spontaneous dissection of vertebral and carotid arteries. Neuroradiology 1991; 33: 111–13.

211. Kirsch E, Kaim A, Engelter S et al. MR angiography in internal carotid artery dissection: improvement of diagnosis by selective demonstration of the intramural haematoma. Neuroradiology 1998; 40: 704–9.

212. Mascalchi M, Bianchi MC, Mangiafico S et al. MRI and MR angiography of vertebral artery dissection. Neuroradiology 1997; 39: 329–40.

213. Brugieres P, Castrec-Carpo A, Heran F et al. Magnetic resonance imaging in the exploration of dissection of the internal carotid artery. J Neuroradiol 1989; 16: 1–10.

214. Kasner SE, Hankins LL, Bratina P, Morgenstern LB. Magnetic resonance angiography demonstrates vascular healing of carotid and vertebral artery dissections. Stroke 1997; 28: 1993–7.

215. Djouhri H, Guillon B, Brunereau L et al. MR angiography for the long-term follow-up of dissecting aneurysms of the extracranial internal carotid artery. AJR Am J Roentgenol 2000; 174: 1137–40.

216. Srinivasan J, Newell DW, Sturzenegger M, Mayberg MR, Winn HR. Transcranial Doppler in the evaluation of internal carotid artery dissection. Stroke 1996; 27: 1226–30.

217. Guillon B, Levy C, Bousser MG. Internal carotid artery dissection: an update. J Neurol Sci 1998; 153: 146–58.

218. Sturzenegger M, Mattle HP, Rivoir A, Baumgartner RW. Ultrasound findings in carotid artery dissection: analysis of 43 patients. Neurology 1995; 45: 691–8.

219. Lucas C, Moulin T, Deplanque D, Tatu L, Chavot D. Stroke patterns of internal carotid artery dissection in 40 patients. Stroke 1998; 29: 2646–8.

220. Biousse V, nglejan-Chatillon J, Touboul PJ, Amarenco P, Bousser MG. Time course of symptoms in extracranial carotid artery dissections. A series of 80 patients. Stroke 1995; 26: 235–9.

221. Krajewski LP, Hertzer NR. Blunt carotid artery trauma: report of two cases and review of the literature. Ann Surg 1980; 191: 341–6.

222. Schievink WI, Piepgras DG, McCaffrey TV, Mokri B. Surgical treatment of extracranial internal carotid artery dissecting aneurysms. Neurosurgery 1994; 35: 809–15.

223. Liu AY, Paulsen RD, Marcellus ML, Steinberg GK, Marks MP. Long-term outcomes after carotid stent placement treatment of carotid artery dissection. Neurosurgery 1999; 45: 1368–73.

224. Malek AM, Halbach VV, Phatouros CC et al. Endovascular treatment of a ruptured intracranial dissecting vertebral aneurysm in a kickboxer. J Trauma 2000; 48: 143–5.

225. Wintemute GJ, Wright MA. Initial and subsequent hospital costs of firearm injuries. J Trauma 1992; 33: 556–60.

226. Max W, Rice DP. Shooting in the dark: estimating the cost of firearm injuries. Health Aff (Millwood) 1993; 12: 171–85.

227. Wintemute GJ. Trauma in transition: trends in death from firearms from motor vehicle injuries. Sacramento, California: Violence Prevention Research Program, 1995.

228. Rao PM, Ivatury RR, Sharma P et al. Cervical vascular injuries: a trauma center experience. Surgery 1993; 114: 527–31.

229. Swan KG, Swan RC. Principles of ballistics applicable to the treatment of gunshot wounds. Surg Clin North Am 1991; 71: 221–39.

230. Hollerman JJ, Fackler ML, Coldwell DM, Ben-Menachem Y. Gunshot wounds: 1. Bullets, ballistics, and mechanisms of injury. AJR Am J Roentgenol 1990; 155: 685–90.

231. Flanigan DP. Civilian vascular trauma. Philadelphia: Lea and Febiger, 1992.

232. Hollerman JJ. Gunshot wounds. Am Fam Physician 1988; 37: 231–46.

233. Roden DM, Pomerantz RA. Penetrating injuries to the neck: a safe, selective approach to management. Am Surg 1993; 59: 750–3.

234. Metzdorff MT, Lowe DK. Operation or observation for penetrating neck wounds? A retrospective analysis. Am J Surg 1984; 147: 646–9.

235. Monson DO, Saletta JD, Freeark RJ. Carotid vertebral trauma. J Trauma 1969; 9: 987–99.

236. Saletta JD, Folk FA, Freeark RJ. Trauma to the neck region. Surg Clin North Am 1973; 53: 73–86.

237. Takayasu M. A case with peculiar changes of the retinal central vessels. Acta Soc Ophthalmol Jpn 1908; 12: 555.

238. Ishikawa K. Natural history and classification of occlusive thromboaortopathy (Takayasu's disease). Circulation 1978; 57: 27–35.

239. Ueda H, Morooka S, Ito I, Yamaguchi H, Takeda T. Clinical observation of 52 cases of aortitis syndrome. Jpn Heart J 1969; 10: 277–88.

240. Kerr GS, Hallahan CW, Giordano J et al. Takayasu arteritis. Ann Intern Med 1994; 120: 919–29.

241. Lagneau P, Michel JB, Vuong PN. Surgical treatment of Takayasu's disease. Ann Surg 1987; 205: 157–66.

242. Maksimowicz-McKinnon K, Clark TM, Hoffman GS. Limitations of therapy and a guarded prognosis in an American cohort of Takayasu arteritis patients. Arthritis Rheum 2007; 56: 1000–9.

243. Jain S, Kumari S, Ganguly NK, Sharma BK. Current status of Takayasu arteritis in India. Int J Cardiol 1996; 54: S111–6.

244. Dabague J, Reyes PA. Takayasu arteritis in Mexico: a 38-year clinical perspective through literature review. Int J Cardiol 1996; 54: S103–9.

245. Lupi-Herrera E, Sanchez-Torres G, Marcushamer J et al. Takayasu's arteritis. Clinical study of 107 cases. Am Heart J 1977; 93: 94–103.

246. Subramanyan R, Joy J, Balakrishnan KG. Natural history of aortoarteritis (Takayasu's disease). Circulation 1989; 80: 429–37.

247. Vanoli M, Daina E, Salvarani C et al. Takayasu's arteritis: A study of 104 Italian patients. Arthritis Rheum 2005; 53: 100–7.

248. Park MC, Lee SW, Park YB, Chung NS, Lee SK. Clinical characteristics and outcomes of Takayasu's arteritis: analysis of 108 patients using standardized criteria for diagnosis, activity assessment, and angiographic classification. Scand J Rheumatol 2005; 34: 284–92.

249. Ishikawa K, Maetani S. Long-term outcome for 120 Japanese patients with Takayasu's disease. Clinical and statistical analyses of related prognostic factors. Circulation 1994; 90: 1855–60.

250. Sharma S, Saxena A, Talwar KK et al. Renal artery stenosis caused by nonspecific arteritis (Takayasu disease): results of treatment with percutaneous transluminal angioplasty. AJR Am J Roentgenol 1992; 158: 417–22.

251. Tyagi S, Verma PK, Gambhir DS et al. Early and long-term results of subclavian angioplasty in aortoarteritis (Takayasu disease): comparison with atherosclerosis. Cardiovasc Intervent Radiol 1998; 21: 219–24.

252. Fields CE, Bower TC, Cooper LT et al. Takayasu's arteritis: operative results and influence of disease activity. J Vasc Surg 2006; 43: 64–71.

7

Intracranial aneurysms and subarachnoid hemorrhage

Michael E Kelly, Peter A Rasmussen and Thomas J Masaryk

Introduction

The term 'aneurysm' comes from the Greek, meaning a 'widening', and it most commonly refers to a pathologic dilatation or outpouching of an artery. The most feared manifestation of this condition exists within the cerebral arteries residing within the subarachnoid space; the most serious sequelae of an aneurysm in these arteries is hemorrhage leading to precipitous, and often fatal, increases in intracranial pressure.

Aneurysms have been recognized since ancient times. Premorbid recognition awaited the routine use of lumbar puncture for diagnosis of subarachnoid hemorrhage and radiography to detect subtle signs of mass effect or calcification.

Successful initial attempts at aneurysm treatment occurred in the late 1800s primarily through the use of parent artery ligation (the 'Hunterian closure').[1] With the introduction of cerebral angiography in 1927 and the progression of surgical techniques, the first successful surgical clipping was performed 10 years later by Dandy.[2] The evolution of surgical clipping was significantly enhanced by the introduction of the bipolar microscope in the 1940s and 1950s and the micro-surgical dissections that were enabled with the gradual acceptance of the operating microscope in the 1960s.[1,3,4] This remained the only primary treatment for the next 35 years, with additional refinements coming in the form of earlier diagnosis of hemorrhage and hydrocephalus with CT scanning (1972), unique exposures, and earlier surgery coupled with aggressive treatment for vasospasm.[5] Over this period, clipping became viewed as safe in skilled hands and durable over the life of the patient.

The digitization of radiology with CT in the early 1970s extended to angiography by the end of that decade.[6] The real-time production of high-contrast subtracted images and implementation of roadmapping marked the transformation of the angiography suite from a diagnostic modality to image-guided minimally invasive surgery. However, even early in the 1980s brave pioneers were exploring possible aneurysm treatments using endovascular methods. The Russian neurosurgeon Serbinenko is widely recognized as the first to be successful;[7] although in North America the popularity was spread by the wider availability of more sophisticated imaging as well as the broader circulation of literature from Debrun, Heishima and Berenstein through the 1980s.[7–10] These early efforts focused on the use of detachable balloons (latex or silicon), which, while elegant for the closure of direct carotid cavernous fistulae, were more cumbersome for the treatment of intracranial aneurysms if one was intent on sparing the parent artery. During this period there were great strides made in the production of variable stiffness micro-catheters and guidewires, which significantly improved access to the intracranial circulation by an endovascular approach.[11]

In the early 1990s, Guglielmi, working with Vinuela and colleagues, described an ingenious device of soft coils mounted on a stylet, which could be positioned, withdrawn, and repositioned in an aneurysm until an optimum configuration was achieved, filling the aneurysm while sparing the parent artery.[12,13] At this point the coil could be electively detached at the leisure of the operator. Serially smaller coils could be nested one within the next much like Russian dolls (a nod to Serbinenko?). These devices have likewise been modified and improved; matched with sophisticated, high-speed biplane digital angiography systems, they now complement surgery by providing lower-risk options for the most difficult surgical lesions.

Etiology

Saccular aneurysms

The majority of intracranial aneurysms are saccular aneurysms. The true cause of saccular aneurysms is not well understood. Saccular aneurysms are focal protrusions that arise at vessel wall weaknesses at major bifurcations of intracranial arteries (Figure 7.1).[14] It is likely that a congenital deficit in the arterial wall predisposes to aneurysm formation secondary to the influences of 'vascular disease' such as hypertension and atherosclerosis. Aneurysms tend to form at arterial branch points or curves in the vessel. Hemodynamic influences and the biologic response of the vessel wall lead to aneurysm formation. If an aneurysm forms along a curve, it tends to form in the direction that the blood would have flowed if the vessel had not altered course.[15]

Other forms of aneurysm

Dissecting (so-called blood blister) aneurysms often form in response to traumatically induced or spontaneous dissection of

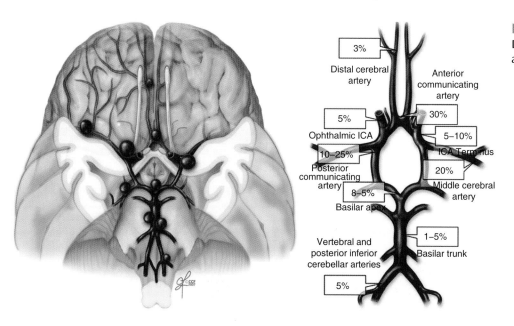

Figure 7.1
Distribution of intracranial aneurysms.

Distal cerebral artery	3%
Anterior communicating artery	30%
Ophthalmic ICA	5%
ICA Terminus	5–10%
Posterior communicating artery	10–25%
Middle cerebral artery	20%
Basilar apex	8–5%
Vertebral and posterior inferior cerebellar arteries	5%
Basilar trunk	1–5%

Table 7.1 Location of aneurysms

Anterior circulation (85–95%)[99]

Anterior communicating complex: 30%[98–100]

Cavernous carotid artery: 3–5%[99–101]

Ophthalmic segment of internal carotid artery: 5%[100]

Posterior communicating artery: 10–25%[98,99]

Middle cerebral artery: 20%[98,99]

Internal carotid artery terminus: 5–10%

Distal anterior cerebral artery: 3%

Posterior circulation (5–15%)[99,102]

Basilar apex (tip): 8–15%[98,99]

Basilar trunk: 1–5%

Posterior inferior cerebellar artery and vertebral artery: 1–5%[99,103]

Epidemiology

Prevalence of unruptured intracranial aneurysms

The overall prevalence of unruptured intracranial aneurysms in the general population is between 0.8% and 6%. These numbers can be derived from numerous studies examining prevalence. Sekhar and Heros[16] published, in 1982, a prevalence rate of 5% in a single-center study. A single-center autopsy study by Inagawa and Hirano examined 10,259 autopsies and found 102 aneurysms in 84 patients, giving a prevalence of 0.8%.[17] Rinkel reported that aneurysms are found in approximately 2% of the population if one considers all the available evidence.[18]

Anatomy and pathophysiology

Anatomy

Saccular aneurysms form around the vessels of the circle of Willis at the base of the brain. Approximately 85–90% of them are found around the anterior circulation (the anterior cerebral artery, the middle cerebral artery, or the internal carotid artery). Posterior circulation aneurysms can arise from the posterior inferior cerebellar artery, the vertebral artery, the basilar artery, the posterior cerebral artery, the superior cerebellar artery, and the basilar apex. The specific locations are shown in Table 7.1 and Figure 7.1. Aneurysms are also classified according to size. Small aneurysms are ≤8 mm in diameter; large are 8–24 mm and giant are ≥25 mm (Figure 7.4).

Pathophysiology

As discussed above, saccular aneurysms that arise at the branch points of the intracranial arteries or off a parent vessel are usually

the intracranial artery. They tend to appear saccular in morphology, but they more often occur at atypical locations on the circle of Willis and large conducting arteries. Fusiform aneurysms can be of two varieties: large or giant saccular aneurysms that are partially thrombosed with a serpentine channel through them to the distal vasculature, or smaller dilatations of the parent vessel in which a large portion of the circumference of the vessel wall is aneurysmal (Figure 7.2). They may have a component that appears saccular, but no obvious neck is apparent. Embolic aneurysms usually form in the distal cerebral vasculature, most commonly the distal middle cerebral territory (the M4 branches). They can form in response to pathologic processes involving the heart (e.g. infective endocarditis, whether bacterial or fungal, or atrial myxomas) (Figure 7.3). All of these other types of aneurysms can cause subarachnoid hemorrhage (SAH).

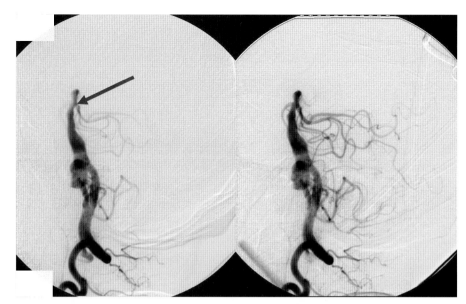

Figure 7.2
Dissecting fusiform aneurysm of the basilar artery. While these rarely produce subarachnoid hemorrhage, they often cause symptoms by virtue of mass effect on the brainstem and adjacent cranial nerves. Additionally, the patulous lumen results in slow flow, which may lead to thrombus formation and symptoms of vertebrobasilar ischemia. Notice on these two successive images the layering of contrast (arrow), due to slow flow.

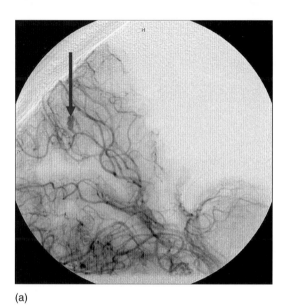
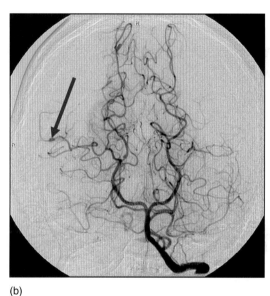

(a)   (b)

Figure 7.3
A 20-year-old heroin addict presented with seizures and fever. Initial CT scan demonstrated edema surrounding a focal area of ischemia in the right occipital lobe. Conventional angiography confirmed the presence of a mycotic aneurysm due to *Staph aureus* (arrow). Follow-up angiography after surgery and 1 week of antibiotics demonstrated resolution of the treated aneurysm, but also showed a second lesion in the posterior temporal branch of the same posterior cerebral artery (arrow).

at a curve and point in the direction of blood flow. The pulsatile flow of the blood leads to wall stress and is believed to cause local destruction of the internal elastic lamina. Turbulent flow within the aneurysm can lead to aneurysm growth. Aneurysms rupture is most often related to size. With the growth of the aneurysm the wall thickness is frequently reduced. This leads to increased wall tension with an increased risk of rupture.[14,16,19]

There are several connective tissue disorders that have been associated with intracranial aneurysm formation: autosomal-dominant polycystic kidney disease (ADPKD), α_1-antitrypsin deficiency, Marfan syndrome, neurofibromatosis type 1, pseudoxanthoma elasticum, and Ehlers–Danlos syndrome type IV.

ADPKD affects between one in 400 and one in 1000 people.[20] It is a systemic disease with cystic involvement of the kidneys, lungs, liver, pancreas, and intracranial vasculature. Rinkel et al.[18]

recently reported a relative risk of 4.4 times the normal population for developing intracranial aneurysms. Gieteling and Rinkel[21] reported that patients with ADPKD have a familial SAH pattern, bleed at a younger age, and are more often men. The most commonly involved site is the middle cerebral artery.[21]

Because of the high rate of aneurysm formation and the increased risk of rupture, screening is recommended for those with ADPKD. Screening can be complicated by poor renal function in these patients. Magnetic resonance angiography (MRA) is generally accepted as the imaging procedure of choice because of improved safety compared with CT angiography (CTA) and conventional intra-arterial digital subtraction angiography (DSA), because of the use of iodinated contrast with CTA and DSA. MRA will reliably detect aneurysms >2 mm in diameter.

Table 7.2 Five-year cumulative rupture rates according to size and location of unruptured aneurysm from the International Study of Unruptured Aneurysm (ISUIA)

	< 7 mm		7–12 mm	13–24 mm	≥ 25 mm
	Group 1*	Group 2**			
Cavernous carotid artery (n = 210)	0	0	0	3.0%	6.4%
AC, MC, IC (n = 1037)	0	1.5%	2.6%	14.5%	40%
Post P comm (n = 445)	2.5%	3.4%	14.5%	18.4%	50%

AC, anterior communicating or anterior cerebral artery; IC, internal carotid artery (not cavernous carotid artery); MC, middle cerebral artery; Post P comm, vertebrobasilar, posterior cerebral arterial system, or the posterior communicating artery
Reprinted with permission from Forbes et al.[35]
*Group 1: patients with no prior history of subarachnoid hemorrhage (SAH).
**Group 2: patients with a history of SAH.

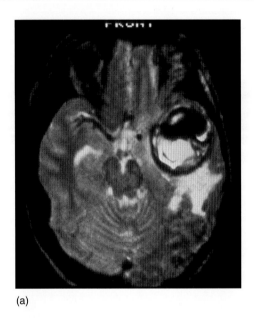

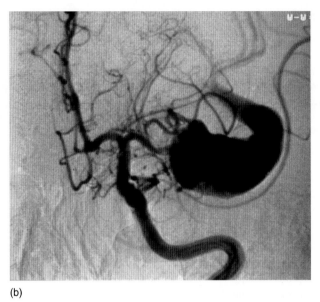

(a)   (b)

Figure 7.4
(a) Axial T2-weighted MRI demonstrating a heterogenous left temporal mass with vasogenic edema secondary to laminated thrombus or blood breakdown products, as well as flow void from a giant fusiform aneurysm of the left middle cerebral artery aneurysm. (b) Confirmatory catheter angiogram.

Aneurysms can also affect multiple family members. It is estimated that 7–20% of patients who suffer from SAH have first- of second-degree relatives with aneurysms.[22–24] The Familial Intracranial Aneurysm (FIA) study is trying to identify genes that may be related to aneurysm development and rupture.[25]

It has also been reported that patients with familial aneurysms have SAH at a younger age than the previous generation.[26] Familial aneurysms are also larger and have a higher prevalence. People with two or more first-degree relatives or three family members (first- or second-degree relatives) should be investigated and offered treatment.

Natural history of aneurysm and the etiology of subarachnoid hemorrhage

Head trauma is the most common cause of SAH.[27,28] Other etiologies include aneurysms, arteriovenous malformations,

peri-mesencephalic hemorrhage, and intracranial carotid and vertebral artery dissection (Figure 7.5).

Intracranial aneurysm rupture accounts for approximately 85% of non-traumatic SAH. The incidence of aneurysmal SAH is between 10 and 15 per 100,000 people per year. This is a generally accepted rate and is derived from pooled data from various studies.[29–34]

Natural history of aneurysms and rupture

There are several risk factors that predispose patients harboring intracranial aneurysms to suffer SAH. Juvela et al.[35] published their results in 142 patients with 181 unruptured aneurysms. They followed these patients until death or SAH or for at least 10 years after the unruptured aneurysm was diagnosed. The median follow-up time was 13.9 years (0.8–30.0 years). During the 1944 patient–years of follow-up study there were 27 first episodes of hemorrhage from a previously unruptured aneurysm, giving

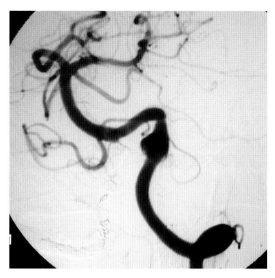

Figure 7.5

A 35-year-old woman with spontaneous dissection of both carotid and both vertebral arteries. The right vertebral dissection was irregular and appeared to be the source of subarachnoid hemorrhage. The right vertebral artery was sacrificed. The remaining left vertebral artery dissection has a prominent, persistent fusiform aneurysm.

an average annual rupture incidence of 1.4%. Fourteen of these bleeding episodes were fatal. The cumulative rate of bleeding was 10% at 10 years after the diagnosis, 26% at 20 years, and 32% at 30 years. The only predictor for the rupture was the size of the aneurysm ($p=0.036$). However, in patients with multiple aneurysms (the main subgroup) the only variable that tended to predict rupture was the age of the patient: risk of rupture was inversely associated with age ($p=0.080$). A new aneurysm was found in six of 31 patients.[35]

The most important study relating to the natural history of aneurysm rupture is by Wiebers et al.[36] This was a prospective multi-center study with centers in the USA, Canada and Europe. The purpose of the study was to assess the natural history of unruptured intracranial aneurysms and also to measure the risks associated with treatment. There were 4060 patients assessed for the study. Of these, 1692 did not have aneurysmal repair and were followed. The 5-year cumulative rupture rate was calculated and is shown in Table 7.2. The authors note that 5-year cumulative rupture rates for patients who did not have a history of SAH with aneurysms located in the internal carotid artery, the anterior communicating, the anterior cerebral artery, or the middle cerebral artery were 0%, 2.6%, 14.5%, and 40% for aneurysms <7 mm, 7–12 mm, 13–24 mm, and ≥25 mm, respectively, compared with rates of 2.5%, 14.5%, 18.4%, and 50%, respectively, for the same size categories involving posterior circulation and posterior communicating artery aneurysms.[36]

Of the treatment group, 1917 had open surgery and 451 had endovascular procedures. These rates were often equaled or exceeded by the risks associated with surgical or endovascular repair of comparable lesions. Poorer surgical outcome was strongly predicted by patient age. Poor outcome with either surgical or endovascular treatment was seen in patients with larger aneurysms and aneurysms in the posterior circulation.[36]

There are several criticisms of this study. Posterior communicating artery aneurysms were placed in the posterior circulation group but are generally considered anterior circulation aneurysms. There were a high number of cavernous segment aneurysms

that cannot cause SAH, and there were a large number of patients excluded from the study. Nonetheless, this is currently the most important study regarding the natural history of unruptured aneurysms and should be considered when advising patients on treatment options.[37]

Besides size and location, described above, there are several other risk factors that can predispose the patient with an unruptured aneurysm to SAH. The highest incidence is seen in older patients (55–60 years). Smoking and hypertension have been associated with an increased risk of SAH.[32] Feigin et al.[38] reviewed 26 prospective cohort studies and identified 306,620 participants. They found that cigarette smoking and systolic blood pressure were the most important risk factors for SAH in the Asia–Pacific region.[38] In the Cooperative study, hypertensive patients had a higher mortality after SAH than normotensive patients.[39] In addition, use of cocaine and its derivatives is a significant risk factor for aneurysmal SAH.

Patients with aneurysmal SAH have a high morbidity and mortality. Approximately one-third of patients will die before reaching the hospital. The overall mortality is around 50%. Hop et al.[40] looked at 21 studies between 1960 and 1992 to try to assess the case–fatality rate. The case–fatality rate ranged from 32% to 67%. The authors also noted a recent decline in the overall case–fatality rate and attributed this to improved management of patients with SAH, which may be attributable to a trend towards early treatment of the aneurysm and advances in neurocritical care.

Clinical presentation of aneurysmal subarachnoid hemorrhage

Patients can present for evaluation secondary to rupture (SAH), headache, mass effect (e.g. a cranial nerve deficit), seizure, or an incidental finding on imaging for some other reason. By far the most common presentation is SAH, usually accompanied by severe headache, nausea, and vomiting. With aneurysm rupture there is a significant and sudden increase in intracranial pressure. Arterial blood is released into the subarachnoid space, where it produces a chemical meningitis. Intracerebral hematoma formation can occur if the aneurysm ruptures from a point on the dome that points toward the brain parenchyma. This presentation is so stereotypical that focal neurologic deficit with or without headache that is associated with nausea or vomiting should be assumed to be hemorrhage in the intracranial compartment until proven otherwise by CT scanning. Over 90% of patients with SAH will complain of headache, and it is usually described as the worst headache of their life. The headache is often accompanied by meningismus and photophobia and the patient will prefer to keep the eyes closed. More profound impact on the level of consciousness can occur with hemorrhage, including lethargy, stupor, and coma. Occasionally, there will be a focal neurologic deficit such as a cranial nerve palsy (e.g. III nerve palsy) or a hemiparesis or visual field defect. Headache without associated hemorrhage is usually new for the non-headache patient and different or more severe for the known cephalgic. The location of the headache will depend on the location of the aneurysm, but it is most commonly seen with posterior communicating artery aneurysms, in which case the headache will be unilateral and retro-orbital. Unruptured aneurysms with

Table 7.3 Hunt–Hess classification of subarachnoid hemorrhage[41]

Grade	Description
1	Asymptomatic, or mild headache and slight nuchal rigidity
2	Cranial nerve palsy (e.g., III, VI), moderate to severe headache, nuchal rigidity
3	Mild focal deficit, lethargy, or confusion
4	Stupor, moderate to severe hemiparesis, early decerebrate rigidity
5	Deep coma, decerebrate rigidity, moribund appearance

Add one grade for serious systemic disease (e.g., hypertension, diabetes nellitus, severe atherosclerosis, chronic obstructive pulmonary disease) or severe vasospasm on arteriography.

Modified classification[41] adds the following:

0	Unruptured aneurysm
1a	No acute meningeal or brain reaction, but with fixed neurologic deficit

Original paper did not consider patient's age, site of aneurysm, or time since bleed; patients were graded on admission and pre-operatively
From Shaibani et al.[41]

Table 7.4 World Federation of Neurological Surgeons Subarachnoid Hemorrhage Grading System

Grade	GCS Score	Major focal deficit*
0[†]		
1	15	–
2	13–14	–
3	13–14	–
4	7–12	+ or –
5	3–6	+ or –

GCS, Glasgow Coma Scale (see Table 7.5)
*aphasia, hemiparesis or hemiplegia (+, present; –, absent)
[†]intact aneurysm
From Teasdale et al.[42]

Table 7.5 Glasgow Coma Score (GCS)[43]

Score*	Best eye opening	Best verbal	Best motor
6	—	—	Obeys
5	—	Oriented	Localizes pain
4	Spontaneous	Confused	Withdraws to pain
3	To speech	Inappropriate	Flexion (decorticate)
2	To pain[†]	Incomprehensible	Extensor (decerebrate)
1	None	None	None[‡]

Technically, this is a scale of *impaired* consciousness, whereas 'coma' implies unresponsiveness
*Range of total points: 3 (worst) to 15 (normal)
[†]When testing eye opening to pain, use peripheral stimulus (the grimace associated with central pain may cause eye closure)
[‡]If no motor response, it is important to exclude spinal cord transection
From Teasdale et al.[43]

associated headache should be treated expeditiously as there is an increased risk of hemorrhage in this setting. Seizures are an uncommon presentation for unruptured aneurysms and are usually secondary to a large or giant aneurysm that exerts mass effect, with accompanying edema, on the temporal lobe. Complete or partial III cranial nerve palsy in a non-diabetic should prompt an immediate imaging evaluation looking for a posterior communicating artery or a superior cerebellar artery aneurysm. Approximately 25% of patients will have preretinal or subhyoid hemorrhages.[41]

The hunt for the etiology of the SAH should culminate in catheter angiography if no aneurysm is disclosed on less invasive imaging studies such as CTA or MRA. Patients are graded clinically using either the Hunt–Hess Scale[42] (Table 7.3) or the World Federation of Neurological Surgeons Subarachnoid Hemorrhage Grading System (WFNS) (Table 7.4).[43] These scales are based on the Glasgow Coma Score (GCS) (Table 7.5).[44]

Direct complications from aneurysmal subarachnoid hemorrhage

Re-bleeding

Re-bleeding is the third most common cause of death from aneurysmal SAH. The rate of re-bleeding is highest within the first 24 hours (4%), with a rate of 1.5% over the first 2 weeks.[39] By 6 months the risk of re-bleeding is 50% without treatment. After 6 months, the re-bleeding rate levels off to approximately 3% per year.[39] When re-rupture does occur it is often fatal or associated with significant neurological deficit.[45] There is an 80% mortality associated with re-bleeding. The goal of early treatment is to prevent re-bleeding by securing the aneurysm by either surgical or endovascular techniques.

Vasospasm

Vasospasm is the leading cause of morbidity and mortality in patients with SAH. The incidence of vasospasm increases with the volume of SAH.[46] Approximately 50–70% of patients will have angiographic evidence of vasospasm, 20–30% will have clinical symptoms from vasospasm, and 10–15% are left with permanent neurological sequelae.[47]

Vasospasm usually occurs within a defined time period after SAH from day 4 to day 14. The etiology of vasospasm is not clear but is related to the release of red blood cells and subsequently oxyhemoglobin into the subarachnoid space. Several other theories also exist.[48–51]

Two forms of vasospasm exist. One is radiographic vasospasm. In this form, the patient has no neurologic symptoms referable to the spasm, but vascular imaging studies such as transcranial Doppler, MRA, or CTA suggest narrowed vessel luminal diameters. Clinical vasospasm represents the form that occurs when patients have new neurologic symptoms in conjunction with imaging studies that suggest narrowed vascular lumen diamters. In addition, other causes of neurologic deterioration such as

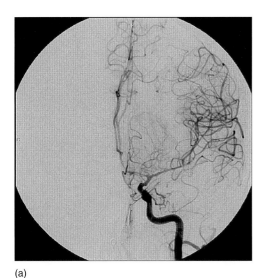

(a)

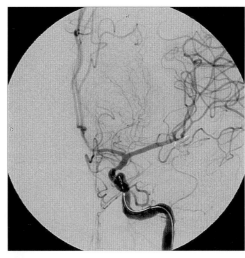

(b)

Figure 7.6
(a) Post subarachnoid hemorrhage with parenchymal hematoma in the left frontal lobe (note the shift of the ipsilateral A2 segment with significant vasospasm of the vessels in the basal cisterns). (b) Post angioplasty the caliber of the A1 and M1 branches are significantly improved.

re-bleeding, hydrocephalus, hypoxemia, hyponatremia, infection, and fever must be ruled out.

Early securing of the aneurysm allows for improved treatment of vasospasm. Treatment of the patient with hypertension, hypervolemia, and hemodilution is often instituted. This is the so-called triple-H therapy. Prophylactic triple-H therapy is instituted in all patients with Hunt–Hess grade 3 and in those with radiographic vasospasm. This treatment consists of keeping the patient on the high end of euvolemia (as measured by central venous pressure) and allowing the systolic blood pressure to seek its own level. At our institution we feel the ideal hematocrit level is in the 32–34 range. If patients develop clinical vasospasm, then active triple-H therapy is instituted. This consists of driving the systolic blood pressure to the 200–220 mmHg range and inserting a Swan–Ganz catheter to achieve a pulmonary capillary wedge pressure (PCWP) in the range of 14–16 mmHg. This must be done expeditiously because no benefit from the treatment of vasospasm is seen if treatment is delayed beyond 4 hours.[52] It should be remembered that patients with clinical vasospasm have a brain at risk of infarction, that this is the clinical correlate of the penumbra concept, and that there is a 'stroke in evolution'. This is a neurologic emergency.

In patients in whom active 'triple-H therapy' fails, intra-arterial administration of nicardipine or another vasodilator with or without balloon angioplasty can be performed (Figure 7.6). Balloon angioplasty has a longer-lasting effect but carries some risk of arterial injury or vessel rupture. Neither of these techniques has been well studied.

Calcium-channel blockers have been studied in aneurysmal SAH. Several large randomized studies have been performed analyzing the effect of nimodipine on vasospasm. The British Aneurysmal Nimodipine Trial (BRANT) showed that there was no significant change in the angiographic appearance of vasospasm, but the rate of poor outcome and stroke decreased from 33% to 20% when nimodipine was given for 21 days after SAH.[53,54] It is standard care to give nimodipine to all patients with aneurysmal SAH. Recent data suggest that good grade patients can have an abbreviated course of nimodipine.[55]

Hydrocephalus

Hydrocephalus is common in patients with aneurysmal SAH (with a rate of 25–70%). The development of hydrocephalus is related to the amount of intraventicular and subarachoid blood. Early treatment of hydrocephalus is performed by external ventricular drainage. It should be considered in all poor grade patients because significant improvement can be observed after such management.

Seizures

Seizures develop in approximately 5% of SAH patients. They usually occur within the first 2 weeks after SAH and have the highest incidence during the first 24 hours. Prophylactic anticonvulsant use remains controversial but is often considered to reduce the risk of seizure before the securing of the aneurysm. Recent data suggest that anticonvulsants should be used for at least 3 days after SAH providing that the aneurysm has been secured.[56]

Diagnosis of aneurysmal subarachnoid hemorrhage

As mentioned above, there is often a high degree of clinical suspicion that prompts further investigations. The first test to be performed is a plain CT scan of the brain. The amount of SAH can be scored using the scale by Fisher et al. (Table 7.6).[46] Figure 7.7 illustrates the CT appearance of a Fisher grade 3 SAH. When this study is performed with a newer-generation scanner within 24 hours of ictus, >97% of SAH can be detected.[39] However, when the diagnosis is delayed and the CT is negative but there is a high degree of clinical suspicion, lumbar puncture is recommended. At our institution, the initial CT is combined with CTA, which is very good at detecting intracranial aneurysms over 2–3 mm in size. Often there is sufficient information obtained from CTA to proceed with treatment planning (Figure 7.8). CTA is used to define the anatomy and often to determine if a patient should undergo surgical clipping or endovascular coil embolization. Surgical clipping of aneurysms can often be performed using CTA alone.

Cerebral angiography remains the gold standard for the diagnosis of intracranial aneurysms. It should be performed when the

Table 7.6 Fisher computed tomography scan classification system for subarachnoid hemorrhage [45]

Fisher grade	Blood on CT*	Score	Vasospasm		
			Angiographic		Clinical vasospasm (DIND)**
			Slight	Severe	
1	No subarachnoid blood detected	11	2	2	0
2	Diffuse or vertical layers <1 mm thick	7	3	0	0
3	Localized clot and/or vertical layer‡ ≥1 mm thick	24	1	23	23
4	Intracerebral or intraventricular clot with diffuse or no SAH	5	2	0	0

SAH, subarachnoid hemorrhage
*Measurements made in the greatest longitudinal and transverse dimension on a CT scan performed within 5 days of SAH in 47 patients
**Delayed ischemic neurological deficits (DINDs)
Reprinted with permission from reference 45.

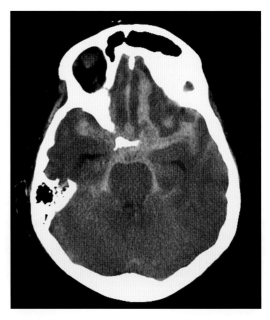

Figure 7.7
(a) CT of a Fisher grade 3 subarachnoid hemorrhage (SAH) from a 10 mm, left ophthalmic artery aneurysm. SAH is seen in the basal cisterns, the subfrontal region, and bilateral Sylvian fissures. Hydrocephalus is present.

plain head CT, the lumbar puncture and the CTA are negative but a high degree of clinical suspicion remains. The angiogram must include all four intracranial vessels and include the external carotid systems as well to search for dural arterial–venous fistulae. Figure 7.8 compares CTA with conventional DSA in a patient with a ruptured right posterior communicating artery aneurysm that was treated with endovascular coiling.

MRI and MRA are also occasionally used in the diagnosis of aneurysmal SAH. They are used in conjunction with CTA and DSA to define anatomy and possible areas of infarction related to the SAH.

Treatment of aneurysmal subarachnoid hemorrhage

Patient selection

Surgical and endovascular techniques are complementary in the management of patients with aneurysmal SAH. The decision on the treatment modality is determined by the patient's age and clinical condition, the aneurysm anatomy, and the operator's experience. Consultation with endovascular and cerebrovascular surgeons is important to decide on the best treatment for the patient.

Presently, patients who present with an aneurysmal SAH are best managed in the setting of a large clinical experience with both endovascular and surgical cases, supported by skilled neurointensivists.[57] Patients are rapidly assessed and examined; measures are taken to ensure adequate airway protection and cardiac stability. Prophylactic phenytoin is given. CT scanning and CTA are performed, and external ventricular drain is

placement performed in patients who have hydrocephalus requiring drainage or who are Hunt–Hess grade 3 or greater.

The majority of middle cerebral artery aneurysms have a wide neck, limiting the potential for acute endovascular coiling, while the location within the Sylvian fissure is readily amenable to surgical exposure and clipping. Otherwise, strategy is guided by the International Subarachnoid Hemorrhage Trial (ISAT), which suggests improved acute clinical outcome with endovascular coiling. However, if successful coiling cannot be performed or is judged too difficult on anatomic grounds, surgery is then performed.

In the 2002 ISAT, a randomized, multi-center studyl compared the safety and efficacy of endovascular coiling to standard neurosurgery clipping for good grade patients after aneurysmal SAH.[58] ISAT has significantly changed the manner in which ruptured aneurysms should be managed. In ISAT, 2143 patients were enrolled at centers mainly from the UK, Europe and Canada. Patients were candidates for the trial when it was deemed that either coiling or clipping were appropriate methods for treatment. The two study groups were similar in baseline characteristics. Endovascular specialists were required to have previously treated 30 or more aneurysms. The experience of the surgeons was not described. The primary outcome was the proportion of patients with a modified Rankin score of 3–6 (dead or disabled) at 1 year. The trial was halted by the steering committee because of a statistically better outcome in the endovascularly treated patients. There were 190 of 801 (23·7%) patients allocated to endovascular treatment that were dependent or dead at 1 year compared with 243 of 793 (30·6%) in the neurosurgical treatment group ($p = 0.0019$). This resulted in a relative and absolute risk reductions in dependency or death of 22·6% (95% CI 8·9–34·2) and 6·9% (95% CI 2·5–11·3) for endovascular versus neurosurgical treatment. The risk of re-bleeding from the ruptured aneurysm after 1 year was 2 per 1276 and 0 per 1081 patient–years for patients allocated endovascular and neurosurgical treatments.

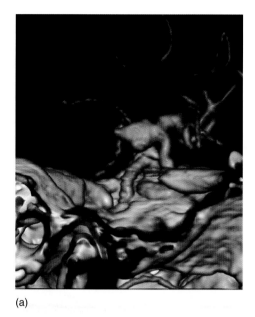

(a)

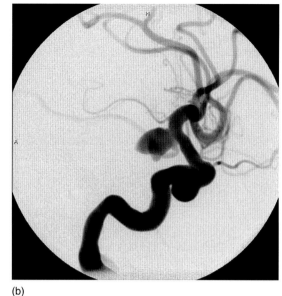

(b)

(c)

Figure 7.8
Comparison between (a) CT angiography and (b) conventional angiography in a 63-year-old woman with subarachnoid hemorrhage from a ruptured right posterior communicating artery aneurysm. (c) This aneurysm was successfully treated with endovascular coil embolization. Note the small thrombus at the neck of the aneurysm. This cleared with time and did not require treatment.

The study concluded that patients with a ruptured intracranial aneurysm for which either surgical clipping or endovascular coiling are acceptable options have an improved outcome in terms of survival free of disability at 1 year with endovascular treatment.

The authors published their 1-year outcomes for 1063 of 1073 patients in the study and 1055 of 1070 patients allocated to neurosurgical treatment.[59] A total of 250 (23·5%) of 1063 patients allocated to endovascular treatment were dead or dependent at 1 year, compared with 326 (30·9%) of 1055 patients allocated to neurosurgery, an absolute risk reduction of 7·4% (95% CI 3·6–11·2, $p = 0.0001$). Nine patients had re-bleeding: seven were in the endovascular group and two were in the surgical group. The risk of epilepsy was significantly lower in the endovascular group. The survival advantage of coiling was maintained for up to 7 years.

The data available to date suggest that the long-term risks of further bleeding from the treated aneurysm are low with either therapy, although somewhat more frequent with endovascular coiling.[60] There are several criticisms of the ISAT study. There was a large percentage of patients that were excluded because either surgery or coiling was the preferred technique (approximately 80%). The majority of the study patients were from the UK and

there was no requirement for the surgeons to have treated a preset number of patients prior to being in the study. The duration of follow-up and use of a mail questionnaire has also been criticized. The durability of coiling is still not known because of the relatively short angiographic follow-up,[61] although initial estimates indicate that re-bleeding rates are unlikely to negate the initial advantages of endovascular treatment over surgical clipping suggested by ISAT.[60]

Surgical clipping

Before the ISAT study, surgical clipping was the standard modality of aneurysm treatment. As emphasized in that study, there is certainly proven durability with surgical clipping. By using an operating microscope and micro-instruments, the majority of anterior circulation aneurysms can be successfully clipped in experienced hands. Once the clip is secured across the neck of the aneurysm and angiography does not reveal any residual aneurysm, the patient is considered cured, although new aneurysms can occur over time.

The Cooperative Study found that patients had a poorer outcome with surgical clipping after SAH when the surgery was performed between day 7 and day 10.[39] This is probably secondary to the peak incidence of vasospasm in these patients. It is not uncommon for patients to present within this window. Our practice is to attempt coiling in these patients. If the patient presents at post-bleed day 7–10 and the aneurysm is not amenable to coiling, we wait until day 11 to proceed with surgical clipping.

Patients who present with acute neurological deterioration from an intracerebral hematoma can be managed in two ways. At our institution, we perform an emergent CTA to define the aneurysm anatomy. In patients with imminent herniation, clot evacuation and aneurysm clipping is performed. In patients who are more stable, we prefer to attempt coiling of the aneurysm followed by surgical evacuation of the aneurysm. Excellent clinical judgment is required in this situation to determine which patients are likely to decompensate, and surgical clot evacuation cannot be delayed.

Specific aneurysms are more likely to be amenable to clipping than coiling. Middle cerebral artery aneurysms are often difficult to coil. This is related to the aneurysm morphology. The majority of these aneurysms are wide-necked and occur at the middle cerebral artery bifurcation. The neck of the aneurysm often incorporates the M2 branches of the middle cerebral artery and the lateral lenticulostriate arteries. In addition, it is often difficult to obtain a safe 'working angle' fluoroscopically to allow the endovascular surgeon to preserve the M2 branches safely. These aneurysms can be formidable to coil and often require adjunctive techniques such as balloon remodeling or stenting. They can be clipped very effectively in expert hands with a lower degree of risk. These aneurysm are more superficial than others, which can makes surgical treatment more straightforward in the setting of an edematous and swollen brain.

Anterior communicating artery aneurysms are another example of aneurysm that often require surgical clipping in preference to coiling. Specific problems related to the coiling of anterior communicating artery aneurysms are the acute angle of the A1 branches of the artery, its wide neck with perforators or branches arising from the neck, and the tortuous carotid anatomy. Posterior directed anterior communicating artery aneurysms are the most difficult to clip because of small anterior communicating artery perforators that are frequently located adjacent to the aneurysm.

Surgical treatment of posterior circulation aneurysm is often more difficult because of limited surgical corridors and injury to brainstem perforators from either the surgical approach or clip placement. This is in contrast to endovascular methods, which work very well for the treatment of posterior circulation aneurysms. This is because of a direct and straight approach up the vertebral artery and into the basilar artery, which facilitates endovascular treatment.

Post-operative or intraoperative angiography should be performed in most patients who undergo aneurym surgery.[62–64] In a consecutive series of 200 patients, intraoperative angiography was deemed to be necessary in 20% of patients.[62] In this study, there was a 0.5% complication rate that was directly attributable to angiography. The authors conclude that, given the frequency of significant disease that remains undetected if intraoperative angiography is used on a selective basis and the low complication rate associated with the procedure, the use of intraoperative angiography should be considered in the majority of aneurysm cases.[62]

Angiography is the best way to ensure complete clipping. The aneurysm can be opened after clipping, but this does not ensure that there is not a significant residual aneurysm.[65] Feuerberg et al. reported a re-bleeding rate of 0.38–0.79% per year from residual aneurysm.[66]

Intraoperative angiography ensures that there is not occlusion of either the parent vessel or a major branch vessel. If it is performed prior to dural closure and immediately after clip application, neurological complications can be reduced. To perform intraoperative cerebral angiography a 5F or 6F sheath is placed into the common femoral artery in the operating room. Depending on the surgeon's room set-up, the right or left groin may be preferred. The sheath is connected to a heparinized saline infusion during the craniotomy. Immediately after placement of the clip, sterile drapes are placed over the craniotomy site and sterile bags are placed over the C-arm. Standard diagnostic catheters are then used to select the vessel of concern. A standard C-arm fluoroscopy unit is used to select the vessel initially and to perform the angiographic runs. Muliple angiographic runs are performed to study completeness of clipping as well as parent and branch vessel patency. If an unsatisfactory clip position is seen, the diagnostic catheter is removed, the clip is immediately readjusted, and repeat angiography is performed.

Endovascular therapy

The Guglielmi Detachable Coil (GDC) was first introduced in 1990.[12,13] There has been a continued increase in the number of aneurysms managed by coil embolization. The addition of adjunctive techniques such as three-dimensional rotational angiography (Figure 7.9), balloon remodeling, stent-assisted coiling, and bioactive coils have further increased the number of aneurysms that can be treated with endovascular techniques. Figure 7.10 illustrates a wide-necked basilar apex aneurysm that was treated with balloon remodeling and Y-stenting with two Neuroform micro-stents.

Anatomic considerations

Aneurysms with a narrow neck are generally considered more suitable for coil embolization. There are several factors that are important for determining whether the patient is a candidate for endovascular coil embolization.[67–69] Aneurysms with a dome to neck ratio of less than 2 have a higher rate of incomplete coil embolization.[67–69] Also related to this are aneurysms with a neck width >4 mm; they also represent a less likely chance of having complete embolization coiling. Aneurysms that are multi-lobulated are more difficult to treat with coil embolization than spherical aneurysms. When the parent or branch vessels are incorporated into the aneurysm, the chances of achieving complete coil occlusion of the aneurysm decrease.[67]

Unstable thrombus and giant aneurysms often have a high rate of re-canalization with coil embolization. A final important anatomical factor relates to the tortuosity of the neck vessels and aorta. The tortuosity can lead to markedly increased difficulty with coiling procedures. This can sometimes be overcome by using extra-long groin sheaths or radial or brachial access for vertebral artery catheterization when the aorta is tortuous.[70–73]

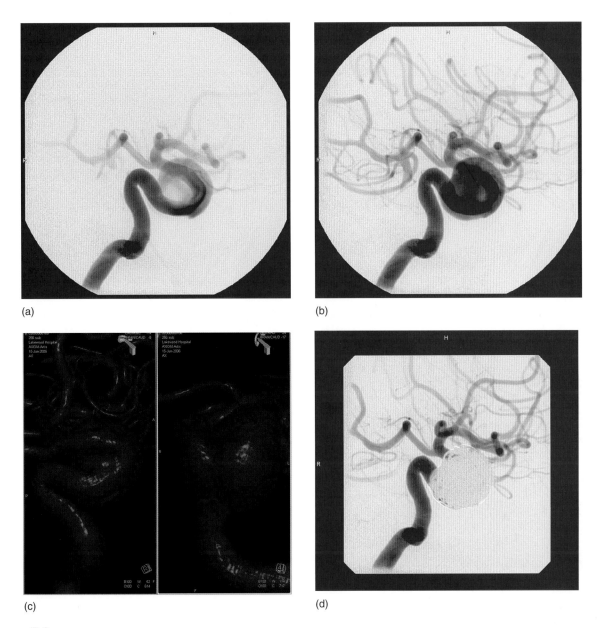

(a)   (b)   (c)   (d)

Figure 7.9
(a) Early and (b) late arterial-phase lateral carotid angiogram showing a large aneurysm of the carotid siphon. Rapid filling precludes optimal demonstration of the neck. (c) Three-dimensional rotational angiography demonstrates the aneurysm neck with high fidelity, facilitating endovascular treatment. (d) Post-coil lateral angiogram.

Technical considerations

Bare platinum coils remain in use today. They consist of a tightly wound platinum wire that is 0.0001–0.003 inches (0.0025–0.0076 mm) in diameter. The coils have a two-dimensional or three-dimensional configuration, depending on the coil type and manufacturer. The coil is deployed into the aneurysm, usually under fluoroscopic roadmap guidance, and then detached. As first described by Guglielmi,[12,13] the detachment of the coil from the pusher wire occurs when an electrical current is passed across the pusher wire–coil junction. The initial coil that is placed should form a basket outlining the wall of the sac of the aneurysm. This is the 'framing coil', and successive coils can then be deployed within this coil.

A newer type of coil has become available in which the platinum coils are covered with a bioactive polymer. An example of this is the Hydrocoil (Microvention, Aliso Viejo, CA). Hydrocoils have a layer of hydrogel polymer around the platinum core. This polymer expands inside the body in a delayed fashion after being hydrated by warm blood. This delay allows for proper coil position and removal if needed. There is a limited working time of approximately 5–7 minutes. After this time, it is not usually possible to remove the coil through the micro-catheter, and often the micro-catheter and coil must be removed from the aneurysm if the position of the coil is unsatisfactory.[74] The fully expanded coils have an increased diameter of 67–107%. This expansion is thought to reduce aneurysm recurrence by increasing packing density and leading to improved endothelization of the aneurysm neck.

Other examples of a bioactive coil are the Matrix coil (Boston Scientific, Fremont, CA) and the Cerecyte coil (Micrus Endovascular, San Jose, CA). The Matrix coil has a platinum core that is covered with a bioactive and bioabsorbable polymer

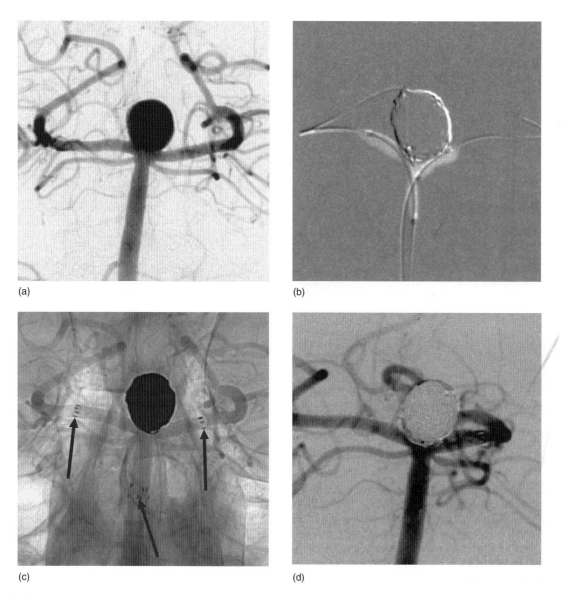

(a)   (b)

(c)   (d)

Figure 7.10

(a) An example of Y-stenting and balloon remodeling for endovascular coiling in a 36 year-old man with an unruptured wide-necked 10 mm basilar apex aneurysm. (b) The patient had bilateral groin access. A micro-catheter has been placed in the aneurysm and a 4 mm × 10 mm Hyperglide balloon (eV3 Neurovascular, Irvine, CA) placed in the right posterior cerebral artery, and a 4 mm × 7 mm Hyperform balloon placed in the left posterior communicating artery, with balloon-assisted coiling of the aneurysm. (c) The native image shows the distal and proximal markers (arrows) of two Neuroform microstents (Boston Scientific, Natick, MA) in a Y-configuration. (d) Final digital subtraction angiogram (left vertebral artery injection) showing complete coil obliteration of the aneurysm. Arrows demonstrate proximal and distal markers of the intersecting stents.

(polyglycolic acid–lactide).[75] The Cerecyte coil has a novel polyglycol acid loaded onto a platinum coil. Neither of these coils expand but are postulated to improve aneurysm thrombosis and healing.

Adjunctive Endovascular Manuevers

The use of an intracranial stent has allowed for wide-necked aneurysms, long the 'contraindication to coiling,' to be effectively treated by endovascular techniques.[76–79] The Neuroform stent (Boston Scientific, Fremont, CA) and the Enterprise Stent (Cordis Neurovascular, Miami Lakes, FL) are approved by the Food and Drug Administration (FDA) for this use in the USA. The stent acts as a bridge to help hold the coils in position inside the aneurysm and to prevent coil herniation into the parent vessel (Figures 7.10, 7.11).

One major disadvantage of the Neuroform stent is the requirement for the patient to be therapeutic on aspirin and clopidogrel in order to prevent serious thromboembolic complications. This limits the application of stenting in patients with acute SAH. Also, patients that require external ventricular drainage after stent placement are at a significantly increased risk of intracerebral hemorrhage from the passage of the drainage catheter through the brain. We prefer to protect the aneurysm dome with coiling and then re-admit patient in the subacute period (2–6 weeks) to perform stent placement and residual aneurysm coiling.

Neuroform stent placement has been described as monotherapy for uncoilable aneurysms (e.g. dissecting pseudoaneurysms) that involve the entire vessel wall. In this case, multiple stents can be placed to help redirect flow through the arterial lumen and away from the aneurysm wall. It is also

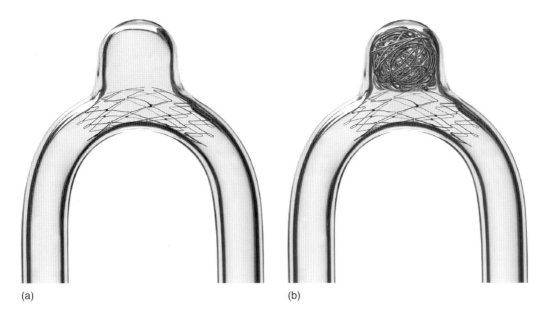

(a)   (b)

Figure 7.11

A clear phantom of a Neuroform stent spanning a wide-neck aneurysm. (b) Neuroform stent with detachable coils.(Courtesy of Boston Scientific, Natick, MA.)

speculated that there is significant endothelial healing that occurs along the stent, and that the previously diseased vessel can remodel over several months.[80,81]

Other novel techniques have been described, such as Y-stent reconstruction of basilar apex aneurysms or other bifurcations aneurysms, trans-posterior communicating artery stenting of basilar apex aneurysms, and trans-anterior communicating artery stenting of carotid terminus aneurysms.[82–85]

Balloon-assisted coiling involves placing a small balloon across the neck of the aneurysm at the point of coil deployment. The balloon helps to mold the coils into the aneurysm and to prevent coil prolapse into the parent vessel. Several authors have reported excellent results with this technique.[86–88] We frequently employ this technique at our institution and find it extremely useful in patients with SAH where stenting is relatively contraindicated with wide necked aneurysms (Figures 7.12, 7.13).

There are several types of balloons available. Two commonly used ones are the Hyperglide and Hyperform balloons (eV3 Neurovascular, Irvine, CA). They are highly compliant balloons that allow for balloon-assisted coiling. The Hyperglide balloon is 4 mm wide and has a length of between 10 mm and 30 mm, depending on the balloon selected. It tends to assume a tubular shape that works well in longer arterial segments such as the internal carotid artery and anterior cerebral artery. The Hyperform balloon is 4 mm × 7 mm is size and is often used at the basilar apex for wide-necked basilar apex aneurysms that may incorporate either of the posterior communicating arteries. It differs from the Hyperglide balloon in that it tends to be more ovoid-shaped and will more readily assume the shape of the space that it is placed within.

Liquid embolic agents for endovascular aneurysm treatment

Onyx (eV3 Neurovascular, Irvine, CA) is a newly available liquid embolic agent approved for pre-surgical embolization of arterial–venous malformations. It is composed of ethylene-vinyl alcohol and micronized tantalum powder suspended in dimethylsulfoxide. Several reports exist of utilizing Onyx to treat intracranial aneurysms.[89–91]

The Cerebral Aneurysm Multi-center European Onyx (CAMEO) trial was undertaken to study the efficacy of Onyx for the treatment of intracranial aneurysms. This multi-center prospective observational study had119 patients with 123 aneurysms that were judged suitable for Onyx treatment.[91] Clinical and angiographic outcomes were recorded at discharge, 3 months, and 12 months. Of 71 aneurysm with available 12-month follow-up, 56 (79%) had complete occlusion. Procedure- or device-related permanent neurologic morbidity at final follow-up was present in eight of 97 patients.[91] Onyx HD 500 has recently been approved by the FDA, which will very likely lead to an increase in the use of Onyx for treatment of intracranial aneurysms. Further studies are needed to determine its final safety and efficacy. Presently this technique is most often employed in North American for vessel sacrifice in peripheral, mycotic aneurysms where the patients are poor candidates (usually because of valvular heart disease) for operative clipping (Figure 7.14).

Deconstructive techniques for treatment of aneurysms

In some instances, parent vessel arterial sacrifice is a viable option over coil embolization or surgical clipping. Proximal arterial ligation often leads to a change in the hemodynamic flow pattern of the aneurysm and can cause thrombosis of the aneurysm. Traditionally, surgical clipping was the mainstay of treatment but endovascular techniques are being used more frequently.[92] Aneurysms of the vertebral artery can often be cured by deliberate occlusion at the site of the aneurysm, with relatively good results.[93] There are several indications for arterial sacrifice. They include symptomatic cavernous internal carotid artery aneurysm, arterial dissections of the anterior or posterior circulation, fusiform aneurysms, and recurrent aneurysms that are not amenable to repeat coiling or surgical treatment. Complications related to this treatment include unintended branch vessel occlusion, thromboembolic events, and stroke from unanticipated poor collateral circulation.

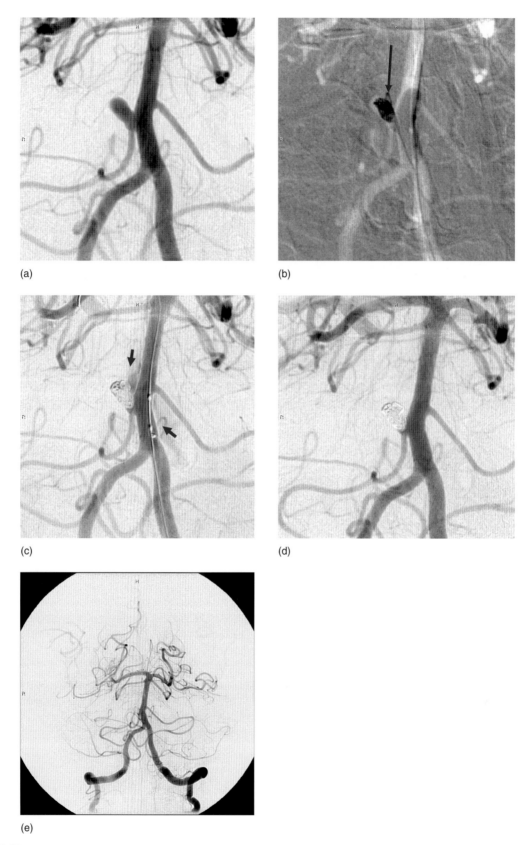

Figure 7.12

(a) Anterior inferior cerebellar artery aneurysm angiogram following subarachnoid hemorrhage. (b) Balloon-assisted coiling demonstrating errant coil loop above the expected location of the aneurysm dome. (c) Post-re-positioning of the coil demonstrating extravasation of contrast (arrows). Heparin was reversed, ventriculostomy opened, balloon re-inflated, and additional soft, smaller coils placed. (d, e) Repeat angiography demonstrates good, brisk filling of the intracranial circulation with no additional extravasation.

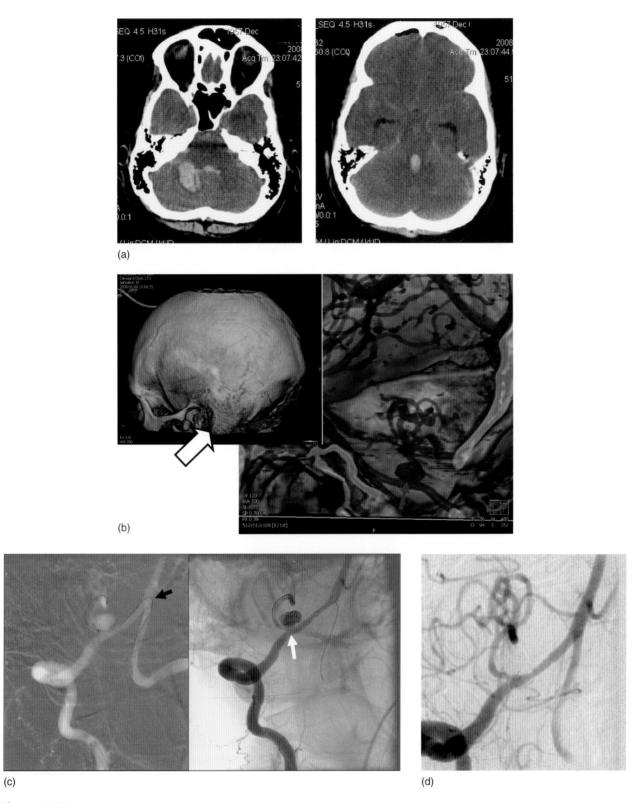

Figure 7.13

(a) CT scan in a 50-year-old women who presented with Hunt–Hess 4 status after a Fischer grade 4 subarachnoid hemorrhage. (b) CT angiogram viewed as through the left mastoid and occiput demonstrating a wide-necked right posterior inferior cerebellary artery (PICA) aneurysm arising from a proximal PICA that supplies both cerebellar hemispheres (a normal variant). (c) The approach to the parent artery by the re-modeling balloon is most direct from above (i.e. across the vertebrobasilar junction) (black arrow), while the aneurysm dome can be directly approached from below via the ipsilateral vertebral artery (white arrow). (d) Post-coil right vertebral angiogram.

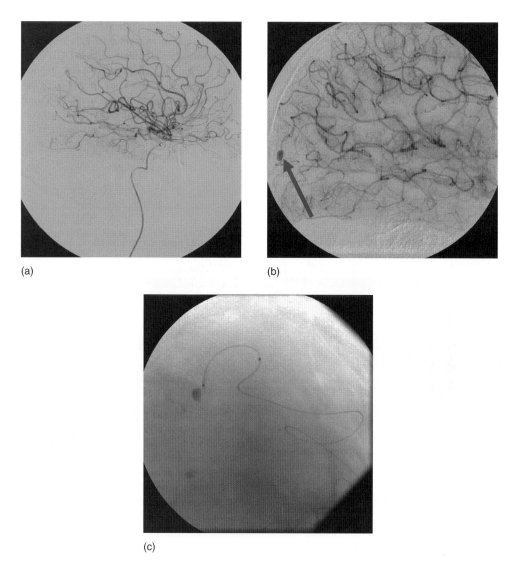

Figure 7.14
(a,b) Lateral view of a conventional carotid angiogram in a patient with endocarditis. While the early arterial phase appears normal, delayed and magnified views demonstrate a mycotic aneurysm. (c) Selective catheterization of a pial pedicle during Onyx embolization.

Prior to undertaking internal carotid artery parent vessel occlusion, the patient can undergo an 'awake temporary balloon test occlusion' to assess collateral supply. Adjunctive methods such as somatosensory evoked potentials, motor evoked potentials, and electroencephalography can be utilized. As technological improvements have been made in endovascular devices, the indications for deconstructive aneurysm treatment have become decreasingly common.

Complications of endovascular aneurysm therapy

Aneurysm rupture

Intraprocedural aneurysm rupture is reported to occur in 2–8% of cases.[94] The result can be catastrophic and life-threatening but this is not always the case. Rupture occurs from protrusion of the coil or micro-catheter or from microwire perforation through the aneurysm dome. Anecdotally, we have seen this more commonly in cases of acute SAH using balloon remodeling where the balloon fixes the coiling catheter in place and does not allow 'unloading' of the forward force of the advancing coil by displacement of the catheter from the aneurysm lumen (i.e. the coil is unloaded by perforating the aneurysm) (see Figure 7.12). When perforation occurs, the following steps should be taken: the heparin (if used) should be reversed immediately with protamine sulfate; coils should be delivered to the remainder of the aneurysm and, if present, a balloon can be inflated across the neck of the aneurysm; and the blood pressure should be lowered to a mean arterial pressure of 60–70 mmHg. The remaining lumen of the aneurysm should be coil occluded as rapidly as possible. If an external ventricular drain is not present this should be considered immediately; if it is present it should be opened at 0 cmH$_2$O.

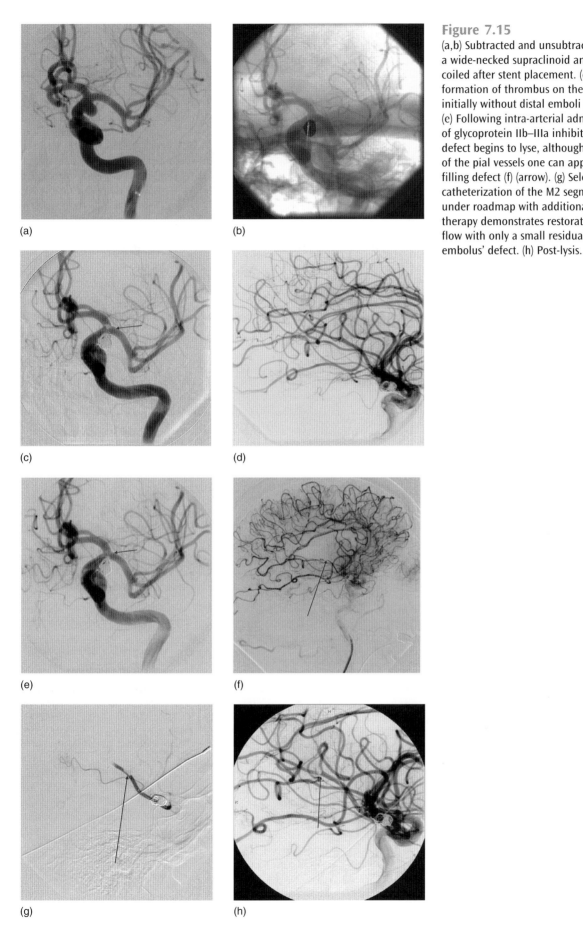

Figure 7.15
(a,b) Subtracted and unsubtracted views of a wide-necked supraclinoid aneurysm, coiled after stent placement. (c) Delayed formation of thrombus on the stent (arrow), initially without distal emboli (d).
(e) Following intra-arterial administration of glycoprotein IIb–IIIa inhibitors, the filling defect begins to lyse, although in the views of the pial vessels one can appreciate a filling defect (f) (arrow). (g) Selective catheterization of the M2 segment under roadmap with additional lytic therapy demonstrates restoration of distal flow with only a small residual 'saddle embolus' defect. (h) Post-lysis.

(a)

(b)

(c)

(d)

(e)

(f)

(g)

(h)

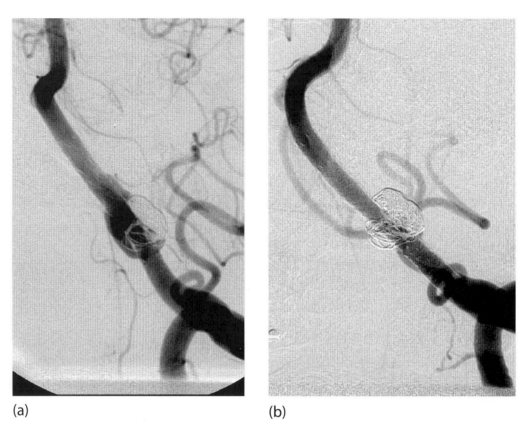

(a)   (b)

Figure 7.16
A 48-year-old man presented with an unruptured left V4 segment vertebral artery aneurysm. The initial treatment was placement of a coronary stent and balloon-assisted coiling. (a) The patient had enlargement of the aneurysm and underwent placement of two Neuroform stents (Boston Scientific, Freemont, California) within the coronary stent. However, the aneurysm continued to enlarge. (b) Immediately following placement of two 4.25 mm × 20 mm Pipeline embolization devices (Chestnut Medical Technologies, Menlo Park, California), there has been complete occlusion of the fusiform aneurysm with restoration of normal vessel anatomy of the V4 segment of the vertebral artery. This result was maintained during serial angiographic follow-up to 1 year. There were no periprocedural or post-procedural complications noted.

Thromboembolic complications

Thromboembolic complications have been reported as occurring in 2.5–28% of patients.[95,96] This risk can be significantly reduced by heparinizing the patient during the procedure and loading the patient with aspirin and clopidrogel in the setting of possible stenting. Difficulty arises in the setting of SAH, when heparinization is more dangerous and loading with aspirin and clopidrogel is relatively contraindicated, especially if there is to be a future placement of an external ventricular drain. In our experience, the risk of thromboemboli is relatively low, and aggressive over-heparinization is not warranted in SAH. When thromboembolic complications arise, they are usually from activation of platelets on the coil surface. Intra-arterial or intravenous glycoprotein IIb–IIIa inhibitors work very effectively to prevent further clot formation, and their use often leads to dissolution of the aggregated platelets.[97] Our strategy in the setting of thromboembolism formation is to ensure that the anticoagulation time is between 250 and 300 seconds and then to administer an intra-arterial IIb–IIIa inhibitor, followed by serial angiographic runs until improvement or at least clot stability is obtained (Figure 7.15). This strategy is safe even in the setting of acute SAH. Patients are then placed on aspirin and occasionally clopidrogel for 2–3 weeks, and also on low-dose intravenous heparin for the next 24 hours. It is vital to follow these patients with transcranial Doppler studies, MRI with diffusion-weighted imaging, and repeat angiography if necessary.

Coils in the parent vessel and misplaced coils

Rarely, a coil can embolize from the aneurysm into the distal circulation. If this situation arises, several measures can be taken. If the coil is small and has embolized distally and it is not occlusive, the patient can be left on aspirin, although there is the risk of more distal embolism. Two devices, the Amplatz Nitinol Microsnare (Microvena, Vadnais Heights, MN) and the Alligator Retrieval Device (Chestnut Medical Technologies, Menlo Park, CA) can both be used to extract coils from the parent vessel.[98,99] As one would expect, this procedure carries an increased risk of vessel perforation and dissection, but if the coil is occluding a major vessel the risk is warranted.

On occasions is there will be one or more coil loops that protrude into the parent vessel. This is usually not clinically significant, and if there is no limitation of flow the patient can be managed conservatively and is usually placed on aspirin with or without clopidogrel for 2–4 weeks. If the patient has been previously loaded on aspirin and clopidogrel, consideration can be given to placing a stent across the aneurysm to attempt to move the prolapsed coil back into position or to trap it against the vessel wall. This strategy increases the risk of the procedure and necessitates post-procedural antiplatelet therapy, which in itself is not risk-free. A final strategy is to place a balloon across the neck of the aneurysm and attempt to drive the loop back into the aneurysm. This technique is moderately successful in our hands.

Post-coiling follow-up strategy and re-canalization

Until the long-term durability of coiling is known, patients should be carefully followed for aneurysm recurrence. At our institution we perform a 6-month angiogram on most patients but have begun to rely on MRA in some patients. If the aneurysm appears to be completely coiled, the patient is followed by MRI or MRA. If there is residual neck or a slight recurrence, the patient undergoes repeat angiography at 1 year and then at 3 years.

Re-canalization of embolized aneurysms has been reported at a wide range of frequencies in the literature, ranging from 10% to 50%, with an average of 20–35%.[100–103] Re-canalization is affected by size, with greater stability seen in small embolized aneurysms and lesser stability in large and giant aneurysms.[101,103] When re-canalization occurs, a decision must be made about re-treatment.

To follow the coiled aneurysms with MRA, we use 1.5 Tesla contrast-enhanced three-dimensional MRA using a three-dimensional ultrafast spoiled gradient-recalled acquisition in the steady state (SPGR) sequence.[104] This sequence provides very clear anatomical definition of the parent vessel. We have found that this sequence will detect re-canalizations >3 mm. The ability to detect aneurysm re-canalization >3 mm is important because this is the size for which we will consider re-treatment. When there is a residual neck, we will generally follow these patients when the neck size is <4 mm.

When recanalization is detected on either angiography or MRA, a decision about for re-treatment must be made. Several factors are important when deciding on re-treatment. The size of the re-canalization is the most important. It is likely that smaller recanalizations can be followed, but they must be carefully followed. Any noticeable change in the degree of re-canalization is an indication for treatment. Large re-canalizations warrant treatment. Re-treatment options include repeat coiling, stent-assisted coiling, and surgical clipping.

Future devices and innovations

There are newer devices on the horizon that will expand the spectrum of aneurysms that can be treated by endovascular techniques. The use of covered stents has been shown to be effective for the definitive treatment of wide-necked aneurysms.[81,105] However, these devices are often stiff and difficult to navigate into the intracranial circulation. The development of newer stents is on the horizon. While not covered these devices have a much higher metal surface area. Also, they are much softer and therefore navigation into the intracranial circulation is easier. When multiple stents are deployed, aneurysm thrombosis can be induced without entering the aneurysm as with coil embolization. However, this may raise some concerns relative to branch vessel or parent vessel thrombosis. These stents are not commercially available.

One example of this kind of stent is the Pipeline Neuroendovascular Device (Chestnut Medical Technologies, Menlo Park, CA). The Pipeline device is a braided, tubular, bi-metallic endoluminal implant. It can occlude both saccular and fusiform aneurysms by disrupting flow along the aneurysm neck or inside the fusiform component of the aneurysm.[106] Currently, the device is not approved for use in the USA by the FDA, but it has been used under an emergency FDA exemption in two patients.[107] Both patients had wide-necked V4 segment vertebral artery aneurysms that had failed other endovascular treatments. (Figure 7.16 shows a patient who had undergone two previous treatments with placement of a coronary stent and balloon-assisted coiling followed by placement of two Neuroform stents when the aneurysm enlarged. After the placement of the three stents and attempted coiling, the aneurysm had further enlargement (see Figure 7.16a). After placement of two Pipeline Emboli Devices, an immediate and complete occlusion of the aneurysm and anatomical reconstruction of the vertebral artery was achieved (see Figure 7.16b). Angiographic follow-up at 6 months and 12 months showed continued cure. The Pipeline device and other new treatment modalities are allowing for the safe and effective treatment of previously untreatable vascular lesions.

Summary

Intracranial aneurysms represent unique surgical and endovascular challenges. Surgical clipping and endovascular coiling should not be viewed as competing techniques but as complementary modalities. Patients are best managed in a setting where both treatments can be readily offered in an unbiased manner.

References

1. Drake CG. Gordon Murray lecture. Evolution of intracranial aneurysm surgery. Can J Surg 1984; 27: 549–55.
2. Dandy WE. Intracranial aneurysms of the internal carotid artery cured by surgery. Ann Surg 1938; 107: 654–9.
3. Greenwood J Jr. Two point coagulation: a follow-up report of a new technic and instrument for electrocoagulation in neurosurgery. Arch Phys Ther 1942; 23: 552–4.
4. McFadden JT. History of the operating microscope: from magnifying glass to microneurosurgery. Neurosurgery 2000; 46: 511.
5. Kassell NF, Torner JC, Jane JA, Halley EC Jr., Adams HP. The International Cooperative Study on the Timing of Aneurysm Surgery. Part 2: surgical results. J Neurosurg 1990; 73: 37–47.
6. Mistretta CA, Crummy AB, Strother CM. Digital angiography: a perspective. Radiology 1981; 139: 273–6.
7. Teitelbaum GP, Larsen DW, Zelman V et al. A tribute to Dr Fedor A Serbinenko, founder of endovascular neurosurgery. Neurosurgery 2000; 46: 462–9.
8. Berenstein A, Ransohoff J, Kupersmith M, Flamm E, Graeb D. Transvascular treatment of giant aneurysms of the cavernous carotid and vertebral arteries. Functional investigation and embolization. Surg Neurol 1984; 21: 3–12.
9. Debrun G, Lacour P, Caron JP et al. Treatment of carotid-cavernous vascular lesions by inflatable and detachable baloon. [in French] Nouv Presse Med 1976; 5: 1294–6.
10. Hieshima GB, Grinnell VS, Mehringer CM. A detachable balloon for therapeutic transcatheter occlusions. Radiology 1981; 138: 227–8.

11. Engelson E. Catheter for guide-wire tracking. United States patent: 4739768. Application number: 06/869597. April 26, 1988.

12. Guglielmi G, Vinuela F, Dion J, Duckwiler G. Electrothrombosis of saccular aneurysms via endovascular approach. Part 2: Preliminary clinical experience. J Neurosurg 1991; 75: 8–14.

13. Guglielmi G, Vinuela F, Sepetka I, Macellari V. Electrothrombosis of saccular aneurysms via endovascular approach. Part 1: Electrochemical basis, technique, and experimental results. J Neurosurg 1991; 75: 1–7.

14. Ferguson GG. Physical factors in the initiation, growth, and rupture of human intracranial saccular aneurysms. J Neurosurg 1972; 37: 666–77.

15. Rhoton AL Jr. Anatomy of saccular aneurysms. Surg Neurol 1980; 14: 59–66.

16. Sekhar LN, Heros RC. Origin, growth, and rupture of saccular aneurysms: a review. Neurosurgery 1981; 8: 248–60.

17. Inagawa T, Hirano A. Autopsy study of unruptured incidental intracranial aneurysms. Surg Neurol 1990; 34: 361–5.

18. Rinkel GJ. Intracranial aneurysm screening: indications and advice for practice. Lancet Neurol 2005; 4: 122–8.

19. Canham PB, Ferguson GG. A mathematical model for the mechanics of saccular aneurysms. Neurosurgery 1985; 17: 291–5.

20. Fick GM, Gabow PA. Natural history of autosomal dominant polycystic kidney disease. Annu Rev Med 1994; 45: 23–9.

21. Gieteling EW, Rinkel GJ. Characteristics of intracranial aneurysms and subarachnoid haemorrhage in patients with polycystic kidney disease. J Neurol 2003; 250: 418–23.

22. Norrgard O, Angquist KA, Fodstad H et al. Intracranial aneurysms and heredity. Neurosurgery 1987; 20: 236–9.

23. Schievink WI, Schaid DJ, Michels VV, Piepgras DG. Familial aneurysmal subarachnoid hemorrhage: a community-based study. J Neurosurg 1995; 83: 426–9.

24. Wills S, Ronkainen A, van der Voet M et al. Familial intracranial aneurysms: an analysis of 346 multiplex Finnish families. Stroke 2003; 34: 1370–4.

25. Broderick JP, Sauerbeck LR, Foroud T et al. The Familial Intracranial Aneurysm (FIA) study protocol. BMC Med Genet 2005; 6: 17.

26. Bailey IC. Familial subarachnoid haemorrhage. Ulster Med J 1993; 62: 119–26.

27. Greene KA, Jacobowitz R, Marciano FF et al. Impact of traumatic subarachnoid hemorrhage on outcome in nonpenetrating head injury. Part II: relationship to clinical course and outcome variables during acute hospitalization. J Trauma 1996; 41: 964–71.

28. Greene KA, Marciano FF, Johnson BA et al. Impact of traumatic subarachnoid hemorrhage on outcome in nonpenetrating head injury. Part I: a proposed computerized tomography grading scale. J Neurosurg 1995; 83: 445–52.

29. Inagawa T, Takahashi M, Aoki H et al. Aneurysmal subarachnoid hemorrhage in Izumo City and Shimane Prefecture of Japan. Outcome. Stroke 1988; 19: 176–80.

30. Ingall TJ, Whisnant JP, Wiebers DO et al. Has there been a decline in subarachnoid hemorrhage mortality? Stroke 1989; 20: 718–24.

31. Pakarinen S. Incidence, aetiology, and prognosis of primary subarachnoid haemorrhage. A study based on 589 cases diagnosed in a defined urban population during a defined period. Acta Neurol Scand 1967; 43 (29 Suppl): 1–8.

32. Sacco RL, Wolf PA, Bharucha NE et al. Subarachnoid and intracerebral hemorrhage: natural history, prognosis, and precursive factors in the Framingham Study. Neurology 1984; 34: 847–54.

33. Sarti C, Tuomilehto J, Salomaa V et al. Epidemiology of subarachnoid hemorrhage in Finland from 1983 to 1985. Stroke 1991; 22: 848–53.

34. Truelsen T, Bonita R, Duncan J et al. Changes in subarachnoid hemorrhage mortality, incidence, and case fatality in New Zealand between 1981–1983 and 1991–1993. Stroke 1998; 29: 2298–303.

35. Juvela S, Porras M, Heiskanen O. Natural history of unruptured intracranial aneurysms: a long-term follow-up study. J Neurosurg 1993; 79: 174–82.

36. Wieber DO, Whisnant JP, Huston J et al. Unruptured intracranial aneurysms: natural history, clinical outcomes, and risks of surgical and endovascular treatment. Lancet 2003; 362: 103–10.

37. Rasmussen PA, Mayberg MR. Defining the natural history of unruptured aneurysms. Stroke 2004; 35: 232–3.

38. Feigin V, Parag V, Lawes CM et al. Smoking and elevated blood pressure are the most important risk factors for subarachnoid hemorrhage in the Asia–Pacific region: an overview of 26 cohorts involving 306,620 participants. Stroke 2005; 36: 1360–5.

39. Nishioka H, Torner JC, Graf CJ et al. Cooperative study of intracranial aneurysms and subarachnoid hemorrhage: a long-term prognostic study. III. Subarachnoid hemorrhage of undetermined etiology. Arch Neurol 1984; 41: 1147–51.

40. Hop JW, Rinkel GJ, Algra A et al. Case–fatality rates and functional outcome after subarachnoid hemorrhage: a systematic review. Stroke 1997; 28: 660–4.

41. Stiebel-Kalish H, Turtel LS, Kupersmith MJ. The natural history of nontraumatic subarachnoid hemorrhage-related intraocular hemorrhages. Retina 2004; 24: 36–40.

42. Hunt WE, Hess RM. Surgical risk as related to time of intervention in the repair of intracranial aneurysms. J Neurosurg 1968; 28: 14–20.

43. Teasdale GM, Drake CG, Hunt W et al. A universal subarachnoid hemorrhage scale: report of a committee of the World Federation of Neurosurgical Societies. J Neurol Neurosurg Psychiatry 1988; 51: 1457.

44. Teasdale G, Jennett B. Assessment of coma and impaired consciousness. A practical scale. Lancet 1974; 2: 81–4.

45. Broderick JP, Brott TG, Duldner JE et al. Initial and recurrent bleeding are the major causes of death following subarachnoid hemorrhage. Stroke 1994; 25: 1342–7.

46. Fisher CM, Kistler JP, Davis JM. Relation of cerebral vasospasm to subarachnoid hemorrhage visualized by computerized tomographic scanning. Neurosurgery 1980; 6: 1–9.

47. Solenski NJ, Haley EC Jr, Kassell NF et al. Medical complications of aneurysmal subarachnoid hemorrhage: a report of the multicenter, cooperative aneurysm study. Participants of the Multicenter Cooperative Aneurysm Study. Crit Care Med 1995; 23: 1007–17.

48. Allen GS, Ahn HS, Preziosi TJ et al. Cerebral arterial spasm—a controlled trial of nimodipine in patients with subarachnoid hemorrhage. N Engl J Med 1983; 308: 619–24.

49. Asano T. Oxyhemoglobin as the principal cause of cerebral vasospasm: a holistic view of its actions. Crit Rev Neurosurg 1999; 9: 303–18.

50. Meguro T, Chen B, Lancon J et al. Oxyhemoglobin induces caspase-mediated cell death in cerebral endothelial cells. J Neurochem 2001; 77: 1128–35.

51. Pluta RM. Delayed cerebral vasospasm and nitric oxide: review, new hypothesis, and proposed treatment. Pharmacol Ther 2005; 105: 23–56.

52. Armonda RA, Thomas JE, Rosenwasser RH. Early and aggressive treatment of medically intractable cerebral vasospasm with pentobarbital coma, cerebral angioplasty and ICP reduction. Neurosurg Focus 1998; 5: e7.

53. Pickard JD, Murray GD, Illingworth R et al. Oral nimodipine and cerebral ischaemia following subarachnoid haemorrhage. Br J Clin Pract 1990; 44: 66–7.

54. Pickard JD, Murray GD, Illingworth R et al. Effect of oral nimodipine on cerebral infarction and outcome after subarachnoid haemorrhage: British aneurysm nimodipine trial. BMJ 1989; 298: 636–42.

55. Toyota BD. The efficacy of an abbreviated course of nimodipine in patients with good-grade aneurysmal subarachnoid hemorrhage. J Neurosurg 1999; 90: 203–6.

56. Chumnanvej S, Dunn IF, Kim DH. Three-day phenytoin prophylaxis is adequate after subarachnoid hemorrhage. Neurosurgery 2007; 60: 99–102; discussion-3.

57. Hoh BL, Rabinov JD, Pryor JC, Carter BS, Barker FG, II. In-hospital morbidity and mortality after endovascular treatment of unruptured

intracranial aneurysms in the United States, 1996–2000: effect of hospital and physician volume. American Journal of Neuroradiology 2003; 24: 1409–20.

58. Molyneux A, Kerr R, Stratton I et al. International Subarachnoid Aneurysm Trial (ISAT) of neurosurgical clipping versus endovascular coiling in 2143 patients with ruptured intracranial aneurysms: a randomised trial. Lancet 2002; 360: 1267–74.

59. Molyneux AJ, Kerr RS, Yu LM et al. International subarachnoid aneurysm trial (ISAT) of neurosurgical clipping versus endovascular coiling in 2143 patients with ruptured intracranial aneurysms: a randomised comparison of effects on survival, dependency, seizures, rebleeding, subgroups, and aneurysm occlusion. Lancet 2005; 366: 809–17.

60. CARAT investigators. Rates of delayed rebleeding from intracranial aneurysms are low after surgical and endovascular treatment. Stroke 2006; 37: 1437–42.

61. Diringer MN. To clip or to coil acutely ruptured intracranial aneurysms: update on the debate. Curr Opin Crit Care 2005; 11: 121–5.

62. Klopfenstein JD, Spetzler RF, Kim LJ et al. Comparison of routine and selective use of intraoperative angiography during aneurysm surgery: a prospective assessment. J Neurosurg 2004; 100: 230–5.

63. Chiang VL, Gailloud P, Murphy KJ et al. Routine intraoperative angiography during aneurysm surgery. J Neurosurg 2002; 96: 988–92.

64. Tang G, Cawley CM, Dion JE, Barrow DL. Intraoperative angiography during aneurysm surgery: a prospective evaluation of efficacy. J Neurosurg 2002; 96: 993–9.

65. Lin T, Fox AJ, Drake CG. Regrowth of aneurysm sacs from residual neck following aneurysm clipping. J Neurosurg 1989; 70: 556–60.

66. Feuerberg I, Lindquist C, Lindqvist M, Steiner L. Natural history of postoperative aneurysm rests. J Neurosurg 1987; 66: 30–4.

67. Kiyosue H, Tanoue S, Okahara M et al. Anatomic features predictive of complete aneurysm occlusion can be determined with three-dimensional digital subtraction angiography. AJNR Am J Neuroradiol 2002; 23: 1206–13.

68. Debrun GM, Aletich VA, Kehrli P et al. Selection of cerebral aneurysms for treatment using Guglielmi detachable coils: the preliminary University of Illinois at Chicago experience. Neurosurgery 1998; 43: 1281–95; discussion 96–7.

69. Vinuela F, Duckwiler G, Mawad M. Guglielmi detachable coil embolization of acute intracranial aneurysm: perioperative anatomical and clinical outcome in 403 patients. J Neurosurg 1997; 86: 475–82.

70. Fessler RD, Wakhloo AK, Lanzino G et al. Transradial approach for vertebral artery stenting: technical case report. Neurosurgery 2000; 46: 1524–7.

71. Levy EI, Boulos AS, Fessler RD et al. Transradial cerebral angiography: an alternative route. Neurosurgery 2002; 51: 335–40.

72. Levy EI, Kim SH, Bendok BR et al. Transradial stenting of the cervical internal carotid artery: technical case report. Neurosurgery 2003; 53: 448–51.

73. Rigatelli G, Magro B, Maronati L et al. An improved technique for gaining radial artery access in endovascular interventions. Cardiovasc Revasc Med 2006; 7: 46–7.

74. Arthur AS, Wilson SA, Dixit S, Barr JD. Hydrogel-coated coils for the treatment of cerebral aneurysms: preliminary results. Neurosurg Focus 2005; 18: E1.

75. Murayama Y, Vinuela F, Ishii A et al. Initial clinical experience with matrix detachable coils for the treatment of intracranial aneurysms. J Neurosurg 2006; 105: 192–9.

76. Fiorella D, Albuquerque FC, Deshmukh VR, McDougall CG. Usefulness of the Neuroform stent for the treatment of cerebral aneurysms: results at initial (3–6-mo) follow-up. Neurosurgery 2005; 56: 1191–201; discussion 201–2.

77. Fiorella D, Albuquerque FC, Deshmukh VR, et al. Endovascular reconstruction with the Neuroform stent as monotherapy for the treatment of uncoilable intradural pseudoaneurysms. Neurosurgery 2006; 59: 291–300; discussion 291–300.

78. Fiorella D, Albuquerque FC, Han P, McDougall CG. Preliminary experience using the Neuroform stent for the treatment of cerebral aneurysms. Neurosurgery 2004; 54: 6–16; discussion-7.

79. Fiorella D, Albuquerque FC, Masaryk TJ, Rasmussen PA, McDougall CG. Balloon-in-stent technique for the constructive endovascular treatment of "ultra-wide necked" circumferential aneurysms. Neurosurgery 2005; 57: 1218–27; discussion-27.

80. Fiorella D, Albuquerque FC, Deshmukh VR et al. In-stent stenosis as a delayed complication of neuroform stent-supported coil embolization of an incidental carotid terminus aneurysm. AJNR 2004; 25: 1764–7.

81. Nelson PK, Sahlein D, Shapiro M et al. Recent steps toward a reconstructive endovascular solution for the orphaned, complex-neck aneurysm. Neurosurgery 2006; 59: S77–S92.

82. Chow MM, Woo HH, Masaryk TJ, et al. A novel endovascular treatment of a wide-necked basilar apex aneurysm by using a Y-configuration, double-stent technique. AJNR Am J Neuroradiol 2004; 25: 509–12.

83. Thorell WE, Chow MM, Woo HH et al. Y-configured dual intracranial stent-assisted coil embolization for the treatment of wide-necked basilar tip aneurysms. Neurosurgery 2005; 56: 1035–40.

84. Cross DT 3rd, Moran CJ, Derdeyn CP et al. Neuroform stent deployment for treatment of a basilar tip aneurysm via a posterior communicating artery route. AJNR Am J Neuroradiol 2005; 26: 2578–81.

85. Moret J, Ross IB, Weill A, Piotin M. The retrograde approach: a consideration for the endovascular treatment of aneurysms. AJNR 2000; 21: 262–8.

86. Cottier JP, Pasco A, Gallas S et al. Utility of balloon-assisted Guglielmi detachable coiling in the treatment of 49 cerebral aneurysms: a retrospective, multicenter study. AJNR Am J Neuroradiol 2001; 22: 345–51.

87. Nelson PK, Levy DI. Balloon-assisted coil embolization of wide-necked aneurysms of the internal carotid artery: medium-term angiographic and clinical follow-up in 22 patients. AJNR Am J Neuroradiol 2001; 22: 19–26.

88. Malek AM, Halbach VV, Phatouros CC et al. Balloon-assist technique for endovascular coil embolization of geometrically difficult intracranial aneurysms. Neurosurgery 2000; 46: 1397–406.

89. Cekirge HS, Saatci I, Geyik S, et al. Intrasaccular combination of metallic coils and onyx liquid embolic agent for the endovascular treatment of cerebral aneurysms. J Neurosurg 2006; 105: 706–12.

90. Weber W, Siekmann R, Kis B et al. Treatment and follow-up of 22 unruptured wide-necked intracranial aneurysms of the internal carotid artery with Onyx HD 500. AJNR Am J Neuroradiol 2005; 26: 1909–15.

91. Molyneux AJ, Cekirge S, Saatci I, Gal G. Cerebral Aneurysm Multicenter European Onyx (CAMEO) trial: results of a prospective observational study in 20 European centers. AJNR Am J Neuroradiol 2004; 25: 39–51.

92. Steinberg GK, Drake CG, Peerless SJ. Deliberate basilar or vertebral artery occlusion in the treatment of intracranial aneurysms. Immediate results and long-term outcome in 201 patients. J Neurosurg 1993; 79: 161–73.

93. Graves VB, Perl J 2nd, Strother CM et al. Endovascular occlusion of the carotid or vertebral artery with temporary proximal flow arrest and microcoils: clinical results. AJNR Am J Neuroradiol 1997; 18: 1201–6.

94. Levy E, Koebbe CJ, Horowitz MB et al. Rupture of intracranial aneurysms during endovascular coiling: management and outcomes. Neurosurgery 2001; 49: 807–11.

95. Koebbe CJ, Veznedaroglu E, Jabbour P et al. Endovascular management of intracranial aneurysms: current experience and future advances. Neurosurgery 2006; 59: S93–102; discussion S3–S13.

96. Pelz DM, Lownie SP, Fox AJ. Thromboembolic events associated with the treatment of cerebral aneurysms with Guglielmi detachable coils. AJNR Am J Neuroradiol 1998; 19: 1541–7.

97. Fiorella D, Albuquerque FC, Han P, McDougall CG. Strategies for the management of intraprocedural thromboembolic complications with abciximab (ReoPro). Neurosurgery 2004; 54: 1089–97; discussion 97–8.

98. Henkes H, Lowens S, Preiss H et al. A new device for endovascular coil retrieval from intracranial vessels: alligator retrieval device. AJNR Am J Neuroradiol 2006; 27: 327–9.

99. Dinc H, Kuzeyli K, Kosucu P et al. Retrieval of prolapsed coils during endovascular treatment of cerebral aneurysms. Neuroradiology 2006; 48: 269–72.

100. Henkes H, Fischer S, Mariushi W et al. Angiographic and clinical results in 316 coil-treated basilar artery bifurcation aneurysms. J Neurosurg 2005; 103: 990–9.

101. Murayama Y, Nien YL, Duckwiler G et al. Guglielmi detachable coil embolization of cerebral aneurysms: 11 years' experience. J Neurosurg 2003; 98: 959–66.

102. Ng P, Khangure MS, Phatouros CC et al. Endovascular treatment of intracranial aneurysms with Guglielmi detachable coils: analysis of midterm angiographic and clinical outcomes. Stroke 2002; 33: 210–17.

103. Raymond J, Guilbert F, Weill A et al. Safety, science, and sales: a request for valid clinical trials to assess new devices for endovascular treatment of intracranial aneurysms. AJNR 2004; 25: 1128–30.

104. Isoda H, Takehara Y, Isogai S et al. MRA of intracranial aneurysm models: a comparison of contrast-enhanced three-dimensional MRA with time-of-flight MRA. J Comput Assist Tomogr 2000; 24: 308–15.

105. Saatci I, Cekirge HS, Ozturk MH, et al. Treatment of internal carotid artery aneurysms with a covered stent: experience in 24 patients with mid-term follow-up results. AJNR Am J Neuroradiol 2004; 25: 1742–9.

106. Kallmes DF, Ding YH, Dai D et al. A new endoluminal, flow-disrupting device for treatment of saccular aneurysms. Stroke 2007; 38: 2346–52.

107. Fiorella D, Woo H, Albuquerque F, Nelson PK. Definitive Reconstruction of Circumferential, Fusiform Intracranial Aneurysms with the Pipeline Embolization Device. Neurosurgery 2008.

108. Rodman KD, Awad AI. Clinical Presentation. In: Awad AI (ed). Current Management of Cerebral Aneurysms. Park Ridge: American Association of Neurological Surgeons, 1993.

109. Greenberg MS. Cerebral aneurysms. In: Green berg MS (ed). Handbook of Neurosurgery, 5th ed. New York: Thieme, 2001.

110. Norwood EG, Kline LB, Chandra-Sekar B, Harsh GR 3rd. Aneurysmal compression of the anterior visual pathways. Neurology 1986; 36: 1035–41.

111. Scialfa G, Vaghi A, Valsecchi F et al. Neuroradiological treatment of carotid and vertebral fistulas and intracavernous aneurysms. Technical problems and results. Neuroradiology 1982; 24: 13–25.

112. Locksley HB. Natural history of subarachnoid hemorrhage, intracranial aneurysms and arteriovenous malformations. Based on 6368 cases in the cooperative study. J Neurosurg 1966; 25: 219–39.

113. Drake CG. The treatment of aneurysms of the posterior circulation. Clin Neurosurg 1979; 26: 96–144.

114. Hunt WE, Kosnik EJ. Timing and perioperative care in intracranial aneurysm surgery. Clin Neurosurg 1974; 21: 79–89.

8

Vascular malformations

Henry Woo, David Fiorella, Michael E Kelly and Thomas J Masaryk

Pial arteriovenous malformations

Classification

Vascular malformations of the central nervous system can be categorized in a number of ways. A simplistic and utilitarian classification is to divide the lesions into those that involve the brain substance and those that that primarily involve the dura. Vascular lesions of the parenchyma are characterized by the McCormick system (recognizing that individual lesions may overlap or occur simultaneously.)[1] This scheme recognizes:

- capillary telangectasias
- slow-flow cavernous malformations
- venous angiomas
- high-flow arteriovenous malformations (AVMs) of the pial arteries.

Capillary telangiectasias

Capillary telangiectasias are composed of small capillary-like blood vessels that resemble normal capillaries surrounded by normal brain parenchyma. They are often small (<1 cm) in diameter, they are poorly marginated, and they occur frequently in the pons. These lesions are clinically silent but are often incidentally discovered as areas of enhancement on MRI (in otherwise normal brain) or at autopsy (Figure 8.1). Capillary telangiectasias may be clinically significant because these lesions are thought by some to represent earlier versions of cavernous malformations; multiple lesions (including cavernous malformations), capillary telangiectasias, and intermediate forms of both have been identified.

Cavernous malformations

Cavernous malformations are composed of cystic vascular spaces lined by a single layer of endothelium. These sinusoidal vessels form a compact mass with no direct arterial in-flow. Cavernous malformations do not have any intervening neural tissue, and this is the major histological feature that differentiates them from capillary telangiectasias. On gross examination these lesions are well-circumscribed areas of reddish-purple discoloration up to a few centimeters in size; they possess a rim of hemosiderin, reactive gliosis, focal areas of calcification, and pockets of blood products in various stages of decay. The paramagnetic and susceptibility effects of these blood breakdown products give these lesions a characteristic appearance on MRI (Figure 8.2).

Clinically these lesions may be asymptomatic, or they may produce headache, a local mass effect, seizures, and occasionally hemorrhage. This last presentation is believed by some to be related to venous drainage. Given that these are 'slow-flow' lesions, the hemorrhage associated with cavernous malformations is usually not catastrophic (unlike that associated with high flow AVMs or intracranial aneurysms). However, location is an important predictor of prognosis. Some patients present with cavernous malformations within the brainstem and deep structures; hemorrhage in these locations, can cause significant clinical problems.

The treatment for cavernous malformations is observational or surgical resection. There is no role for endovascular embolization of these lesions.

Developmental venous anomalies

Developmental venous anomalies (DVAs) are the most commonest vascular anomaly of the brain. They are composed of low-flow anomalous veins separated by normal brain. Typically there are a number of smaller veins, which are described as a *caput medusae* that coalesce into a prominent single draining vessel. This configuration often produces a characteristic appearance on MRI (Figure 8.3). The clinical significance of DVAs arises because they can be associated with cavernous malformations. In the absence of an associated cavernous malformation, these anomalies are asymptomatic and are viewed by some as incidental, anatomic variants of normal venous drainage.

Arteriovenous malformations

AVMs comprise a spectrum developmental anomalies, with a unique, but poorly understood vascular pathophysiology.[2-5] The *sine qua non* of AVM pathology is arterial shunting to draining veins in the absence of capillaries. The pathologic hallmarks of arterioles feeding directly to nidal vessels have a distinctive correlate of angiographic shunting (Figure 8.4).[6-8] Variability of lesions,

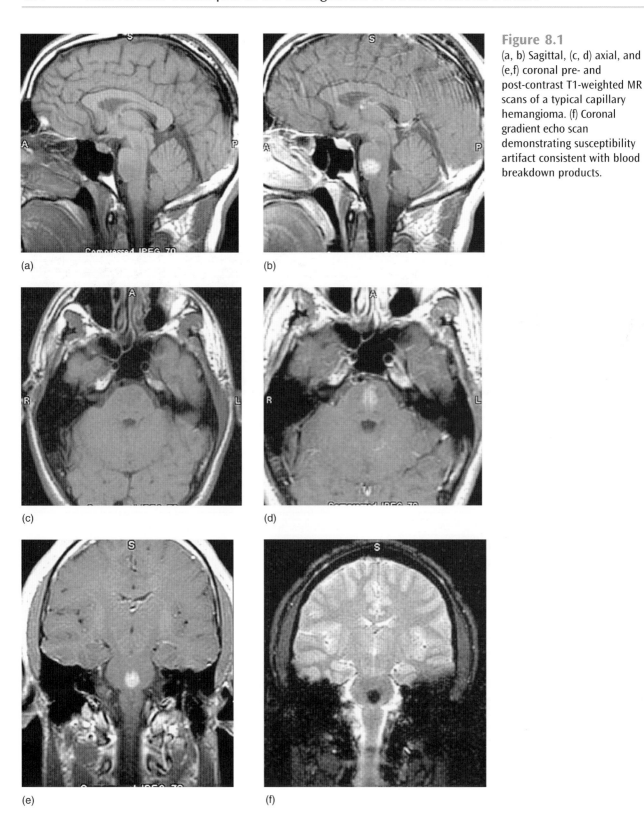

(a)

(b)

(c)

(d)

(e)

(f)

Figure 8.1
(a, b) Sagittal, (c, d) axial, and (e,f) coronal pre- and post-contrast T1-weighted MR scans of a typical capillary hemangioma. (f) Coronal gradient echo scan demonstrating susceptibility artifact consistent with blood breakdown products.

which can be quite dramatic, can be appreciated as a spectrum, ranging from a compact, tight nidus without significant intervening brain parenchyma to diffuse, reticulated anastamotic channels with a lobar or even hemispheric distribution. Regardless of where an AVM falls on this spectrum, the propensity for it to bleed has histologic and pathologic correlates in microscopic areas of hemosiderin and gliosis (even in the absence of an apoplectic event) as well as macroscopic features such as arterial aneurysms and central venous drainage.[7,9,10]

Historical perspective

From Rokitansky and Virchow's first descriptions of AVMs in the 1800s, their management has continually challenged physicians.[11] While reports exist of surgical excision of intracranial AVMs as early as the turn of the last century,[11,12] Cushing and Dandy both commented on the frequency of poor surgical outcomes.[13,14] Nevertheless, Cushing and Bailey presciently recognized, even in the 1920s, that the complexity of such lesions would require a

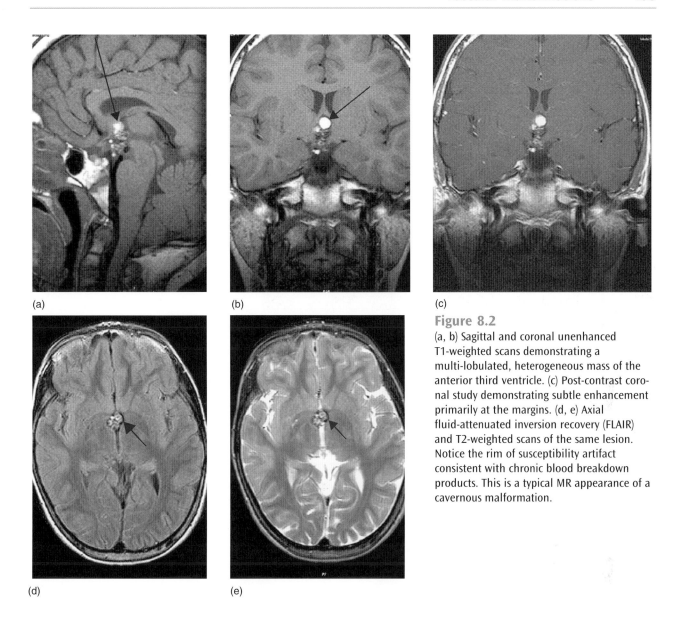

(a)   (b)   (c)

(d)   (e)

Figure 8.2
(a, b) Sagittal and coronal unenhanced T1-weighted scans demonstrating a multi-lobulated, heterogeneous mass of the anterior third ventricle. (c) Post-contrast coronal study demonstrating subtle enhancement primarily at the margins. (d, e) Axial fluid-attenuated inversion recovery (FLAIR) and T2-weighted scans of the same lesion. Notice the rim of susceptibility artifact consistent with chronic blood breakdown products. This is a typical MR appearance of a cavernous malformation.

better understanding of their natural history as well as the thoughtful application of multiple treatment modalities.[15] Since that time, remarkable advances in technology have given cerebrovascular specialists surgical, endovascular, and radiosurgical tools that allow for safer and more efficacious treatment for many intracranial AVMs. And yet, in many ways, pial AVMs remain among the most formidable cerebrovascular lesions to manage. Optimal management continues to demand an experienced multidisciplinary team approach, as well as an honest assessment of the natural history of a given lesion.

Epidemiology

Pial vascular malformations are considered developmental anomalies whose clinical evolution is influenced by vascular anatomy, hemodynamics and, growth factors.[2,4] Although occasional cases are associated with other abnormalities (e.g. Osler–Weber–Rendu disease, Wyburn-Mason and the Sturge–Weber syndrome)[16–18] (Figure 8.5), AVMs are not regarded as familial, and the overwhelming majority of cases are sporadic. The prevalence of AVMs is estimated at approximately 0.01% of the general population, but reported rates range from 0.001% to 0.52%.[1,19–22] There is a slight male preponderance, with a reported male to female ratio ranging from 1:1 to 2:1.[20]

AVMs can occur throughout the brain and have three morphologic components:[1]

- the feeding artery or arteries;
- the draining vein(s); and
- the dysplastic nidus or abnormal connection between arteries and veins, which without an intervening capillary bed results in a precipitous pressure sump serving to reinforce the lesion.

AVMs are commonly classified using the Spetzler–Martin classification system (Table 8.1), which is based on three radiologic characteristics:[23]

- the size of the AVM;
- the location and therefore the eloquence of the surrounding brain; and
- the pattern of venous drainage, either deep or superficial.

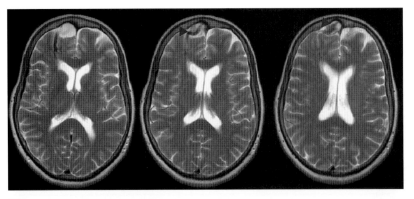

(a)

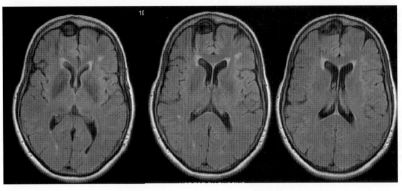

(b)

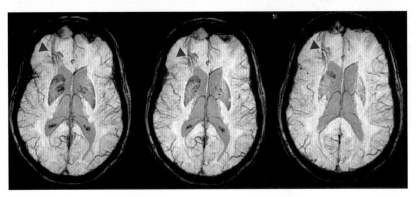

(c)

Figure 8.3

(a) Axial T2-weighted, (b) axial FLAIR and (c) axial gradient echo studies at 3.0T demonstrating a typical *caput medusa* and prominent anterior draining vein (arrowhead) connecting to the superior sagittal sinus. The prominence of the venous structures on the gradient echo studies is a function of deoxyhemaglobin and the high field strength (not hemorrhage or chronic blood breakdown products.)

Upon initial presentation, 30% of AVMs are < 3 cm in size, 60% are between 3–6 cm, and the remainder are > 6 cm in size.[24] In approximately 15–20% of AVMs, an associated intracranial aneurysm will be found.[24]

Clinical presentation and natural history

AVMs are relatively uncommon lesions.[25] As such, the literature describing the natural history of AVMs is limited and is composed predominantly of retrospective analyses of selected populations (e.g. people not undergoing surgery, patients with symptoms other than hemorrhage at presentation), yielding biased and relatively variable estimates of the rate of hemorrhage and its associated consequences.[26] Typically, AVMs may present as hemorrhage,

seizure disorder, or migraine-like headache; in addition, they may be discovered incidentally during imaging. Rarely, progressive neurologic deficits are thought to arise from a 'steal phenomenon' with diversion of blood away from viable brain tissue, or from venous stasis and hypertension, both leading to chronic ischemia.[27]

AVMs of the brain are the third most common cause of intracranial hemorrhage and a common cause of parenchymal hemorrhage in young adults.[28] A first hemorrhage most commonly occurs in patients between 20 and 40 years of age.[19,20,27,29,30] The initial presenting symptom is a hemorrhage in 42–72% of patients, a seizure in 33–46%, a headache in 14–34%, and a progressive neurologic deficit in 21–23%.[27,29–31] Large AVMs, those > 7 cm³, are more likely to present with a seizure (72%) than with a hemorrhage (28%), whereas smaller AVMs, those < 7 cm³, are more likely to present with a hemorrhage (75%) than a seizure (25%).[32] In those cases where the initial presentation is a hemorrhage, larger AVMs tend to have a higher risk of re-bleeding.[20,27]

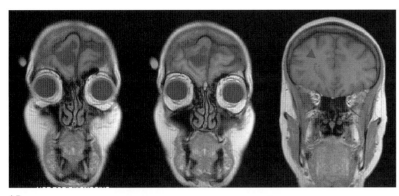

(d)

Figure 8.3 (*Continued*)
(d, e) Pre- and post-contrast T1-weighted
studies as well as (f) axial post-contrast scans
demonstrating a typical pattern of a
developmental venous anomaly.

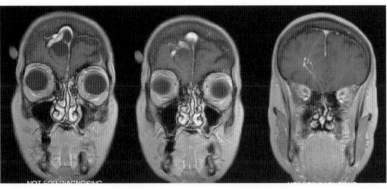

(e)

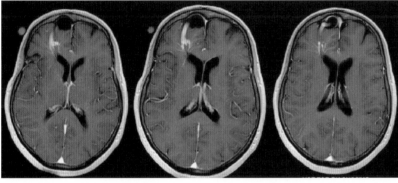

(f)

Most estimates approximate a 2–4% per year risk of hemorrhage.[30,33] In the year immediately after a symptomatic hemorrhage, the risk of re-bleeding is generally thought to be considerably higher, of the order of 6–18% per year, gradually returning toward the 2–4% baseline with time.[33–36] The annual mortality risk of AVM hemorrhage is 0.9–1%, but it decreases after 15 years from the last hemorrhage.[27] With each episode of hemorrhage, there is a 20% risk of a major neurologic deficit and a 10% risk of mortality.[20,24,27,31] The risk of a neurologic deficit is decreased if the hemorrhage has a subarachnoid component.[27]

The location of the AVM correlates with the risk of epilepsy. The risk of seizures is highest in those patients with AVMs located in the frontal lobes (75%), lowest in the occipital lobes (0%), and intermediate in the parietal (57%) and temporal lobes (29%).[37] In one study of 545 patients, 44% of initial seizures were non-focal.[20] Seizures can in general be controlled with medical therapy alone. Piepgras et al.[38] in a series of 102 patients, reported that 83% were seizure-free 2 years post-operatively. There were only four patients whose seizures were the same or worse compared with their pre-operative state. It also appears that seizures may improve after radiosurgery.[39]

The relationship of pregnancy and the risk of hemorrhage from an AVM is a controversial one. Horton et al.[40] in their retrospective analysis of 451 women who had 540 pregnancies, reported 17 intracranial hemorrhages. For patients harboring unruptured AVMs, they calculated an annual hemorrhage rate of 3.5% for pregnant women and 3.1% rate for non-pregnant women of childbearing age. The conclusion was that pregnancy was not a significant risk factor for hemorrhage in women with unruptured AVMs. However, there are numerous reports that suggest that once an AVM has hemorrhaged during pregnancy, the risk of recurrent hemorrhage is significantly increased.[41] While there are reports of mothers having undergone successful surgical removal of their AVMs during pregnancy, higher-grade lesions at eloquent locations are best managed conservatively, with special precautions taken at the time of delivery.[40]

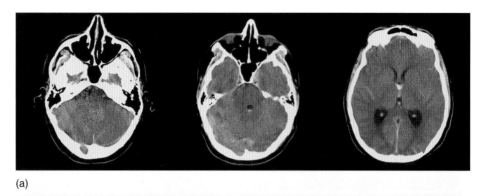

(a)

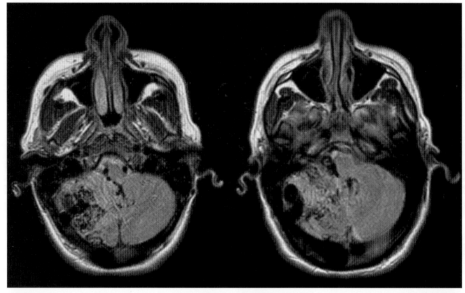

(b)

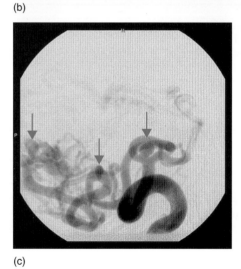

(c)

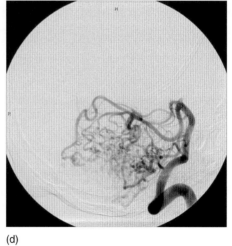

(d)

Figure 8.4
(a) A series of axial CT scans demonstrating acute blood in the third ventricle and Sylvian fissures, and along the leaves of the tentorium (arrowheads). Note the subtle vessels seen end-on in the pre-pontine cistern. Note too the absence of parenchymal hemorrhage and lack of mass effect on the brainstem. (b) Axial fluid-attenuated inversion recovery (FLAIR) images through the posterior fossa demonstrating serpiginous flow voids in the cerebellum consistent with a high flow lesion. Subarachnoid blood or protein can been seen as subtle areas of high signal in the cerebrospinal fluid spaces on FLAIR. (c) Lateral view from a diagnostic angiogram; ipsilateral vertebral artery injection demonstrating a markedly enlarged posterior inferior cerebellar artery (PICA) with several aneurysms along the major feeder. Given the lack of parenchymal hemorrhage this was the suspected source of bleeding. (d) Contralateral PICA demonstrating steal from the inferior and superior vermian branches.

Diagnosis

Computed tomography

As with aneurysmal subarachnoid hemorrhage, the mainstay for the correct diagnosis of an AVM at the time of presentation is often a CT scan with and without contrast. CT readily detects hemorrhage and it is also very sensitive for calcification that is frequently associated with AVMs (Figure 8.6).[24,27,42] On a non-contrast enhanced CT scan, areas of acute hemorrhage or calcification will appear as hyperdense regions with or without surrounding hypodensity representing edema. In cases without acute hemorrhage or calcification, the lesion may appear as isodense, but with contrast enhancement the AVM will enhance intensely, typically in a 'serpentine' pattern as the abnormal and dilated vessels fill with contrast material.[24]

Magnetic resonance imaging

Cranial MRI is more sensitive for detecting unruptured AVMs than CT.[42] On MRI, hemorrhages will have varying signal

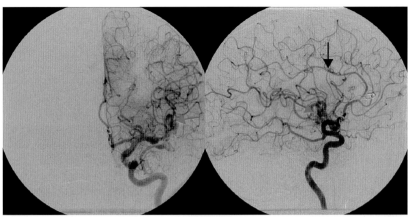

(a)

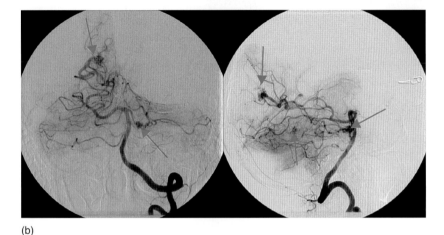

(b)

Figure 8.5
(a) Anterior–posterior (AP) and lateral left internal carotid artery injection in a patient with Osler–Weber–Rendu syndrome. The patient has multiple intracranial aneurysms (see registration artifact from prior surgical clipping) and has evolved multiple pial arterial–venous malformations (AVMs) over time. Two small AVMs are seen in these views in the left temporal lobe (red arrow) and near the midline of the frontal lobe (black arrow). (b) AP and lateral left vertebral artery injections demonstrating malformations in the right occipital lobe and the superior cerebellum bilaterally (arrows).

Table 8.1 Features of pial vs dural arterial-venous malformations (AVM)

Pial	Dural
Congenital	Acquired
Hemorrhage risk	Venous infarction risk
Primary RX surgery/radiosurgery	Primary RX endovascular
	■ Aggressive embolization of venous drainage
	■ Secondary attack of arterial pedicle
Endovascular RX as adjuvant	Surgery/radiosurgery as secondary RX
■ Primarily attack of arterial pedicles	
■ Strictly avoid venous embolization	

Table 8.2 The Spetzler–Martin scale for evaluating risk of neurologic deterioration following surgery for arterial–venous resection

Characteristic	Points assigned
Size of lesion	
Small (<3 cm)	1
Medium (3–6 cm)	2
Large (>6 cm)	3
Location	
Non-eloquent site	0
Eloquent site (sensorimotor, language, visual cortex, hypothalamus, thalamus, brainstem, cerebellar nuclei, or regions directly adjacent to these structures)	1
Direction of venous drainage	
Superficial	0
Deep (any)	1

From Spetzler and Martin.[54]

intensities depending on the age of the hematoma and the oxidation state of the hemoglobin within the lesion. Vessels within the AVM will appear as hypointense 'flow voids' on spin-echo scans and are not typical of the normal vascular anatomy of the affected region of the brain (see figure 8.4).[24] In addition, MRI allows for the accurate localization of associated normal and abnormal brain tissue, including white matter tracts (using diffusion tensor tractography or DTI), which is crucial for the adequate determination of eloquence as defined in the Spetzler–Martin scale and which is often able to assess the dominant venous drainage.[23]

Functional imaging

Functional studies, such as xenon CT, single-photon computed tomography (SPECT), and positron emission tomography (PET) have also been used to study the risk of AVM hemorrhage, infarction, or normal perfusion pressure breakthrough.[24,43] Functional imaging has also helped to document the variability and

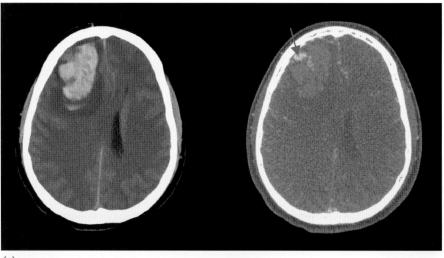

(a)

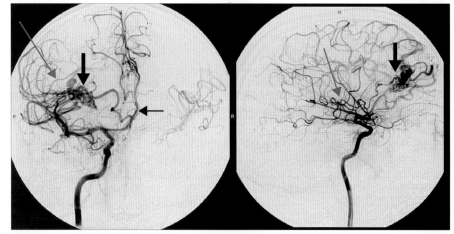

(b)

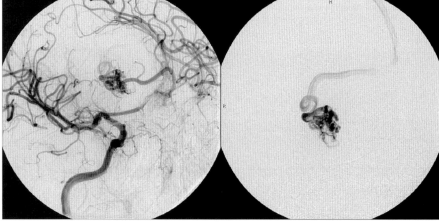

(c)

Figure 8.6
(a) Unenhanced and enhanced CT scans in a young patient with acute hemorrhage. A wide window demonstrates central enhancement of the compressed nidus AVM. (b) AP and lateral views of a right internal carotid angiogram demonstrating downward mass effect on the Sylvian triangle (red arrow) and midline shift of the anterior cerebral artery vessels from the hematoma (black arrow). A small focal nidus corresponds to the area of enhancement on the CT scan with cortical venous drainage (thick black arrows), Spetzler–Martin grade II AVM. (c) Oblique internal carotid artery (ICA) and microcatheter views of the nidus. There is the suggestion of small nidal aneurysms.

plasticity of the motor and language cortex in patients with an AVM. As a result, estimating the location of functional cortex by anatomic landmarks alone is inadequate. Previously, the only method of defining the exact location of functional tissue was by intraoperative stimulation; however, recent developments of functional imaging modalities can now offer a pre-operative assessment of the proximity of an AVM to eloquent cortex and fiber tracts. The most common techniques are functional MRI (fMRI), magnetoencephalography (MEG, or magnetic source imaging), PET scanning superimposed on MRI images, and superselective Wada testing.[44–48]

Catheter angiography

Conventional four-vessel cerebral angiography remains the gold standard for the assessment AVMs. Angiography is able to define

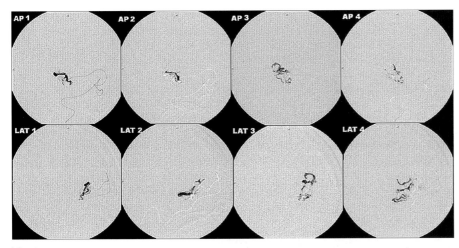

(d)

Figure 8.6 (*Continued*)
(d) From left to right, 'Start–stop' serial microcatheter shots during 'plug–push' Onyx injection. Lower view is from corresponding ipsilateral ICA injection. (e) Post embolization lateral angiogram and corresponding radiograph of the Onyx cast. Note the lack of visible shunting. (f) Oblique radiograph of Onyx cast and corresponding ICA angiogram pre-embolization.

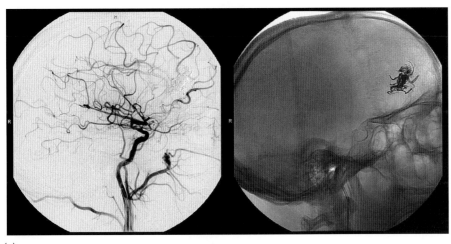

(e)

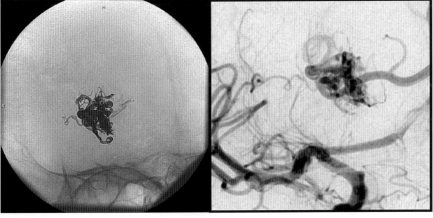

(f)

AVM features that relate to natural history as well as treatment planning. It is important to emphasize that MRA is not an adequate substitute for conventional angiography.[24] The cerebral angiogram clearly delineates the three morphologic substrates of an AVM: the feeding arteries, the nidus, and the draining veins.

The feeding arteries for cortical AVMs can arise from:

- the superficial pial arterial system (i.e. the anterior cerebral artery, the middle cerebral artery, or the posterior cerebral artery);

- the deep perforating vessels, such as the lenticulostriates, the anterior or posterior choroidal arteries, or the thalamo-perforators; and

- high-flow lesions parasitizing supply from the normal meningeal arteries.

The relationship of the feeding arteries to the AVM is crucial for clinical decision-making. The feeding arteries may have proximal branches that supply normal parenchyma before supplying the nidus, or they may be en-passage vessels that provide branches to the nidus before continuing to supply normal brain.

Approximately 15–20% of patients with an AVM harbor underlying aneurysms (see figure 8.4).[49–51] The majority of these lesions are 'flow related' and form secondary to the hemodynamic stress placed on the feeding vessels, but they may also be seen at or within the nidus. The former may regress with removal of the offending malformation.[9,22,52] These later aneurysms are often implicated as a source of hemorrhage.[10,49]

Only angiography is able to delineate the true nidus of an AVM. The nidus is a network of dysplastic vessels and is in general the source of hemorrhage. The nidus itself can be compact and may contain components that are more fistulous in nature, while lesions may present as a diffuse nidus, with poorly delineated margins and intervening gliotic parenchyma.

The high-flow state of AVMs lead to dilated and arterialized draining veins. The draining veins can be superficial or deep and may demonstrate stenoses or varices. The presence of stenoses is associated with an increased risk of hemorrhage[10,53] as is exclusively deep drainage (where the rigid straight sinus effectively limits venous capacity).[54]

The development of micro-catheter technology and digital subtraction angiography has made navigation into nearly all intracerebral vessels possible. Superselective angiography not only provides greater anatomic detail, but also provides a route for embolization and functional testing with sodium amytal.

Classification, grade and treatment strategy

Numerous grading systems have been devised to characterize lesions and stratify surgical risk.[54–56] The risk of surgical intervention has been directly related to the angiographic architecture of the particular lesion: the size of the AVM, the location and therefore the eloquence of the surrounding brain, and the pattern of venous drainage, either deep or superficial.[23] This relationship is best characterized with the Spetzler–Martin grading system (see Table 8.1).

In prospective studies, the Spetzler–Martin grade demonstrated a reliable correlation with surgical outcome. Hamilton and Spetzler[57] reported operative morbidity and mortality rates for the resection of grade I and II AVMs (< 1%) and grade III AVMs (< 3%) to be very low. However, much higher morbidity rates were observed for grade IV and V AVMs, reaching 31% and 50%, respectively, in the early post-operative period, and subsequently improving to 22% and 17%, respectively, at the time of the follow-up examination. Heros et al.[58] reported a similar relationship between Spetzler–Martin grade and outcome. These data form the foundation for most management decisions regarding AVM therapy. Therapeutic options for AVMs include observation, embolization, stereotactic radiosurgery, microsurgery, or various combinations of these.[59]

In general, for grade I and II AVMs, the risk of hemorrhage far outweighs the risk of surgical resection. As such, these lesions are generally treated with surgical resection. For grade I lesions, because of the low operative morbidity and mortality, pre-operative embolization is not frequently pursued, given that the risk of the embolization procedure may approach or even surpass the risk of surgery. In some instances, stereotactic radiosurgery, rather than surgical resection, is used for treatment of a grade II lesion. The most common example would be a small grade II AVM in a highly eloquent region. Stereotactic radiosurgery is also utlized in lesions that have not presented with previous

hemorrhage. Small low-grade hemorrhagic lesions in non-eloquent regions are less desirable for radiosurgery because of the risk of hemorrhage while waiting for the AVM nidus to obliterate (usually 2–3 years).

Grade III AVMs represent a complex and heterogeneous group, each requiring an individualized assessment. The heterogeneity of this category led Lawton[60] to stratify these lesions further into three additional angioarchitectural subcategories, with low (2.9%), intermediate (7.1%), and high (14.8%) risk of post-surgical death or new deficit. Most of these lesions are treated with either radiosurgery or pre-operative embolization followed by surgical resection. When these lesions are approached surgically, pre-operative embolization frequently plays an important role.

The surgical resection of grade IV and V AVMs is generally associated with a risk of operative morbidity and mortality that exceeds the risks associated with the natural history of the lesion. Han et al.[61] analyzed outcomes in a series of 73 consecutive patients with grade IV and V AVMs. These authors recommended no treatment for most patients in this group (55 out of 73) and reported a relatively low risk of hemorrhage in these patients (1% per year). Conversely, accumulating data suggest that partial AVM resection does not reduce, but rather increases, the risk of future hemorrhage. Han et al.[61] observed a hemorrhage rate of 10.4% in patients with grade IV and grade V AVMs after partial treatment, compared with a 1% risk in patients with no previous treatment. Miyamota et al.[62] found an annual risk of hemorrhage of 14.6% in patients who underwent palliative treatment of cerebral AVMs. Wikholm et al.[63] observed an increased rate of hemorrhage and death in patients undergoing partial treatment that resulted in less than 90% nidal obliteration. In accordance with these observations, treatment for grades IV and V AVMs is recommended only in patients with progressive neurological deficits attributable to repeated hemorrhage or disabling symptoms, such as intractable seizures. If treatment is undertaken, the goal should be to achieve cure and not simply to reduce the AVM size. The use of multimodality treatment in patients with grades IV and V AVMs can improve eventual cure rates and patient outcomes.

Role of endovascular therapy

The role of neuroendovascular therapy in the management of brain AVMs depends ultimately on the overall treatment plan. In general, five scenarios make up the vast majority of rational management strategies (listed here from most to least common):

1. Pre-operative embolization: embolization as a precursor to complete curative surgical resection
2. Targeted therapy: embolization to eradicate a specific bleeding source
3. Pre-radiosurgery embolization: embolization as a precursor to radiation therapy
4. Curative embolization: embolization for attempted cure
5. Palliative embolization: embolization to palliate symptoms attributed to shunting.

Pre-operative embolization

AVM embolization is most frequently performed as a precursor to curative surgical resection. Before initiating the neuroendovascular

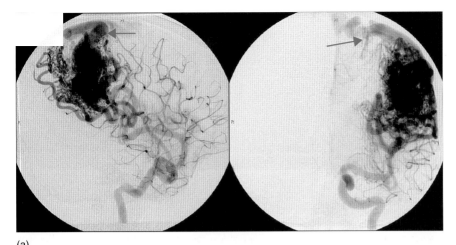

(a)

(b)

Figure 8.7

(a) Anterior–posterior and lateral left internal carotid artery injections demonstrating a larger parietal arteriovenous malformation in the dominant hemisphere. Based on the size and location this would be a high-risk surgical lesion (Spetzler–Martin grade IV). However, venous drainage is cortical (arrows), the number of feeding pedicles is relatively limited, and the nidus is relatively 'tightly packed', features that make this lesion more amenable to endovascular treatment. (b) Post-embolization radiographs demonstrating Onyx cast.

portion of AVM therapy, it is critical that the interventionists have a complete understanding of the overall plan for, as well as the goals of, the embolization. This understanding is predicated on maintaining open lines of communication with the vascular neurosurgeon who will be performing the resection (or the radiosurgical treatment). The risks of microsurgical resection, as defined by the Spetzler–Martin category of the lesion, should be clear before the procedure. It is important to weigh these risks against those involved with each catheterization and each embolization.

In general, the primary goal of the embolization is to decrease the blood supply to the malformation, thereby decreasing the level of technical difficulty and associated morbidity of surgical resection. A successful embolization is effective in reducing the size of the AVM nidus, occluding deep feeding vessels that are difficult to access and control surgically, reducing intraoperative hemorrhage, and providing better delineation of a surgical resection plane (Figure 8.7).

The neuroendovascular operator must always be cognizant of the surgical approach and the complication rate associated with the resection of any particular lesion and must make every attempt to ensure that the risks of the embolization do not exceed those of the surgical resection (e.g. pre-operative embolization of a grade II AVM that is associated with a very low operative morbidity). The goal of the vascular neurosurgeon must be to achieve a complete, curative resection of the AVM.

The efficacy of modern AVM embolization using n-butylcyanoacrylate (NBCA) has been demonstrated in several clinical studies. Jafar et al.[64] demonstrated that pre-operative embolization reduced the operative morbidity of large AVMs to a level similar to that of smaller AVMs that were not embolized before surgery. DeMerritt et al.[65] reported similar results, with pre-operative embolization of large AVMs improving post-surgical outcomes in comparison with a control group of smaller AVMs that were not embolized.

Targeted therapy

With few exceptions, all treatment strategies for AVM management should ultimately be directed toward the complete eradication of the lesion. However, in some patients with grades IV and V AVMs that are not amenable to surgical resection, partial treatment targeted to eliminate an identified bleeding source is undertaken.

Aneurysms are identified in association with AVMs in 7–20% of cases.[10,52,66,67] Aneurysms may be located on vessels that are remote from the nidus, on a feeding vessel (flow-related aneurysms), or within the nidus itself. In addition, intranidal pseudoaneurysms – composed of an organized hematoma that communicates with the intravascular space – may form after AVM hemorrhage. The presence of an aneurysm represents a risk factor for intracranial hemorrhage in patients with AVMs.[10,49] Although both intra- and extranidal aneurysms are risk factors for intracranial hemorrhage in patients with AVMs, the increased risk of hemorrhage in the setting of an extranidal aneurysm may be attributed to aneurysm rupture rather than hemorrhage from the AVM nidus itself.[66]

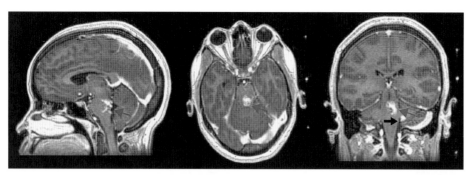

(a)

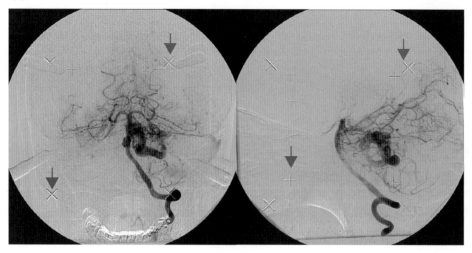

(b)

Figure 8.8
(a) Sagittal, axial, and coronal post-contrast three-dimensional magnetization prepared rapid-gradient echo T1-weighted scans used for stereotactic radiosurgical planning demonstrate an AVM nidus at the floor of the fourth ventricle (red arrows). Feeding vessels arise deep from the basilar artery; black arrow designates the central draining vein.
(b) Anterior–posterior and lateral left vertebral artery angiogram performed with Leksell fiducial head frame (red arrows demonstrate examples of fiducials; there should be nine in each field of view) prior to radiosurgery. The size, shape, and location of this lesion make it a prototypical example of radiosurgery indications.

Remote and feeding vessel aneurysms can usually be identified by conventional angiography. Nidal aneurysms may occasionally be visualized on conventional angiographic views. Often, however, only superselective angiography performed using high frame rates can demonstrate these lesions. Nidal aneurysms are frequently obscured by overlying vessels and varices or other portions of the AVM nidus on conventional angiographic views. As such, when an unresectable AVM hemorrhages one or more times, endovascular exploration for a nidal aneurysm represents a reasonable strategy. In these cases, if the AVM is not to be resected, a targeted embolization may be undertaken to eradicate the aneurysm either with a liquid embolic agent (in the case of a nidal aneurysm) or coils (in the case of a proximal, flow-related aneurysm or remote aneurysm).

Pre-radiosurgery embolization

Stereotactic radiosurgery is often used for focal AVMs (i.e. with a tight nidus) located deep within eloquent areas of the brain (Figure 8.8). The success of radiotherapy is inversely proportional to the size of the AVM nidus to be treated.[68] AVMs with nidal volumes less than 10 ml (diameter < 3 cm) [69] are frequently curable by radiosurgery, with rates of cure at 2 years estimated at between 80% and 88%.[70,71] Often the characteristics that make a lesion difficult to treat surgically may limit endovascular treatment (see figure 8.8). Nevertheless, despite the eloquent location there may be circumstances in which the size of the nidus is unfavorably large for radiosurgery and portions of the lesion may be accessible by endovascular means. The theoretical goal of embolization in this setting would be to reduce the size of the AVM

nidus into a target size that is more amenable to radiosurgical ablation. In this setting, the use of a more permanent embolisate, such as NBCA (see below), is mandatory to avoid recanalization of portions of the AVM that have been embolized but not included in the radiation field. Additional goals of pre-radiosurgical embolization would include targeted therapy for components predisposed to hemorrhage (i.e. nidal or feeding vessel aneurysms) and the ablation of large arteriovenous fistulae that are typically more refractory to the effects of radiotherapy.

Despite the straightforward rationale for pre-radiosurgical embolization, very little data exist to support this approach. This is related in part to the extended latency period (2–3 years) required for radiotherapy to have a definitive effect. Of the available case series, many were conducted in the late 1980s and early 1990s, and many used particulate embolysates (e.g., polyvinyl alcohol). The use of a temporary embolisate for the permanent eradication of a component of AVM is contraindicated at this time, given the availability of more durable agents. In this category, the largest series was reported by Gobin et al.,[72] who described their experience with 125 patients undergoing embolization (predominantly with NBCA) as a precursor to radiosurgery. These authors were able to achieve total occlusion in 11.2% of AVMs after embolization alone, with an additional 76% of lesions reduced sufficiently in size to undergo radiotherapy. A 65% rate of total occlusion was observed after radiotherapy in patients undergoing combined treatment. More recently, Henkes et al.[73] reported a series of 30 patients undergoing combined embolization and radiotherapy, observing a less impressive 47% obliteration rate in a series of 30 patients. However, in this study, most of the treated AVMs were of very high grade. From the existing data, no compelling evidence exists to justify or refute the usefulness of preradiosurgical embolization.

Embolization for cure

Embolization for cure of pial arteriovenous malformations is the exception rather than the rule of endovascular therapy. Several key variables determine which cases are amenable to complete endovascular obliteration: 1) the experience of the operator, 2) the type of embolic agent, and 3) the angiographic architecture of the target.

Given the uncommon nature of such lesions (0.01% of the general population)[74] and the variability in performance of different embolic agents, it is no surprise that the experience of the operator is a key determinant in the declaration of 'cure.' This is perhaps most evident in the use of NBCA where operator selectable parameters of sequencing of target pedicles, proximity of catheter placement, local hemodynamics under anesthesia, ratio of the mixture of acrylic monomer with radiographic contrast, and speed of injection provide tremendous variability in the success of filling the malformation nidus with embolic material (while at the same time minimizing venous or proximal arterial occlusion.)[75]

It is generally accepted that liquid embolic agents (NBCA or ethylene vinyl alcohol) provide the best opportunity of 'casting' or completely filling the AVM nidus while creating a durable seal of the arterial feeding vessels.[76,77] Choice of agent in any given case is often dependent on experience of the operator, local anatomy, and hemodynamics. As noted by Wikholm et al NBCA has a steep learning curve with embolic injections occurring over seconds to minutes.[78,79] Alternatively ethylene vinyl alcohol injections may be more controlled, occasionally protracted (hours), which may prove problematic for extremely large lesions.[77,80–82]

Finally, the architecture of the nidus itself is a key determinant of success. The accessibility of the arterial pedicle to catheterization has obvious implications for the injection of embolic agent; however the degree of arteriovenous shunting and proximity of eloquent brain will also affect the aggressiveness of the injection. Finally, much like treatment with stereotactic radiosurgery, the compactness or density of the nidus in relation to the endovascular access of feeding pedicles will greatly affect the degree of obliteration of the malformation.

Small series with lengthy follow-up estimate the rate of complete obliteration of pial arteriovenous malformations at 16-49%.[77,82,83]

Palliative embolization

Palliative embolization is controversial, but some investigators theorize that large AVMs may cause progressive neurological deficits, intellectual deterioration, or debilitating headaches as sequelae of the shunting of blood away from physiologically normal brain (i.e. a steal phenomenon).[69,74] Given that the lesions responsible for this type of phenomenon are large and typically unresectable, some investigators have advocated partial embolization in an attempt to reduce the severity of arterial–venous shunting and to improve perfusion pressure in the surrounding functional brain parenchyma.[61] Although no large clinical series exist to support this strategy, several case reports have described success in small numbers of patients.[75,76] Fox et al.[77] reported improvement in limb weakness in three patients after subtotal embolization of large AVMs located near the motor cortex, attributing the improvement to a reduction in cerebrovascular steal.

Endovascular techniques

The success of endovascular therapy of AVMs depends on the equipment utilized, the embolic agents employed, the quality of the angiographic equipment, and the experience and clinical judgment of the endovascular surgeon.

The embolization is performed in a neuroradiologic suite or operating room that is equipped with biplanar fluoroscopy. Ideally the patient is awake, facilitating neurologic assessment during the procedure, although in practice the long procedure times, the requirement for precise roadmap, and the discomfort of intracranial catheterization preclude this. A transfemoral route is used, and a 5–8 guiding catheter is positioned in the internal carotid or vertebral artery, depending on the vascular supply of the AVM. A micro-catheter is used for superselective catheterization of the feeding arterial pedicles.

Microcatheters

Small size is a requisite for access of these potentially diminutive arteries. Catheters capable of reaching the distal cerebral arteries range in size from 2.3F to 3.0F. Two general types are available: an over-the-wire system and a flow-directed system. Both of these catheter types have a hydrophilic coating that improves their performance and the ease with which they can be advanced up a vessel. Over-the-wire catheters require vessels to be accessed with a steerable micro-guidewire and then the catheter to be advanced over the wire until the desired location is reached. Because AVMs usually have high-flow feeding pedicles, the preferential blood flow to these vessels may be used to the operator's advantage by using a catheter that has an extremely floppy, low-mass, bulb-shaped tip. Such flow-directed catheters move like a sail in the wind and are drawn to the nidus by the flow of blood. Flow-directed techniques work best for accessing the nidus during the early stages of embolization while there is still a high-flow state through the AVM and its feeders. As the embolization proceeds and the shunt decreases, the ease with which these catheters 'sail' to the nidus diminishes.

Guidewires

Like microcatheters, microguidewires also need to be small (0.010–0.014 inches; 0.25–0.36 mm) and flexible. Generally, a balance must be struck between the stiffness of the wire (which supports forward pushing or 'stripping' of the catheter) and the softness of the tip to reduce the risk of vessel perforation. Usually manufactured from stainless steel or nitinol, the wire provides torque-ability to steer the wire into the desired vessels despite having to navigate several bends through tortuous vessel loops. Movements of guidewire-supported microcatheters are flow-independent and consequently these systems are best suited for accessing small feeders arising from a more proximal, main vessel trunk.

Embolic agents

Before delivering embolic material to an AVM, the operator needs to assess the risk of causing a permanent neurologic deficit. Angiography through the microcatheter after it has achieved its final position will reveal whether any normal brain is being perfused distal to the tip of the microcatheter. If there is any question as to whether functional brain will be embolized, some advocate that provocative neurologic challenge can be performed by injecting amobarbital through the microcatheter.[47] Careful examination of the patient's neurologic function subserved by the portion of the brain in question is then performed. If there are no deficits, embolization will very likely not lead to a significant neurologic deficit, although in the setting of high-flow lesions some would question the validity of the test (shunting producing false negative results).

Embolic agents (see Chapter 4) can be categorized into two main groups: liquids and particles. The cyanoacrylates ('glues') are the prototypical liquid embolic agents, and they are the only agents that currently can lead to a permanent endovascular cure. The most widely used cyanoacrylate, cyanoacrylate NBCA, exists as a liquid that polymerizes immediately upon contact with an ionic solution containing free hydrogen ions. Because of its low viscosity, it can be injected through the smallest of microcatheters (i.e. flow-directed catheters), a limitation in delivering the larger particulates.

The technique of glue embolization requires a careful knowledge of the polymerization characteristics of the agent, the rate of blood flow through the nidus, the degree of pedicle occlusion by the microcatheter, and the rate of material delivery through any given microcatheter.[78–80] Endovascular cure demands that the entire AVM nidus be occluded, including the components nearest the venous side, or else the nidus will recruit a new arterial supply. Because NBCA polymerizes so rapidly, an agent must be added that will retard its polymerization rate. The oily contrast medium lipiodol is used for this purpose, and it has the added advantage of opacifying the otherwise radiotransparent NBCA, allowing for visualization under fluoroscopy. By varying the ratios of the components, an experienced physician can mix a cocktail that will penetrate the entire nidus before polymerizing without reaching the draining vein. Should the draining vein be occluded, the blood pressure head within the nidus may rise to high levels that cannot be supported by the fragile walls of the dysplastic AVM vessels, resulting in rupture and hemorrhage. In addition, great care must be taken to avoid gluing the microcatheter to the nidus, usually an irretrievable situation (although limited experience would suggest that this complication is much less catastrophic).[8]

Despite their complexities and potentially serious complications, cyanoacrylates have been useful in reducing the size of selected AVMs before stereotactic radiosurgery because of their adhesive properties. Other non-permanent embolic agents (i.e., particulates) cannot fulfill this role, since the AVM nidus will recannulate within a few weeks after their delivery. In contrast, particulates are somewhat safer and easier to use and are particularly helpful as an adjunct to open surgical therapy.

Particulates are manufactured from a variety of materials and come in a range of sizes. The smallest are polyvinyl alcohol (PVA) particles that are engineered in sizes ranging from 50 μm to 1500 μm and are injected as a suspension in radiographic contrast media. The exact size used depends on the rate of flow through the nidus and the presence of intranidal shunts and fistulae. If too much polyvinyl traverses the nidus without lodging in it, an inflammatory pulmonary reaction can develop, with transient pulmonary failure.[82] To minimize this complication, intranidal shunts can be partially occluded by mixing the polyvinyl alcohol with fibrillary collagen or by using platinum coils. When delivered to small feeding pedicles, they will lead to thrombosis and occlusion of the vessel.

More recently a novel polymer, Onyx (eV3, Irvine, California) has been approved for the pre-surgical embolization of AVMs of the brain. Onyx is an ethylene vinyl alcohol copolymer that is dissolved in dimethylsulfoxide (DMSO) and precipitates as the DMSO diffuses away. This agent lacks the adhesive quality of cyanoacrylates, and has more predictable set-up, making it safer to use. The procedure of Onyx embolization requires that a stable 'plug' of Onyx be established at the catheter tip to prevent reflux. The process of establishing the plug is critical. Multiple small injections followed by waiting between 30 and 120 seconds are necessary to allow precipitation to occur. Once the plug is stable, the material will penetrate into the AVM nidus, often with excellent results (see figure 8.7). As with NBCA, care must be taken to ensure that the venous outflow of the nidus is not occluded.

Staging treatment

The number of embolizations that can be performed during a single session varies with the preference of the operator, the anatomy of the lesion, and the strategy for additional treatment. One potential risk of over-embolization of a large lesion is hemorrhage related to normal perfusion pressure breakthrough – the sequelae of an abrupt reduction in arterial–venous shunting and a sudden increase in the perfusion pressure of the adjacent normal brain parenchyma with impaired autoregulatory capacity.[32,83]

In a patient with a large AVM scheduled for surgical resection on the next morning, one might perform between five and seven NBCA injections during a single session. Given the much larger volume of Onyx that can be injected from a single catheter position, the number of pedicles catheterized and the volume of embolic agent injected is much more variable and is assessed on a case-by-case basis. If multiple vascular distributions provide supply to the lesion (e.g. the right internal carotid and vertebrobasilar arteries) and multiple sessions are to be performed, it is our preference to embolize within only one vascular distribution during any given session. In general, for AVMs larger than 3cm, it is preferable to have at least two sessions of embolization scheduled.

Dural arteriovenous malformations and fistulae

Dural arterial–venous malformations or dural arterial–venous fistulae (DAVFs) are acquired lesions consisting of one or more fistulous connections within the leaflets of the dura mater. They account for 10–15% of cranial arteriovenous malformations.[84,85] Here these lesions will be referred to as DAVFs because the term 'malformation' is a misnomer: malformation implies a congenital etiology when, in fact, the majority, if not all of these lesions, are acquired.

Etiology and pathogenesis

Given the variable locations and complexity of DAVFs, there may be multiple etiologic factors responsible for fistula formation. Most lesions appear in the middle-aged or the elderly, far later in life than typical pial AVMs. Specific factors are known to predispose to fistula formation, including sinus thrombosis, trauma, and surgery. There are several cases of documented sinus thrombosis with subsequent fistula formation associated with the involved sinus.[86–89] In such cases, the primary cause of sinus thrombosis may be a generalized hypercoagulable state or an infection of a major sinus such as the mastoid or sphenoid sinus. It is thought that the fistula occurs during the phase of attempted re-canalization and neovascularization within the sinus. Given these circumstances, it is reasonable to test for a nascent hypercoaguable state in these patients.

Conversely, not all DAVFs are associated with thrombosis or stenosis of a major dural sinus. Venous hypertension within a sinus may lead to the development of a DAVF.[90–92] In a recent histopathologic study of DAVFs, the presence of 30 µm 'crack-like' vessels within the dural sinus wall was described, and it was postulated that steno-occlusive disease of the venous sinuses triggers the development of these vessels. In this scenario, subsequent sinus thrombosis is then an epiphenomenon that occurs as a result of turbulent flow and sinus wall thickening.[93] Additionally, conditions associated with vascular frailty, such as fibromuscular dysplasia, neurofibromatosis type I, and Ehlers–Danlos syndrome, have been associated with DAVFs.[94–98]

Clinical presentation and anatomic considerations

The clinical presentation of DAVFs is highly varied and is primarily determined by the location of the fistula and the subsequent pattern of venous drainage. Other factors include the degree of AV shunting, the presence of venous hypertension, and the presence of venous stenoses or ectasias (Figure 8.9). The two most common locations are the transverse sigmoid sinus and the cavernous sinus (Figures 8.9, 8.10, 8.11),[99,100] followed by the deep venous system, the superior sagittal sinus, the superior petrosal sinus, the ethmoidal sinus, the marginal sinus, and the inferior petrosal sinus. The reason for this discordant distribution has not been clearly established. A delay in the development of the external carotid territory and the presence of numerous emissary veins near the skull base have been proposed as two possible causative mechanisms.[101] Theoretically, any site along the dura mater is a potential source for fistula formation. The primary factor in determining the aggressive, morbid behavior of a DAVF, however, is the presence of leptomeningeal venous drainage, which can engender venous hypertension, progressive neurologic deficit, infarction, and hemorrhage.[102]

Lesions involving the transverse sigmoid sinus are the most common (occurring in 38% of cases of DAVF).[100] The clinical picture can range from an asymptomatic lesion to overt hemorrhage. Common symptoms may include a simple pulsatile bruit or a headache. If there has been longstanding venous hypertension and swelling, the presentation can mimic transient ischemic attacks or ischemic infarctions of the adjacent brain parenchyma.[103] The arterial supply typically occurs through transmastoid branches of the occipital, posterior auricular and middle meningeal branches of the external carotid artery, neuromeningeal branches of the ascending pharyngeal artery, branches of the vertebral artery (including the posterior meningeal artery, and the artery of the falx cerebelli), and the meningeal branches of the carotid siphon (see figure 8.12). A complete evaluation of the venous drainage system should include the identification of any downstream stenosis or any occlusion of the ipsilateral transverse sigmoid sinus, the presence of flow across the torcula, and the presence of cortical venous drainage. Particular attention should paid to the direction of flow in the vein of Labbé and its point of insertion, since it

has significant implications for the endovascular options for treatment. If the vein of Labbé flows in a retrograde fashion, its origin in the sinus can be occluded from a transvenous approach. If the flow is antegrade, occlusion of its origin can exacerbate the venous hypertension, leading to a worsening of symptoms and possible hemorrhage.

Lesions involving the cavernous sinus frequently manifest themselves with ocular pathology (see Figures 8.10, 8.11). The classic signs of orbital venous hypertension include pulsatile exophthalmos, chemosis, conjunctival injection, and glaucoma resulting in vision loss. A progressive cavernous sinus syndrome can also cause extraocular muscle paresis (especially involving cranial nerves III and VI), a decline in visual acuity, optic neuropathy, and proptosis. These are all indications for treatment. Tinnitus and ocular bruits are also relative indications. The arterial supply for a cavernous sinus lesion can include branches from the inferolateral or meningohypophyseal trunk, branches of the middle or accessory meningeal artery, the artery of the foramen rotundum, and the ascending pharyngeal artery, among others. A large draining superior ophthalmic vein can be easily identified on MRI, and surgical access into this vein provides a route for potential therapy. Access into the cavernous sinus via the inferior petrosal sinus provides yet another, more convenient route for endovascular therapy (see figure 8.10). Again, particular attention should be paid to the venous phase of the diagnostic angiogram, including intracranial cortical venous drainage from the cavernous sinus into the superficial and deep Sylvian systems (see figure 8.11).

Rarely, patients may present with lesions of the marginal sinus. Symptoms depend on the pattern of venous drainage. Those with jugular venous drainage typically present with large fistulae and symptoms of pulsatile tinnitus and other posterior circulation phenomena.[100] Those with retrograde venous drainage via the inferior petrosal sinus may present in the same fashion as those with cavernous sinus fistulae, with variable degrees of ophthalmologic symptoms.[104] In either case, direct treatment of the nidus may involve a risk to lower cranial nerves and may cause potentially significant morbidity.[104]

Ethmoidal DAVFs typically derive supply from the anterior and posterior ethmoidal branches of the ophthalmic artery and may recruit supply from the distal branches of the internal maxillary artery. The drainage is almost always into pial veins along the floor of the anterior cranial fossa and, ultimately, into the superior sagittal sinus. As a result, the most common presentation of an ethmoidal DAVF is a frontal lobe hemorrhage. Occasionally, drainage can occur into the cavernous sinus, which leads to chemosis, proptosis, and elevated intraocular pressures. These are one of the few types of DAVF that have a male preponderance and for which surgical coagulation of the vein is the preferred method of treatment because of the associated low morbidity and high cure rate.[105]

Superior sagittal sinus DAVFs are rare and are varied in their presentation. Because of the distant location between the superior sagittal sinus and the auditory apparatus, early detection secondary to a pulsatile tinnitus is rare. The presentation, therefore, is predominantly secondary to hemorrhage (subarachnoid, subdural, or intraparenchymal), headache, or symptoms resulting from venous hypertension. The arterial supply is generally derived from branches of the middle meningeal artery, the anterior falcine artery off the ophthalmic artery, or the posterior meningeal artery. Frequently, the arterial supply will be bilateral. Should endovascular therapy fail to achieve complete obliteration, surgical excision should be considered. If surgical excision is performed, care must be taken to identify the patterns of cerebral venous drainage to prevent exacerbation of the venous hypertension.

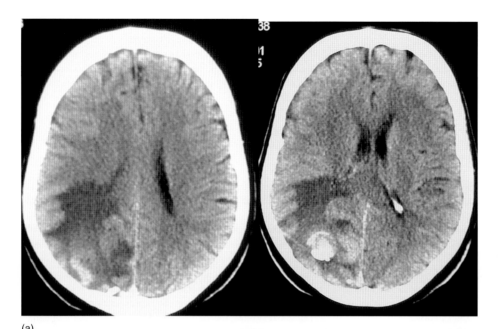

(a)

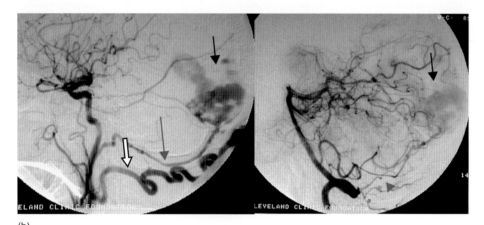

(b)

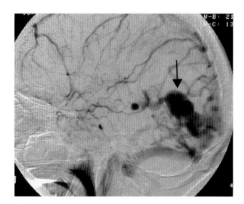

(c)

Figure 8.9

(a) Axial CT scans of a 59-year-old man with a new, gradual-onset headache and hemianopsia demonstrate vasogenic edema and mass effect in the right occipital lobe. Dystrophic calcification is seen centrally. (b) Lateral angiographic views of the right common carotid and right vertebral arteries demonstrate dural AVM fed by the posterior auricular artery (red arrow), the occipital artery (open arrow), and the dural vertebral artery (red arrowhead) with intracranial cortical venous drainage (black arrows). (c) Delayed view of the right common carotid artery injection demonstrating cortical venous stasis and slow flow (black arrow). Following successful transarterial embolization, the veins collapsed and the vasogenic edema as well as the symptoms completely resolved.

Patients with lesions involving the superior petrosal sinus, also referred to as tentorial DAVFs, generally present with hemorrhage or mass effect from dilated veins. The arterial supply typically arises from the artery of Bernasconi and Cassinari off the meningohypophyseal trunk, the inferolateral trunk, and the petrosal and petrosquamosal branches of the middle meningeal artery. The venous drainage usually involves the superior petrosal sinus and the pontine and perimesencephalic veins. Even if endovascular treatment fails to obliterate the fistula, it can aid in its local-

ization of the fistula on post-procedure axial imaging and it can minimize the amount of blood loss during surgical resection.[106]

In summary, the location and pattern of venous drainage are the key components in determining the clinical presentation of a DAVF. The arterial supply is largely determined by the location of the fistula, and the venous drainage and degree of venous hypertension indicate the potential for a malignant clinical course. The overall angiographic anatomy aids in determining whether endovascular therapy by transarterial, transvenous,

Table 8.3 Revised Djindjian classification of dural arterial–venous fistulae

Type I	Antegrade drainage into a sinus
Type IIa	Reflux into the sinus (retrograde flow)
Type IIb	Reflux into cortical veins
Type IIa+b	Reflux into both sinus and cortical veins
Type III	Direct cortical venous drainage without venous ectasia
Type IV	Direct cortical venous drainage with venous ectasias
Type V	Spinal venous drainage

From Cognard et al.[107]

Table 8.4 Borden classification of dural arterial–venous fistulae

Type I		Drainage into the dural venous sinus
Type II		Drainage into the dural venous sinus with retrograde drainage into subarachnoid veins
Type III		Drainage into subarachnoid veins
	Subtype a	Simple fistula
	Subtype b	Multiple fistulas

or a combined treatment can obliterate the fistula, and endovascular therapy is generally the first line of therapy for the majority of these lesions. Should the endovascular approach fail to cure the lesion, it can aid in localization of the fistula on axial CT imaging and minimize the amount of blood loss during surgical resection.

Diagnostic Imaging

The preliminary diagnosis of a DAVF is based on its clinical presentation. CT, CT angiography, MRI, and magnetic resonance angiography often support the clinical diagnosis by revealing engorged cortical veins, sinus stenosis or occlusion, hemorrhage, osseous changes from hypertrophied and ectatic vessels, or vasogenic edema from venous hypertension. All patients with clinical and radiographic evidence suggestive of a DAVF should undergo cerebral angiography. If a DAVF is revealed, a thorough angiographic evaluation should be obtained to delineate the fistula location, the arterial feeders, the sinus drainage, the cortical venous drainage, any occlusions, stenoses or ectasias, and the blood flow dynamics. A complete angiographic evaluation may require evaluation and careful analysis of both internal and external carotid arteries both vertebral arteries and possibly the ascending and deep cervical systems.

Classification

There are numerous classification schemes for DAVFs, the most useful and modern are the revised Djindjian classification scheme proposed by Cognard[107] (Table 8.3) and the Borden classification scheme[108] (Table 8.4), which are both based on that initial scheme. No matter the classification system, they all focus on the patterns of venous drainage and the clinical implications of presentation, treatment, and prognosis associated with them.

Treatment strategies

The decision to treat a DAVF depends primarily on the clinical presentation of the patient and the angiographic characteristics of the fistula, especially on the venous side (see Figures 8.10, 8.11, 8.12). A simple fistula draining into a sinus in a patient with a mild bruit or one who is asymptomatic is best served with conservative or compression therapy.[109] It is important to continue to follow the clinical course of these patients since DAVFs can progress to a more malignant state. If a pulsatile bruit resolves, it is an indication for repeat angiography, because the sinus may have thrombosed and the venous drainage may be redirected into the leptomeningeal or deep venous system, a finding that portends a more aggressive course of therapy.

There is a subset of patients who are symptomatic (commonly with a bruit) and whose activities of daily living are affected, but who do not harbor aggressive angiographic features. In these cases, a subtotal obliteration or a subtotal angiographic occlusion of the DAVF can palliate the symptoms. An aggressive angiographic cure may not be required and may even impose unnecessary risks.[110]

The treatment goal for any patient presenting with hemorrhage, symptoms of cortical venous hypertension or significant ocular pathology or vision loss should be to achieve complete obliteration of the lesion. Even the asymptomatic patient whose fistula demonstrates significant cortical venous pathology should be considered for aggressive treatment. In this high-risk population, there is little evidence to support the notion that incomplete obliteration reduces the risk of hemorrhage, venous infarction, or visual loss.

Compression therapy

A small percentage of DAVFs involving the transverse sigmoid sinus or the cavernous sinus can be treated with compression therapy. This involves compression of the involved occipital artery or the carotid artery (carotid atherosclerosis must first be excluded) with the contralateral hand for 30 minutes several times a day. For small fistulas, this may promote thrombosis in up to 30% of cases.[109]

Endovascular treatment

Transvenous embolization of fistulae was popularized by Halbach et al. and it has been used with good success and is especially effective in the treatment of transverse and cavernous sinus DAVFs.[103,110–112] Venous access into the transverse sinus is generally not an issue; and, even if the sinus is occluded at the level of the sigmoid sinus or jugular bulb, access into the involved sinus can be obtained by crossing the torcula. Consideration of the venous drainage of the fistula itself as well as the drainage of normal cerebral tissue is paramount in minimizing risk

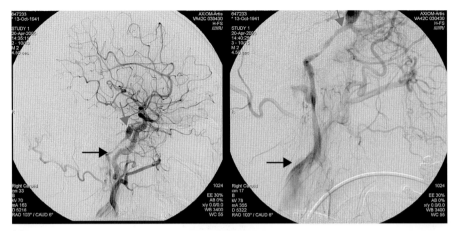

(a)

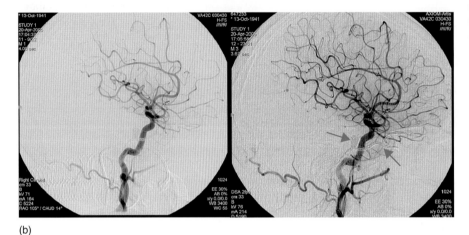

(b)

Figure 8.10
(a) Early and delayed right common carotid artery injection demonstrating early arterial–venous shunting to the cavernous sinus (red arrow) due to a dural fistula fed by small branches of the internal maxillary artery and dural branches of the carotid siphon. Of particular note is the large inferior petrosal sinus, which connects to the internal jugular vein well below the foramen magnum (black arrow). (b) Lateral right common carotid angiogram following inferior petrosal venous access and coil embolization of the ophthalmic veins and cavernous sinus. In the absence of venous outflow to perpetuate the shunt, the lesion is no longer present. Misregistration artifact denotes the presence of the venous coils (red arrows)

(see Figures 8.11, 8.12). Care must be taken not to re-route the pattern of venous drainage into the cortical veins, which can exacerbate venous hypertension (see figure 8.9). For transverse sinus fistulae, particular attention must be paid to the vein of Labbé. If flow in this vein is antegrade, embolization cannot proceed across the origin of the vein without compromising normal venous drainage. However, if it is retrograde, occlusion across the vein of Labbé is ultimately tolerated and indeed may be required to provide a definitive cure.

There are many methods of occluding the sinus with balloons or coils. Advocates of balloon occlusion[113] espouse the advantage of possible balloon test occlusion of the sinus. Unlike arterial infarction, however, venous infarction generally does not occur for hours, and occasionally days, after the permanent occlusion. A short temporary period of balloon occlusion therefore does not suggest that the patient will tolerate long-term occlusion. Indeed, clinical symptoms (especially with cavernous sinus lesions) may transiently worsen following transvenous embolization, requiring frequent monitoring and adjunctive pharmacologic treatment (e.g. corticosteroids). Furthermore, placement of a detachable balloon against the blood flow into a sinus may not be technically feasible in every case and certainly will not be possible for Borden Type III DAVFs, in which the drainage occurs directly into subarachnoid veins (see figure 8.9).

The alternative to balloons is coil occlusion. Unfortunately, even dense packing with coils may not permanently occlude the fistula and further thrombosis within the coil mass itself may be required. Currently, we favor coil embolization of the sinus,

which will decrease the degree of shunting, occasionally augmented by transarterial embolization of select pedicles.

The initial results of transarterial treatment of DAVFs were suboptimal, owing to the low rates of cure and the subsequent recruitment of collaterals.[103,110,111,114] The difficulty in curing DAVFs transarterially probably resulted from the use of polyvinyl alcohol particles and proximal occlusion of feeding pedicles during NBCA injections.[115] Embolization with polyvinyl alcohol may result in re-canalization, while transarterial embolization with liquid agents may not traverse the fistulous connection into the venous side and may permit the re-appearance of smaller collaterals, which may be more difficult to catheterize selectively. An additional consideration is the potential for dangerous overt or occult anastomoses between the external carotid artery and the internal carotid or vertebral arteries; or ischemic cranial nerve palsies could also preclude a safe and effective embolization. In a recent series of 21 patients treated transarterially under flow-arrest conditions, cures were demonstrated in all fistulae without complications.[116] Although the definite curative embolization occurred under flow-arrest conditions, a significant portion of these patients underwent adjunctive embolization with polyvinyl alcohol or NBCA or previous transvenous coiling of the recipient venous structure. This served to devascularize the collateral inflow to minimize NBCA fragmentation, prevent systemic venous embolization, and increase the probability of polymerization within the pathologic shunt itself. This illustrates the complex angioarchitectural spectrum of DAVFs and the expertise in multimodality treatments required to engender treatment safe and effective.

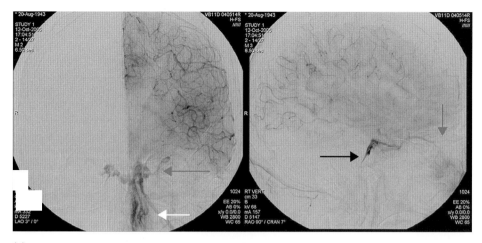

(a)

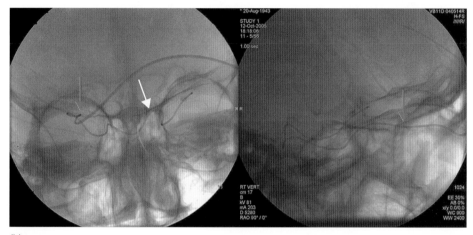

(b)

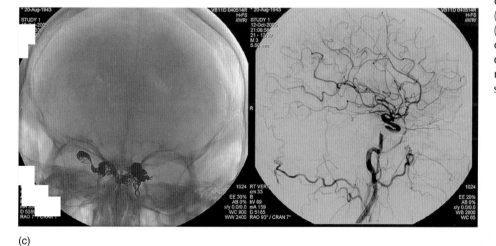

(c)

Figure 8.11
(a) Anterior–posterior (AP) and lateral left carotid artery injection in an elderly woman demonstrating early filling of the cavernous sinus and superior ophthalmic veins consistent with a dural carotid cavernous fistula. The AP view hints at a patent inferior petrosal sinus (white arrow), this is actually the angular vein, which is extracranial and lies over the maxilla. The lateral view demonstrates the inferior petrosal sinus to be occluded. (b) While orbital catheterization via the angular vein has been reported, the angulation at the trochlea typically makes this an arduous task. An accommodating and skilled ophthalmologic surgeon can obtain direct access to the orbit via the superior ophthalmic vein (red arrow) cut-down, as shown here in the AP and lateral radiographs. As is often the case with these lesions, the arterial supply as well as the venous drainage may be bilateral, and it may require bilateral coiling. Note the micro-catheter accessing the side opposite the cut-down via the circular sinus (white arrow). (c) AP radiograph (left) and lateral left common carotid artery angiogram (right) demonstrating bilateral coil mass as well as cessation of shunting.

Recently, reports have appeared using Onyx for transarterial embolization of dural AVFs.[117–121] Accessibility of the feeding pedicles in conjunction with a higher threshold for reflux (of less concern outside the pial circulation) probably accounts for the excellent penetration of the fistula and the good clinical results.[118] Nevertheless, one must remain vigilant in the event of cortical venous reflux, a since this may pose a risk of intracranial hemorrhage.[119]

Surgical treatment

Unlike pial AVMs of the brain or spinal cord, the venous drainage of a DAVF can frequently be safely ligated, excised, or occluded prior to occlusion of all the arterial pedicles.[122] However, profuse bleeding can occur during the exposure and bone flap elevation, owing to the arterialized dura, the pedicles, and drainage into the intradiploic vascular channels. Sinus skeletonization or

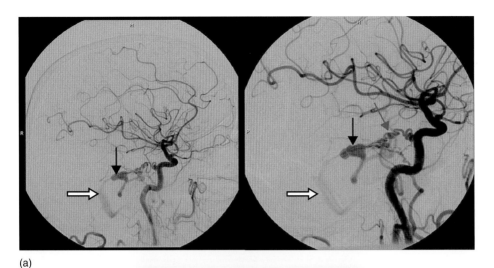

(a)

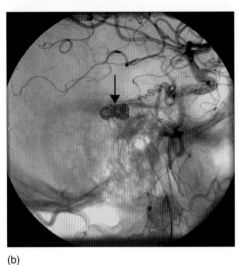

(b)

Figure 8.12
(a) Lateral carotid angiograms demonstrating a tentorial dural arterial–venous malformation fed from the tentorial branch of the internal carotid artery (red arrow), a solitary draining varix (black arrows), with ultimate communication to the sigmoid sinus (open arrow).
(b) Unsubtracted carotid angiogram post-coiling of the varix (arrow) demonstrating occlusion of the shunt.

excision of DAVFs should be reserved for those cases in which endovascular therapy has failed to effect a cure but has at least decreased the flow to reduce blood loss. Surgical access of a recipient venous structure, such as the superior ophthalmic vein for cavernous DAVFs, to deliver endovascular materials continues to play a significant role. As previously mentioned, for ethmoidal DAVFS[105] and some petrosal sinus DAVFS, surgical excision of the draining vein is the primary treatment modality.

In a recent series, 34 patients with primarily transverse sigmoid, superior sagittal, or superior petrosal sinus DAVFs were cured by surgical treatment.[122] The authors separated their patient population into two groups depending on whether the fistulous drainage occurred purely through leptomeningeal veins (non-sinus fistulae) or whether the fistula drained into a sinus with retrograde flow into the leptomeningeal circulation (sinus fistulae). In the former scenario, the surgical treatment required a disconnection of the draining veins at the point where they exited the dural wall of the sinus. In the latter, a surgical excision of the involved sinus segment after preoperative embolization represented a safe and definitive treatment because this segment did not serve to drain the normal cerebrovasculature. Their cure rate was 100%, and there were no instances of mortality or permanent morbidity. Again, the treatment goals were determined by a careful evaluation of the venous anatomy, and the importance of pre-operative embolization was emphasized.

Radiosurgery

The role of stereotactic radiosurgery in the treatment of DAVFs is continuing to develop, and the experience with this modality is growing.[123–129] Owing to the complex nature of DAVFs and the relatively small number of patients in each series, the rate of angiographic obliteration is still uncertain. It does appear, however, that the complication rates of the initial treatment are relatively low. However, there is the possibility of hemorrhage or symptomatic clinical events that could occur from the time of treatment until obliteration is obtained. This may be untenable for patients who present with hemorrhage, significant venous hypertension, or high-risk angiographic profiles.

Owing to the relative efficacy of endovascular and surgical treatment of these lesions, we view stereotactic radiosurgery as the third-line treatment modality. There will be, however, a relatively small patient population in whom endovascular or surgical treatment may be extremely difficult or risky, including the elderly population with significant comorbidities, and in such patients stereotactic radiosurgery may play a role.

Conclusions

DAVFs comprise a highly complex series of lesions, both clinically and angiographically. The clinical presentation can range from being asymptomatic to causing devastating intracranial hemorrhage. The location of the fistula is a primary factor in determining the method of presentation. Angiographically, the pattern of venous drainage is the main factor in determining the ultimate prognosis. The goal of therapy for any DAVF that exhibits or displays cortical venous drainage or cause ocular compromise should be angiographic obliteration and cure. The method of treatment will be highly individualized to the angiographic architecture of each DAVF, and can consist of endovascular therapy, surgery, or a combination of methods to achieve the appropriate treatment goal and to minimize risk.

In general, we feel that the endovascular approach is the primary mode of therapy for transverse sinus, cavernous, superior sagittal, and petrosal sinus fistulas and that surgery is the primary mode of therapy for ethmoidal DAVFs. Stereotactic radiosurgery should be reserved for lesions where endovascular or surgical options have failed or would subject the patient to inordinate risk. The importance of a multidisciplinary approach to these highly complex lesions cannot be over-emphasized, and such an approach yields the safest and most effective outcomes.

References

1. McCormick WF. Pathology of vascular malformations of the brain. In: Wilson CB, Stein BM, eds. Intracranial Vascular Malformations. Baltimore: Williams and Wilkins, 1984: 44–63.
2. Mullan S, Mojtahedi S, Johnson DL, Macdonald RL. Embryological basis of some aspects of cerebral vascular fistulas and malformations. J Neurosurg 1996; 85: 1–8.
3. Hashimoto T, Wu Y, Lawton MT et al. Coexpression of angiogenic factors in brain arteriovenous malformations. Neurosurgery 2005; 56: 1058–65.
4. Koizumi T, Shiraishi T, Hagihara N et al. Expression of vascular endothelial growth factors and their receptors in and around intracranial arteriovenous malformations. Neurosurgery 2002; 50: 117–24.
5. Merrill MJ, Oldfield EH. A reassessment of vascular endothelial growth factor in central nervous system pathology. J Neurosurg 2005; 103: 853–68.
6. Kida Y, Kobayashi T, Tanaka T et al. Seizure control after radiosurgery on cerebral arteriovenous malformations. J Clin Neurosci 2000; 7: 6–9.
7. Meng JS, Okeda R. Histopathological structure of the pial arteriovenous malformation in adults: observation by reconstruction of serial sections of four surgical specimens. Acta Neuropathol (Berl) 2001; 102: 63–8.
8. Chin LS, Raffel C, Gonzalez-Gomez I, Giannotta SL, McComb JG. Diffuse arteriovenous malformations: a clinical, radiological, and pathological description. Neurosurgery 1992; 31: 863–8.
9. Redekop G, Terbrugge K, Montanera W, Willinsky R. Arterial aneurysms associated with cerebral arteriovenous malformations: classification, incidence, and risk of hemorrhage. J Neurosurg 1998; 89: 539–46.
10. Marks MP, Lane B, Steinberg GK, Chang PJ. Hemorrhage in intracerebral arteriovenous malformations: angiographic determinants. Radiology 1990; 176: 807–13.
11. Yasargil MG. Microneurosurgery. New York: Thieme, 1984.
12. Forster DM, Steiner L, Hakanson S. Arteriovenous malformations of the brain. A long-term clinical study. J Neurosurg 1972; 37: 562–70.
13. Cushing H. The Harvey Cushing Collection of Books and Manuscripts. New Haven: Yale University Department of the History of Science and Medicine, 1943.
14. Dandy WE. Selected Writings of Walter Dandy. Springfield: Thomas, 1957.
15. Cushing H, Bailey P. Tumors arising from blood vessels of the brain. Springfield: Charles C. Thomas Publishing, 1928.
16. Kikuchi K, Kowada M, Sasajima H. Vascular malformations of the brain in hereditary hemorrhagic telangiectasia (Rendu–Osler–Weber disease). Surg Neurol 1994; 41: 374–80.
17. Laufer L, Cohen A. Sturge-Weber syndrome associated with a large left hemispheric arteriovenous malformation. Pediatr Radiol 1994; 24: 272–3.
18. Luo CB, Lasjaunias P, Bhattacharya J. Craniofacial vascular malformations in Wyburn-Mason syndrome. J Chin Med Assoc 2006; 69: 575–80.
19. ApSimon HT, Reef H, Phadke RV, Popovic EA. A population-based study of brain arteriovenous malformation: long-term treatment outcomes. Stroke 2002; 33: 2794–800.
20. Perret G, Nishioka H. Report on the cooperative study of intracranial aneurysms and subarachnoid hemorrhage. Section VI. Arteriovenous malformations. An analysis of 545 cases of cranio-cerebral arteriovenous malformations and fistulae reported to the cooperative study. J Neurosurg 1966; 25: 467–90.
21. Brown RD Jr, Wiebers DO, Torner JC, O'Fallon WM. Incidence and prevalence of intracranial vascular malformations in Olmsted County, Minnesota, 1965 to 1992. Neurology 1996; 46: 949–52.
22. Al-Shahi R, Fang JS, Lewis SC, Warlow CP. Prevalence of adults with brain arteriovenous malformations: a community based study in Scotland using capture-recapture analysis. J Neurol Neurosurg Psychiatry 2002; 73: 547–51.
23. Spetzler RF, Martin NA. A proposed grading system for arteriovenous malformations. J Neurosurg 1986; 65: 476–83.
24. Misra M, Aletich VI, Charbel FT et al. Multidisciplinary approach to arteriovenous malformations. In: Kaye AH BP, editor. Operative Neurosurgery. London: Churchill Livingstone, 2000, 1138–51.
25. Berman MF, Sciacca RR, Pile-Spellman J et al. The epidemiology of brain arteriovenous malformations. Neurosurgery 2000; 47: 389–96.
26. Al-Shahi R, Warlow CP. Quality of evidence for management of arteriovenous malformations of the brain. Lancet 2002; 360: 1022–3.
27. Wilkins RH. Natural history of intracranial vascular malformations: a review. Neurosurgery 1985; 16: 421–30.
28. Chicoine MR, Darcy RG. Clinical aspects of subarachnoid hemorrhage. In: Weilch KMA CLWBSB, ed. Primer on cerebrovascular diseases. San Diego: Academic Press, 1997: 425–32.
29. Brown RD Jr, Wiebers DO, Torner JC, O Fallon WM. Frequency of intracranial hemorrhage as a presenting symptom and subtype analysis: a population-based study of intracranial vascular malformations in Olmsted Country, Minnesota. J Neurosurg 1996; 85: 29–32.
30. Crawford PM, West CR, Chadwick DW, Shaw MD. Arteriovenous malformations of the brain: natural history in unoperated patients. J Neurol Neurosurg Psychiatry 1986; 49: 1–10.
31. Ondra SL, Troupp H, George ED, Schwab K. The natural history of symptomatic arteriovenous malformations of the brain: a 24-year follow-up assessment. J Neurosurg 1990; 73: 387–91
32. Spetzler RF, Hargraves RW, McCormick PW et al. Relationship of perfusion pressure and size to risk of hemorrhage from arteriovenous malformations. J Neurosurg 1992; 76: 918–23.
33. Mast H, Young WL, Koennecke HC et al. Risk of spontaneous haemorrhage after diagnosis of cerebral arteriovenous malformation. Lancet 1997; 350: 1065–8.
34. Graf CJ, Perret GE, Torner JC. Bleeding from cerebral arteriovenous malformations as part of their natural history. J Neurosurg 1983; 58: 331–7.
35. Itoyama Y, Uemura S, Ushio Y et al. Natural course of unoperated intracranial arteriovenous malformations: study of 50 cases. J Neurosurg 1989; 71: 805–9.
36. Jane JA, Kassell NF, Torner JC, Winn HR. The natural history of aneurysms and arteriovenous malformations. J Neurosurg 1985; 62: 321–3.
37. Waltimo O. The relationship of size, density and localization of intracranial arteriovenous malformations to the type of initial symptom. J Neurol Sci 1973; 19: 13–9.
38. Piepgras DG, Sundt TM Jr, Ragoowansi AT, Stevens L. Seizure outcome in patients with surgically treated cerebral arteriovenous malformations. J Neurosurg 1993; 78: 5–11.

39. Flickinger JC, Kondziolka D, Pollock BE, Lunsford LD. Radiosurgical management of intracranial vascular malformations. Neuroimaging Clin N Am 1998; 8: 483–92.

40. Horton JC, Chambers WA, Lyons SL, Adams RD, Kjellberg RN. Pregnancy and the risk of hemorrhage from cerebral arteriovenous malformations. Neurosurgery 1990; 27: 867–71.

41. Robinson JL, Hall CS, Sedzimir CB. Arteriovenous malformations, aneurysms, and pregnancy. J Neurosurg 1974; 41: 63–70.

42. Lewis AI, Sathi SR, Tew JM. Intracranial vascular malformations. In: Grossman RG, Loftus CM ed. Principles of Neurosurgery. Philadelphia: Lippincott-Raven, 1999.

43. Batjer HH, Devous MD Sr. The use of acetazolamide-enhanced regional cerebral blood flow measurement to predict risk to arteriovenous malformation patients. Neurosurgery 1992; 31: 213–7.

44. Baumann SB, Noll DC, Kondziolka DS et al. Comparison of functional magnetic resonance imaging with positron emission tomography and magnetoencephalography to identify the motor cortex in a patient with an arteriovenous malformation. J Image Guid Surg 1995; 1: 191–7.

45. Leblanc R, Meyer E. Functional PET scanning in the assessment of cerebral arteriovenous malformations. Case report. J Neurosurg 1990; 73: 615–9.

46. Maldjian J, Atlas SW, Howard RS et al. Functional magnetic resonance imaging of regional brain activity in patients with intracerebral arteriovenous malformations before surgical or endovascular therapy. J Neurosurg 1996; 84: 477–83.

47. Rauch RA, Vinuela F, Dion J et al. Preembolization functional evaluation in brain arteriovenous malformations: the ability of superselective Amytal test to predict neurologic dysfunction before embolization. AJNR Am J Neuroradiol 1992; 13: 309–14.

48. Turski PA, Cordes D, Mock B et al. Basic concepts of functional magnetic resonance imaging and arteriovenous malformations. Magn Reson Imaging Clin N Am 1998; 6: 801–10.

49. Brown RD Jr, Wiebers DO, Forbes GS. Unruptured intracranial aneurysms and arteriovenous malformations: frequency of intracranial hemorrhage and relationship of lesions. J Neurosurg 1990; 73: 859–63.

50. Miyasaka K, Wolpert SM, Prager RJ. The association of cerebral aneurysms, infundibula, and intracranial arteriovenous malformations. Stroke 1982; 13: 196–203.

51. Perret G, Nishioka H. Report on the cooperative study of intracranial aneurysms and subarachnoid hemorrhage. IV. Cerebral angiography. An analysis of the diagnostic value and complications of carotid and vertebral angiography in 5,484 patients. J Neurosurg 1966; 25: 98–114.

52. Lasjaunias P, Piske R, Terbrugge K, Willinsky R. Cerebral arteriovenous malformations (C. AVM) and associated arterial aneurysms (AA). Analysis of 101 C. AVM cases, with 37 AA in 23 patients. Acta Neurochir (Wien) 1988; 91: 29–36.

53. Miyasaka Y, Yada K, Ohwada T et al. An analysis of the venous drainage system as a factor in hemorrhage from arteriovenous malformations. J Neurosurg 1992; 76: 239–43.

54. Spetzler RF, Martin NA. A proposed grading system for arteriovenous malformations. J Neurosurg 1986; 65: 476–83.

55. Luessenhop AJ, Rosa L. Cerebral arteriovenous malformations. Indications for and results of surgery, and the role of intravascular techniques. J Neurosurg 1984; 60: 1–14.

56. Luessenhop AJ, Gennarelli TA. Anatomical grading of supratentorial arteriovenous malformations for determining operability. Neurosurgery 1977; 1: 30–5.

57. Hamilton MG, Spetzler RF. The prospective application of a grading system for arteriovenous malformations. Neurosurgery 1994; 34: 2–6.

58. Heros RC, Korosue K, Diebold PM. Surgical excision of cerebral arteriovenous malformations: late results. Neurosurgery 1990; 26: 570–7.

59. Rosenblatt S, Lewis AI, Tew JM. Combined interventional and surgical treatment of arteriovenous malformations. Neuroimaging Clin N Am 1998; 8: 469–82.

60. Lawton MT. Spetzler-Martin Grade III arteriovenous malformations: surgical results and a modification of the grading scale. Neurosurgery 2003; 52: 740–8.

61. Han PP, Ponce FA, Spetzler RF. Intention-to-treat analysis of Spetzler-Martin grades IV and V arteriovenous malformations: natural history and treatment paradigm. J Neurosurg 2003; 98: 3–7.

62. Miyamoto S, Hashimoto N, Nagata I et al. Posttreatment sequelae of palliatively treated cerebral arteriovenous malformations. Neurosurgery 2000; 46: 589–94.

63. Wikholm G, Lundqvist C, Svendsen P. The Goteborg cohort of embolized cerebral arteriovenous malformations: a 6-year follow-up. Neurosurgery 2001; 49: 799–805.

64. Jafar JJ, Davis AJ, Berenstein A, Choi IS, Kupersmith MJ. The effect of embolization with N-butyl cyanoacrylate prior to surgical resection of cerebral arteriovenous malformations. J Neurosurg 993; 78: 60–9.

65. DeMeritt JS, Pile-Spellman J, Mast H et al. Outcome analysis of preoperative embolization with N-butyl cyanoacrylate in cerebral arteriovenous malformations. AJNR Am J Neuroradiol 1995; 16: 1801–7.

66. Kim EJ, Halim AX, Dowd CF et al. The relationship of coexisting extranidal aneurysms to intracranial hemorrhage in patients harboring brain arteriovenous malformations. Neurosurgery 2004; 54: 1349–57.

67. Murayama Y, Vinuela F, Ulhoa A et al. Nonadhesive liquid embolic agent for cerebral arteriovenous malformations: preliminary histopathological studies in swine rete mirabile. Neurosurgery 1998; 43: 1164–75.

68. Kwon Y, Jeon SR, Kim JH et al. Analysis of the causes of treatment failure in gamma knife radiosurgery for intracranial arteriovenous malformations. J Neurosurg 2000; 93: 104–6.

69. Batjer HH, Devous MD Sr, Seibert GB et al. Intracranial arteriovenous malformation: relationships between clinical and radiographic factors and ipsilateral steal severity. Neurosurgery 1988; 23: 322–8.

70. Lunsford LD, Kondziolka D, Flickinger JC et al. Stereotactic radiosurgery for arteriovenous malformations of the brain. J Neurosurg 1991; 75: 512–24.

71. Steiner L, Lindquist C, Adler JR et al. Clinical outcome of radiosurgery for cerebral arteriovenous malformations. J Neurosurg 1992; 77: 1–8.

72. Gobin YP, Laurent A, Merienne L et al. Treatment of brain arteriovenous malformations by embolization and radiosurgery. J Neurosurg 1996; 85: 19–28.

73. Henkes H, Nahser HC, Berg-Dammer E et al. Endovascular therapy of brain AVMs prior to radiosurgery. Neurol Res 1998; 20: 479–92.

74. Marks MP, Lane B, Steinberg G, Chang P. Vascular characteristics of intracerebral arteriovenous malformations in patients with clinical steal. AJNR Am J Neuroradiol 1991; 12: 489–96.

75. Kusske JA, Kelly WA. Embolization and reduction of the "steal" syndrome in cerebral arteriovenous malformations. J Neurosurg 1974; 40: 313–21.

76. Luessenhop AJ, Mujica PH. Embolization of segments of the circle of Willis and adjacent branches for management of certain inoperable cerebral arteriovenous malformations. J Neurosurg 1981; 54: 573–82.

77. Fox AJ, Girvin JP, Vinuela F, Drake CG. Rolandic arteriovenous malformations: improvement in limb function by IBC embolization. AJNR Am J Neuroradiol 1985; 6: 575–82.

78. Brothers MF, Kaufmann JC, Fox AJ, Deveikis JP. n-Butyl 2-cyanoacrylate—substitute for IBCA in interventional neuroradiology: histopathologic and polymerization time studies. AJNR Am J Neuroradiol 1989; 10: 777–86.

79. Gounis MJ, Lieber BB, Wakhloo AK, Siekmann R, Hopkins LN. Effect of glacial acetic acid and ethiodized oil concentration on embolization with N-butyl 2-cyanoacrylate: an in vivo investigation. AJNR Am J Neuroradiol 2002; 23: 938–44.

80. Spiegel SM, Vinuela F, Goldwasser JM, Fox AJ, Pelz DM. Adjusting the polymerization time of isobutyl-2 cyanoacrylate. AJNR Am J Neuroradiol 1986; 7: 109–12.

81. Zoarski GH, Lilly MP, Sperling JS, Mathis JM. Surgically confirmed incorporation of a chronically retained neurointerventional

microcatheter in the carotid artery. AJNR Am J Neuroradiol 1999; 20: 177–8.

82. Sorimachi T, Koike T, Takeuchi S et al. Embolization of cerebral arteriovenous malformations achieved with polyvinyl alcohol particles: angiographic reappearance and complications. AJNR Am J Neuroradiol 1999; 20: 1323–8.

83. Cronqvist M, Wirestam R, Ramgren B et al. Endovascular treatment of intracerebral arteriovenous malformations: procedural safety, complications, and results evaluated by MR Imaging, including diffusion and perfusion imaging. AJNR Am J Neuroradiol 2006; 27: 162–76.

84. Newton TH, Cronqvist S. Involvement of dural arteries in intracranial arteriovenous malformations. Radiology 1969; 93: 1071–8.

85. Nishijima M, Takaku A, Endo S et al. Etiological evaluation of dural arteriovenous malformations of the lateral and sigmoid sinuses based on histopathological examinations. J Neurosurg 1992; 76: 600–6.

86. Chaudhary MY, Sachdev VP, Cho SH et al. Dural arteriovenous malformation of the major venous sinuses: an acquired lesion. AJNR Am J Neuroradiol 1982; 3: 13–9.

87. Houser OW, Campbell JK, Campbell RJ, Sundt TM Jr. Arteriovenous malformation affecting the transverse dural venous sinus—an acquired lesion. Mayo Clin Proc 1979; 54: 651–61.

88. Kuhner A, Krastel A, Stoll W. Arteriovenous malformations of the transverse dural sinus. J Neurosurg 1976; 45: 12–9.

89. Obrador S, Soto M, Silvela J. Clinical syndromes of arteriovenous malformations of the transverse-sigmoid sinus. J Neurol Neurosurg Psychiatry 1975; 38: 436–51.

90. Herman JM, Spetzler RF, Bederson JB, Kurbat JM, Zabramski JM. Genesis of a dural arteriovenous malformation in a rat model. J Neurosurg 1995; 83: 539–45.

91. Lawton MT, Jacobowitz R, Spetzler RF. Redefined role of angiogenesis in the pathogenesis of dural arteriovenous malformations. J Neurosurg 1997; 87: 267–74.

92. Terada T, Higashida RT, Halbach VV et al. Development of acquired arteriovenous fistulas in rats due to venous hypertension. J Neurosurg 1994; 80: 884–9.

93. Hamada Y, Goto K, Inoue T et al. Histopathological aspects of dural arteriovenous fistulas in the transverse-sigmoid sinus region in nine patients. Neurosurgery 1997; 40: 452–6.

94. Bahar S, Chiras J, Carpena JP, Meder JF, Bories J. Spontaneous vertebro-vertebral arterio-venous fistula associated with fibromuscular dysplasia. Report of two cases. Neuroradiology 1984; 26: 45–9.

95. Deans WR, Bloch S, Leibrock L, Berman BM, Skultety FM. Arteriovenous fistula in patients with neurofibromatosis. Radiology 1982; 144: 103–7.

96. Graf CJ. Spontaneous carotid-cavernous fistula. Ehlers-Danlos syndrome and related conditions. Arch Neurol 1965; 13: 662–72.

97. Halbach VV, Higashida RT, Dowd CF, Barnwell SL, Hieshima GB. Treatment of carotid-cavernous fistulas associated with Ehlers-Danlos syndrome. Neurosurgery 1990; 26: 1021–7.

98. Schievink WI, Piepgras DG. Cervical vertebral artery aneurysms and arteriovenous fistulae in neurofibromatosis type 1: case reports. Neurosurgery 1991; 29: 760–5.

99. Malek AM, Halbach VV, Higashida RT et al. Treatment of dural arteriovenous malformations and fistulas. Neurosurg Clin N Am 2000; 11: 147–66, ix.

100. McDougall CG, Halbach VV, Dowd CF et al. Dural arteriovenous fistulas of the marginal sinus. AJNR Am J Neuroradiol 1997; 18: 1565–72.

101. Houser OW, Baker HL Jr, Rhoton AL Jr, Okazaki H. Intracranial dural arteriovenous malformations. Radiology 1972; 105: 55–64.

102. Awad IA, Little JR, Akarawi WP, Ahl J. Intracranial dural arteriovenous malformations: factors predisposing to an aggressive neurological course. J Neurosurg 1990; 72: 839–50.

103. Halbach VV, Higashida RT, Hieshima GB et al. Dural fistulas involving the cavernous sinus: results of treatment in 30 patients. Radiology 1987; 163: 437–42.

104. Turner RD, Gonugunta V, Kelly ME, Masaryk TJ, Fiorella DJ. Marginal sinus arteriovenous fistulas mimicking carotid cavernous fistulas: diagnostic and therapeutic considerations. AJNR Am J Neuroradiol 2007; 28: 1915–18..

105. Halbach VV, Higashida RT, Hieshima GB et al. Dural arteriovenous fistulas supplied by ethmoidal arteries. Neurosurgery 1990; 26: 816–23.

106. Tomak PR, Cloft HJ, Kaga A et al. Evolution of the management of tentorial dural arteriovenous malformations. Neurosurgery 2003; 52: 750–60.

107. Cognard C, Gobin YP, Pierot L et al. Cerebral dural arteriovenous fistulas: clinical and angiographic correlation with a revised classification of venous drainage. Radiology 1995; 194: 671–80.

108. Borden JA, Wu JK, Shucart WA. A proposed classification for spinal and cranial dural arteriovenous fistulous malformations and implications for treatment. J Neurosurg 1995; 82: 166–79.

109. Higashida RT, Hieshima GB, Halbach VV, Bentson JR, Goto K. Closure of carotid cavernous sinus fistulae by external compression of the carotid artery and jugular vein. Acta Radiol Suppl 1986; 369: 580–3.

110. Barnwell SL, Halbach VV, Higashida RT, Hieshima G, Wilson CB. Complex dural arteriovenous fistulas. Results of combined endovascular and neurosurgical treatment in 16 patients. J Neurosurg 1989; 71: 352–8.

111. Halbach VV, Higashida RT, Hieshima GB et al. Dural fistulas involving the transverse and sigmoid sinuses: results of treatment in 28 patients. Radiology 1987; 163: 443–7.

112. Halbach VV, Higashida RT, Hieshima GB, Mehringer CM, Hardin CW. Transvenous embolization of dural fistulas involving the transverse and sigmoid sinuses. AJNR Am J Neuroradiol 1989; 10: 385–92.

113. Roy D, Raymond J. The role of transvenous embolization in the treatment of intracranial dural arteriovenous fistulas. Neurosurgery 1997; 40: 1133–41.

114. Grossman RI, Sergott RC, Goldberg HI et al. Dural malformations with ophthalmic manifestations: results of particulate embolization in seven patients. AJNR Am J Neuroradiol 1985; 6: 809–13.

115. Quisling RG, Mickle JP, Ballinger W. Small particle polyvinyl alcohol embolization of cranial lesions with minimal arteriolar-capillary barriers. Surg Neurol 1986; 25: 243–52.

116. Nelson PK, Russell SM, Woo HH. Alastra AJ, Vidovich DV. Use of a wedged microcatheter for curative transarterial embolization of complex intracranial dural arteriovenous fistulas: indications, endovascular technique, and outcome in 21 patients. J Neurosurg 2003; 98: 498–506.

117. Arat A, Inci S. Treatment of a superior sagittal sinus dural arteriovenous fistula with Onyx: technical case report. Neurosurgery 2006; 59: ONSE169–70.

118. Carlson AP, Taylor CL, Yonas H. Treatment of dural arteriovenous fistula using ethylene vinyl alcohol (onyx) arterial embolization as the primary modality: short-term results. J Neurosurg 2007; 107: 1120–5.

119. Cognard C, Januel AC, Silva NA Jr, Tall P. Endovascular treatment of intracranial dural arteriovenous fistulas with cortical venous drainage: new management using Onyx. AJNR Am J Neuroradiol 2008; 29: 235–41.

120. Nogueira RG, Dabus G, Rabinov JD et al. Preliminary experience with Onyx embolization for the treatment of intracranial dural arteriovenous fistulas. AJNR Am J Neuroradiol 2008; 29: 91–7.

121. Suzuki S, Lee DW, Jahan R, Duckwiler GR, Vinuela F. Transvenous treatment of spontaneous dural carotid-cavernous fistulas using a combination of detachable coils and Onyx. AJNR Am J Neuroradiol 2006; 27: 1346–9.

122. Collice M, D Aliberti G, Arena O et al. Surgical treatment of intracranial dural arteriovenous fistulae: role of venous drainage. Neurosurgery 2000; 47: 56–66.

123. Friedman JA, Pollock BE, Nichols DA et al. Results of combined stereotactic radiosurgery and transarterial embolization for dural arteriovenous fistulas of the transverse and sigmoid sinuses. J Neurosurg 2001; 94: 886–91.

124. Guo WY, Pan DH, Wu HM et al. Radiosurgery as a treatment alternative for dural arteriovenous fistulas of the cavernous sinus. AJNR Am J Neuroradiol 1998; 19: 1081–7.

125. Lewis AI, Tomsick TA, Tew JM Jr. Management of tentorial dural arteriovenous malformations: transarterial embolization combined with stereotactic radiation or surgery. J Neurosurg 1994; 81: 851–9.

126. Maruyama K, Shin M, Kurita H, Tago M, Kirino T. Stereotactic radiosurgery for dural arteriovenous fistula involving the superior sagittal sinus. Case report. J Neurosurg 2002; 97: 481–3.

127. O'Leary S, Hodgson TJ, Coley SC, Kemeny AA, Radatz MW. Intracranial dural arteriovenous malformations: results of stereotactic radiosurgery in 17 patients. Clin Oncol (R Coll Radiol) 2002; 14: 97–102.

128. Onizuka M, Mori K, Takahashi N et al. Gamma knife surgery for the treatment of spontaneous dural carotid-cavernous fistulas. Neurol Med Chir (Tokyo) 2003; 43: 477–82.

129. Pan DH, Chung WY, Guo WY et al. Stereotactic radiosurgery for the treatment of dural arteriovenous fistulas involving the transverse-sigmoid sinus. J Neurosurg 2002; 96: 823–9.

9

Venous disease: dural sinus thrombosis and occlusion

Raymond D Turner IV and Thomas J Masaryk

Intracranial venous anatomy

Normal anatomy

Intracranial venous anatomy is functionally complex, with significant variations in size, drainage patterns, and anastomoses. Stenosis and occlusion of intracranial veins may be asymptomatic or may result in significant neurological deficit, diffuse parenchymal edema with coma, and even death. This chapter approaches the intracranial venous system as several inter-related components:

- the central or deep venous drainage of the hemispheres and posterior fossa;
- the cortical venous drainage, systems; and
- the dural sinuses.

The deep venous system of the cerebral hemispheres is concerned with craniopetal venous drainage of deep cerebral white matter and basal ganglia and can be divided at two separate levels:

- the internal cerebral vein, the basal vein (of Rosenthal), and the vein of Galen, and
- the transcerebral (medullary) venous system (Figures 9.1 and 9.2).

The internal cerebral vein originates at the interventricular foramen of Monro, where it is formed by the confluence of the septal, anterior caudate, ventricular, choroidal, and terminal (thalamostriate) subependymal veins, although anatomical variation in this region is common.[2] The internal cerebral veins run posteriorly to become united in the rostral quadrigeminal cistern to form the great cerebral vein of Galen.

The basal vein of Rosenthal originates deep within the Sylvian fissure, near the medial part of the anterior temporal lobe, and of can receive drainage from the insula, the cerebral peduncles, and multiple cortical (temporal) tributaries. The basal vein courses posteriorly, curving around the cerebral peduncles to its junction with the vein of Galen or the internal cerebral vein. The basal vein has important anastamoses, with its openings into the deep middle cerebral vein anteriorly, the vein of Galen posteriorly, and the petrosal veins inferiorly.

Paired with the basal vein is the posterior mesencephalic vein. The anterior pontomesencephalic vein runs along the anterior surface of the pons and commonly drains superiorly via the peduncular vein into the posterior mesencephalic vein, which in turn runs around the upper midbrain to drain into the great cerebral vein of Galen.

The vein of Galen is a short, unpaired, midline structure that curves posteriorly beneath the splenium of the corpus callosum. It unites with the inferior sagittal sinus at the tentorial apex to form the straight sinus. Deep venous drainage of the posterior fossa includes the precentral cerebellar vein and the superior vermian vein, which typically drain to the vein of Galen.

Despite a highly variable appearance, several large cortical veins can often be identified individually and include:

- the superficial middle cerebral vein
- the superior anastomotic vein of Trolard
- the inferior anastomotic vein of Labbé.

These last two anastomotic veins are often in a reciprocal relationship such that if one is dominant, the other is usually hypoplastic or absent.

The superficial middle cerebral vein runs anteriorly along the lateral (Sylvian) fissure and receives smaller veins draining the lateral surface of the hemisphere. This large vein curves around the anterior temporal pole and either drains medially into the cavernous sinus or inferiorly into the pterygoid plexus. Anastomotic channels allow the superficial middle cerebral vein to drain in other directions. These include the superior anastomotic vein of Trolard, which opens into the superior sagittal sinus, and the inferior anastomotic vein of Labbé, which opens into the transverse sinus.

Dural venous sinuses are enclosed between the periosteal and meningeal layers of dura, and they lack valves. The superior sagittal sinus lies along the attached border of the falx cerebri and extends from the foramen cecum to the torcula herophili. As it extends posteriorly, the superior sagittal sinus increases in caliber as it collects the superficial cerebral veins draining the cerebral convexities. Arachnoid granulations, contained within venous lacunae, are found protruding into the superior sagittal sinus along its course and may produce normal filling defects on imaging studies. The inferior sagittal sinus lies along the inferior free margin of the falx cerebri and drains the falx, the anterior part of the corpus callosum, and medial aspects of

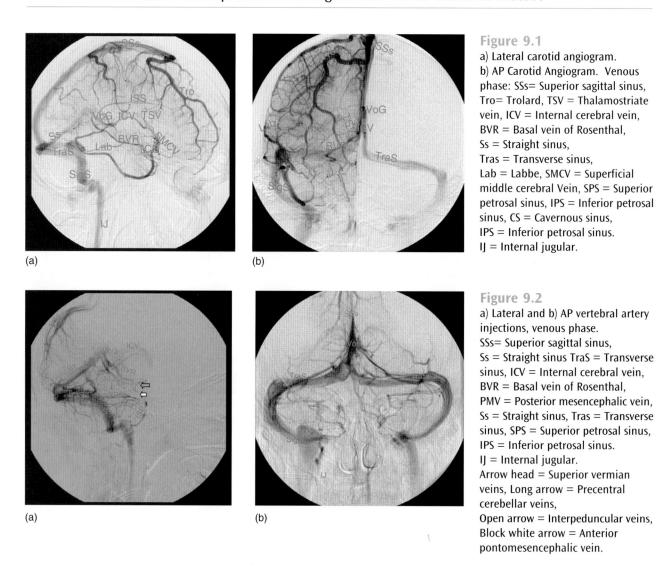

(a)   (b)

Figure 9.1
a) Lateral carotid angiogram.
b) AP Carotid Angiogram. Venous phase: SSs= Superior sagittal sinus, Tro= Trolard, TSV = Thalamostriate vein, ICV = Internal cerebral vein, BVR = Basal vein of Rosenthal, Ss = Straight sinus, Tras = Transverse sinus, Lab = Labbe, SMCV = Superficial middle cerebral Vein, SPS = Superior petrosal sinus, IPS = Inferior petrosal sinus, CS = Cavernous sinus, IPS = Inferior petrosal sinus. IJ = Internal jugular.

(a)   (b)

Figure 9.2
a) Lateral and b) AP vertebral artery injections, venous phase.
SSs= Superior sagittal sinus, Ss = Straight sinus TraS = Transverse sinus, ICV = Internal cerebral vein, BVR = Basal vein of Rosenthal, PMV = Posterior mesencephalic vein, Ss = Straight sinus, Tras = Transverse sinus, SPS = Superior petrosal sinus, IPS = Inferior petrosal sinus. IJ = Internal jugular.
Arrow head = Superior vermian veins, Long arrow = Precentral cerebellar veins, Open arrow = Interpeduncular veins, Block white arrow = Anterior pontomesencephalic vein.

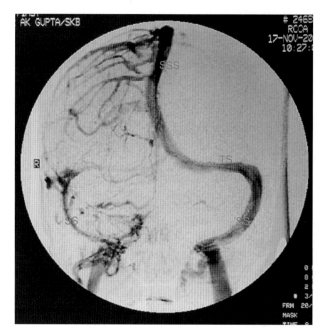

Figure 9.3
Normal variant. Hypoplasia of the right transverse sinus.

the cerebral hemispheres. The inferior sagittal sinus extends posteriorly and is joined by the great cerebral vein of Galen to form the straight sinus.

The transverse sinuses lie along the attached margin of the tentorium cerebelli within a groove on the inner table of the occipital bone. Each transverse sinus courses anterolaterally and, on reaching the base of the petrous portion of the temporal bone, turns inferomedially to form the sigmoid sinus that lies in the sigmoid sulcus of the temporal bone.

The transverse sinuses are commonly asymmetric, with the right transverse sinus being dominant in the majority of cases (Figure 9.3). Other common variations include a unilateral atretic segment[3,4] and normal intraluminal filling defects resulting from arachnoid granulations, similar to those seen in the superior sagittal sinus.[4–7] In addition to receiving drainage from the straight and superior sagittal sinuses, the inferior vermian veins (paramedian veins that course posterosuperiorly along the inferior vermis) drain into the transverse sinuses.

The cavernous sinuses are situated on each side of the sphenoid body. Each cavernous sinus is a multi-compartmental extradural space that extends from the superior orbital fissure to the petrous portion of the temporal bone (Figure 9.4). This sinus encloses the cavernous segment of the internal carotid artery and the abducens nerve, whereas the lateral wall of the sinus contains the oculomotor, trochlear, and ophthalmic divisions of the trigeminal nerves (cranial nerve V) between its dural leaves. The inferior petrosal sinus extends from the posterior aspect of the cavernous sinus, which it drains, and runs posterolaterally in a groove along the petro-occipital fissure, where it terminates, usually, by joining the jugular bulb.

The superior petrosal sinus extends from the posterior aspect of the cavernous sinus to the transverse sinus, running along the attachment of the tentorium cerebelli to the petrous part of the temporal bone. The petrosal vein lies in the cerebellopontine angle cistern and received drainage from the anterior cerebellar veins, in addition to other venous tributaries from the pons and medulla, before emptying into the middle portion of the superior petrosal sinus.

The sphenoparietal sinus lies along the lesser wing of sphenoid and drains usually to the superficial middle cerebral (Sylvian) vein into the cavernous sinus. Less common variations include the sphenoparietal sinus bypassing the cavernous sinus to drain into the pterygoid plexus or the inferior petrosal or transverse sinus (Figure 9.5).

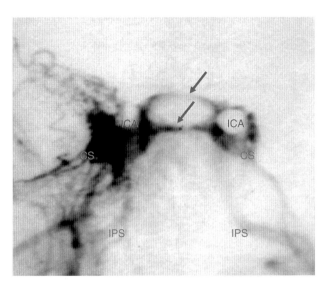

Figure 9.4
Cavernous sinus venogram. ICA = Filling defects from internal carotid arteries. Arrows = Circular sinus, CS= Cavernous sinus, IPS = Inferior petrosal sinus.

Anatomic variants

Variations in venous anatomy are not uncommon, with some important variations relating to transverse sinus dominance, superior sagittal sinus variants, and great vein of Galen bulbous prominence (Figures 9.6–9.10). As noted above, there is frequently dominance of one of the transverse sinuses, with the right transverse sinus more commonly being larger, it is believed to be responsible for the majority of drainage from the superior sagittal sinus. The left transverse sinus is smaller and it is more often responsible for deep venous drainage from the straight sinus. Hypoplasia and aplasia of the transverse sinus is common, with asymmetry found in 31% of patients.[8] The superior sagittal sinus may be hypoplastic, particularly the anterior third, and non-fusion of the superior sagittal sinus posteriorly has also been reported (Figure 9.6).[9] The accessory straight sinus (the Falcine sinus), which connects the great vein of Galen to the superior sagittal sinus, normally regresses by the fifth gestational month; however it may persist and form a bulbous prominence of the vein of Galen.[9] These variations, along with the common variations in anastomoses and drainage patterns, make predicting the consequences of venous occlusion, particularly in the elective setting such as during surgery, difficult.

Venous anomolies

Calvarial venous malformations are rarely isolated; most are associated with diffuse adjacent venous malformations. Involvement of the cranial vault is particularly common in large venous malformations that are located in the temporal–parietal regions. The thickness of the involved calvarium may be increased calvarially, usually caused by the extension of the venous malformation within the diploic space potentially separating the inner and outer tables. If the calvarium is involved, palpation of the area may reveal a bony defect or irregularity. Involvement of the calvarial diploic space in extensive cervical facial venous malformations is frequently associated with sinus pericranii and intracranial developmental venous anomalies.[10]

Sinus pericranii represents a communication between the intracranial and extracranial venous circulations, often associated with an extracranial vascular malformation.[1,10–14] The classic presentation of this condition has been described as a round,

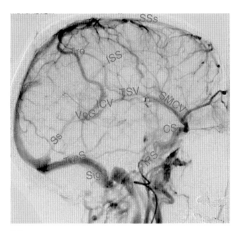

(a)

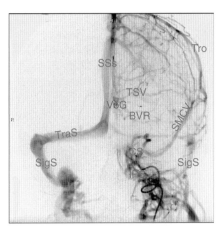

(b)

Figure 9.5
a) Lateral and b) AP view of normal variant venous drainage. Enlarged Trolard and superficial middle cerebral vein drain temporal and parietal lobes with corresponding hypoplasia of the ipsilateral vein of Labbé and transverse sinus.

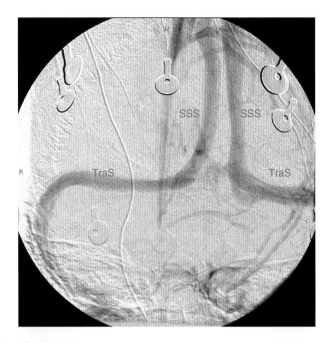

Figure 9.6
Normal variant. Duplicate superior sagittal sinus.

flocculent, non-pulsatile and compressible soft tissue mass, which becomes more prominent with crying or coughing. Sinus pericranii has also been described in patients with craniosynostosis and other skull base anomalies.[15,16] Sinus pericranii has been classified as being either 'closed' or 'draining'; most sinus pericranii associated with a venous malformations are draining, in which the intracranial circulation can drain to extracranial veins. Diagnosis of sinus pericranii is usually made clinically; imaging is performed to confirm the diagnosis and to investigate the extent of the venous malformation.

Venous physiology

It is important to remember the relationship between developmental venous anatomy, cerebrospinal fluid (CSF) production and resorption, and the complex relationship between intracranial venous pressure, brain water, and CSF. Arachnoid granulations are involved in the reabsorption of CSF. Arachnoid granulations bulge into the dural sinuses; the villi open in conditions of raised CSF pressure, and close in conditions of raised venous pressure.[17] They may represent only one route of CSF drainage. Alternative pathways may exist, including

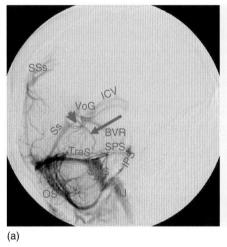

(a)

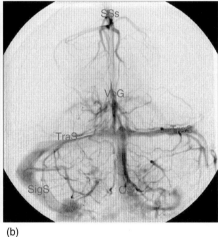

(b)

Figure 9.7
a) Lateral and Townes view.
b) Normal variant. Posterior fossa venogram demonstrating an occipital sinus (OS). Ss = Straight sinus, Long arrow = Precentral cerebellar vein,
Arrowhead = Superior vermian vein. SPS = Superior petrosal sinus, IPS = Inferior petrosal sinus.

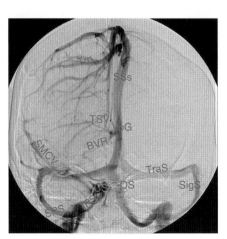

(a)   (b)

Figure 9.8
a) Lateral and b) AP carotid Injection, venous phase. Normal variant occipital sinus.

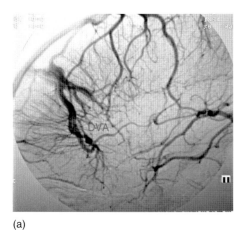

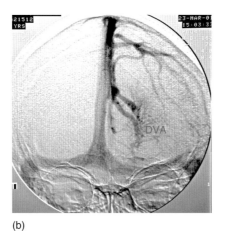

(a)   (b)

Figure 9.9
a) Lateral and b) AP venous phase
of a frontal venous angioma (VA).

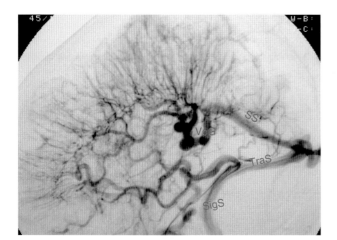

Figure 9.10
Holo-hemispheric venous angioma.

drainage through perineural sheaths, transcranial routes (e.g. the emissary veins and in the cribriform plate), and by way of the lymphatics in the nasal mucosa. Hence there is a complex in relationship between the veins, the routes of venous drainage, venous hemodynamics, and drainage of brain water and CSF. Arachnoid granulations are poorly formed a birth, being visible by the 35th week of life. They develop in infancy and continue to develop throughout life. Povlishok and Levine have postulated that the cerebral venous system is probably important for CSF absorption at birth (Figure 9.11).[18]

Dural sinus thrombosis

Cerebral venous sinus thrombosis (CVST) accounts for 1–2% of strokes in adults, although the exact incidence is unknown.[19] It most often affects young adults and children, with a particular predilection for females since the introduction of oral contraception, particularly third generation contraceptives containing gestodene or desogestrel.[20,21] The superior, transverse, and sigmoid sinuses are most often involved, and there is a wide variability in the presentation. Efficient and accurate diagnosis is critical to beginning treatment; however, despite aggressive management, mortality rates range from 5 to 30%.[22,23]

Risk factors

Any process that triggers a pro-thrombotic state can increase the risk of developing CVST. Risk factors for hypercoagulability can be found in nearly 85% of patients.[24] Head injury or obstetrical delivery can precipitate CVST in patients with genetic risk factors, such as antithrombin deficiency, protein C and protein S deficiency, factor V Leiden mutation, or prothrombin mutation.[21,25–30] Pregnancy, particularly the peri-partum and post-partum period, is associated with the development of CVST in about 12 cases per 100,000 deliveries.[31,32]

The use of oral contraceptives requires a special mention. Before their introduction, CVST affected men and women equally.[33] However since that time, there has been a noticeable shift in the incidence to young woman, with recent studies finding women of childbearing age accounting for up to 70–80% of the newly diagnosed cases.[27,34] In addition, there is good evidence to support the pro-thrombotic side effects of oral contraceptives.[35]

Lumbar punctures and the subsequent drainage of spinal fluid may also trigger CVST.[36] The exact mechanism is unclear, but it is suspected that the lowered intracranial pressure causes downward herniation, which deforms the venous system and triggers thrombosis.

Infections also precipitate a pro-thrombotic state, and thus any severe infection systemically increases the risk of CVST.[27] More specifically, intracranial infections such as cerebritis, subdural empyema, and sinus infections have a predilection for triggering thrombosis, owing to proximity of the site of infection to the cerebral veins. Although less common in the era of modern antibiotic treatment, this mechanism is still occasionally seen involving the transverse sinus or middle fossa in children with otitis media or mastoiditis. The overall frequency of sinus infections triggering thrombosis has been on the decline, with recent studies placing it at 6–12%.[26,37]

Inflammatory disease such as systemic lupus erythematosus, Wegener's granulomatosis, sarcoidosis, inflammatory bowel disease, and Behçet's disease all have the potential to increase acute phase reactants and increase the risk of thrombosis.[38–41] Hematological conditions, such as polycythemia, thrombocythemia, leukemia, and anemia can be associated with CVST.[21,31,32,42–44] Acquired prothombotic conditions include nephrotic syndrome, antiphospholipid syndrome, homocysteinemia, and pregnancy.[30,45] Dehydration also has the ability to trigger CVST by increasing hematocrit and blood viscosity.[27] Lastly, neoplasms of all types have been linked to an increased risk of thrombosis (Figure 9.12).[27]

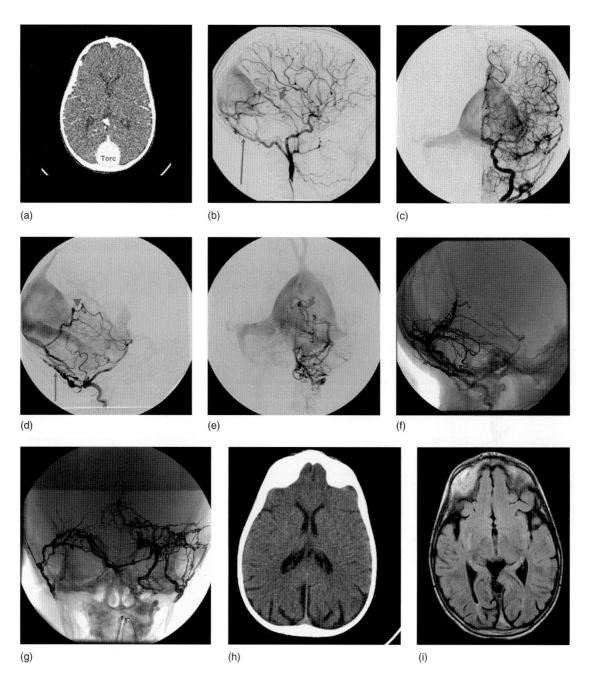

(a)   (b)   (c)

(d)   (e)   (f)

(g)   (h)   (i)

Figure 9.11
a) Contrast CT of a 2 year old with a dural fistula enlarging the straight sinus and vein of Galen (VoG). Notice CSF spaces over convexity. b,c) AP and lateral carotid injection demonstrating dural arterial supply with shunting. d,e) Lateral and AP vertebral injection demonstrating dural supply from left vertebral artery as well as dural supply from the left posterior cerebral arteries (of Davidoff and Schecter). Retrograde filling of sagittal sinus suggests venous hypertension. f, g) Post-onyx embolization plain film. h, i) Post-embolization CT and FLAIR MRI demonstrate markedly decreased size of the torcula/ VoG as well as increased CSF spaces likely due to the reduced flow/ pressure on the venous side with corresponding changes in CSF reabsoprtion.

Pathophysiology

Occlusion of cerebral veins impedes arterial outflow and causes venous hypertension, leading to edema and venous infarcts and hemorrhages. Venous hypertension is related to the inability to balance the outflow of venous blood with the inflow of arterial blood. This imbalance can trigger tedema and intracranial hypertension. The edema associated with CVST can be either cytotoxic or vasogenic.[46,47] Cytotoxic edema is irreversible and is caused by

ischemia related to to poor oxygen delivery from the arterial side. Vasogenic edema is caused by a reversible disruption in the blood–brain barrier, with extravasation of blood plasma into the interstitial space. Communicating hydrocephalus and intracranial hypertension can also develop from the inability to maintain the normal CSF absorption in the setting of dural sinus thrombosis.[26]

Venous hypertension can decrease the normal transit of blood through the intracranial circulation; if impaired significantly, this

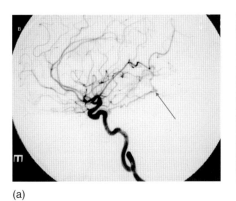

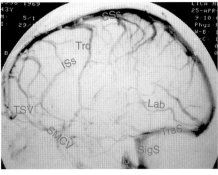

Figure 9.12
Lateral a) arterial and b) venous phase of a RICA angiogram arising at the tentorial apex at the midline, posteriorly. Arterial phase demonstrates a large feeding trunk from the artery of Berasconi-Casanari (red arrows) secondary to a meningioma. The lesion has occluded the ICV and VOG.

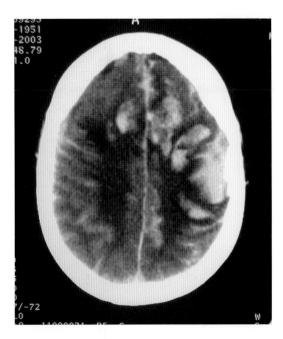

Figure 9.13
Typical paramedian, bilateral hemorrhage post-SSs thrombosis.

can lead to venous infarction. These infarcts can develop anywhere upstream from the occlusion, and in association with the venous hypertension, they can also lead to venous hemorrhages (Figure 9.13). Since the superior sagittal sinus and transverse sinuses are most often affected, these infarctions and hemorrhages are typically paramedian or temporal in location and are often multiple or bilateral.

Clinical manifestations

Severe headache is the most common symptom associated with CVST, affecting almost 90% of the patients. It is often slow in onset, increasing over days; however, abrupt onset has been noted.[48] Patients may also present with a seizure or stroke-like symptoms, such as hemiparesis or aphasia. Seizures are focal in 50% of the cases. Deep sinus thrombosis of the straight sinus can cause thalamic disturbances such as mutism, amnesia, and delirium.[49] Patients may present in or progress to a moribund state if intracranial pressures are high. Focal disturbances such as ocular paresis, proptosis, and chemosis have been described with cavernous

sinus thrombosis. Patients who have intracranial hypertension alone may present only with headaches and papillema on fundoscopic examination.

Diagnosis

Owing to the wide-ranging and often vague symptoms associated with CVST, diagnosis can be difficult and time-consuming.[34] A detailed history to identify risk factors is crucial. Patients who present with unusual headaches with or without neurological manifestions, particularly when associated with risk factors, warrant detailed investigation. Young people without vascular risk factors but with stroke-like symptoms and patients, with intracranial hypertension should also have CVST considered in the differential diagnosis. Patients with unusual hemorrhages both in appearance and location on CT imaging may have an associated cerebral venous thrombosis.

Imaging is crucial to the diagnosis of CVST.[26] Non-contrasted CT imaging may or may not reveal hyperdensity of the occluded vein. The classic description is the 'cord sign' on non-contrasted imaging; however, beam-hardening artifact from the temporal bone may obscure the transverse and sigmoid sinuses. Contrasted CT imaging may or may not reveal the 'empty delta' sign, which results from a void of contrast as a result of the presence of a thrombus surrounded by the enhancing dura of the dural sinus. CT venography will also show an absence in opacification of the sinus.[50] Other non-specific imaging characteristics include generalized or focal brain edema, hypodensity secondary to venous infarction, hemorrhage (intracerebral and/or subarachnoid), and dural enhancement secondary to venous congestion.[22,51] The use of multi-row detector CT angiography has increased the sensitivity and specificity of identifying CVST in one recent study to 100%.[52]

MRI is currently the diagnostic study of choice in children because of its capacity to visualize flow, thrombus, infarction, and any underlying abnormality without ionizing radiation.[22,53–57] MRI will reveal a hyperdensity of T1- and T2-weighted scans at the location of the thrombus. However, depending on the age of the clot, the thrombus may be isointense on T1-weighted imaging during the first few days after its formation or ever after 1 month.[54,58] Additionally, MRI has the advantage of extremely high sensitivity to the parenchymal changes seen in CVST. Cortical and subcortical high-signal intensity lesions on fluid attenuation inversion-recovery sequences and T2-weighted imaging may be highly suggestive of CVST when the lesions do not correspond to

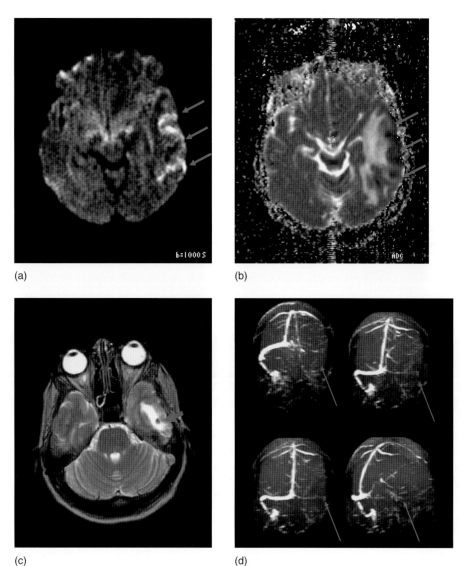

(a)

(b)

(c)

(d)

Figure 9.14
a) Diffusion tensor and b) ADC map demonstrating injury to the left temporal lobe (arrows).
c,d) T2 weighted scan confirms left temporal edema, with a small focal dark area (hemorrhage, arrowhead) above middle ear and mastoid infection. 2D TOF MRA demonstrates ipsilateral transverse- signmoid occlusion.

an arterial territory.[59] Restricted diffusion on diffusion-weighted imaging with a decreased apparent diffusion coefficient (ADC) value is often associated with arterial infarction and a permanent neurological deficit. Diffusion techniques have been used in CVT to differentiate reversible ischemic tissue from irreversible ischemia; ADC is normal or increased) (Figure 9.14).[60–64]

The major advantage of two-dimensional time of flight MR angiography is that it does not require contrast administration and is sensitive to slow flow with relatively short acquisition times. The orientation of the acquisition plane is selected to be perpendicular to the main direction of flow and is typically coronal when imaging the intracranial venous system.[65,66] Spatial pre-saturation pulses are commonly applied either above or below each slice to reduce signal from overlapping arteries or veins and thereby select for flow in one direction or the other. Its main disadvantages include an insensitivity to in-plane flow, patient motion causing vessel misregistration among the slices, and high signal from substances with short T1 values (e.g. thrombus).[66,67] Advances using gadolinium-enhanced MR venography techniques have improved conspicuity and observer agreement, primarily by eliminating the variables of flow direction and mis-registration of two-dimensional slices.[68] MR venography in combination with MRI increases the sensitivity of the diagnosis.[65]

Conventional catheter angiography remains the gold standard for diagnosing cerebrovascular lesions, however, it is rarely needed to diagnose CVST with current MR and CT capabilities.[26,54] Absence in opacification and delayed transit time are both seen. However, absent or hypoplastic transverse sinus may be a normal variant and indistinguishable from transverse sinus thrombosis.[22] Angiography is reserved for those patients whose diagnosis is in doubt after non-invasive imaging, or in those who warrant endovascular intervention.

Treatment

Since the presenting symptoms of CVST can range from a mild headache to a comatose state with herniation or intracerebral hemorrhage, the first intervention should be to stabilize the patient. This may require giving hydration and analgesics, treating increased intracranial pressure, or performing a decompressive craniectomy.[69] Once the patient has been stabilized, investigating the underlying cause of the CVST (e.g. infection, oral contraceptive medications) should be addressed and treatment initiated. Presentations with an altered level of

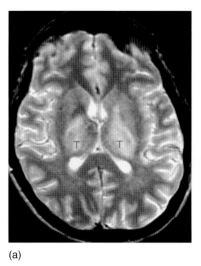

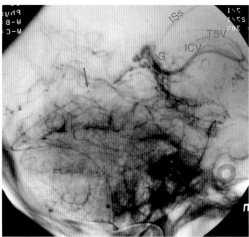

(a)   (b)

Figure 9.15
a) Axial T2 image demonstrating high signal in the thalamus.
b) Lateral angiogram in a patient with straight sinus thrombosis. Catheter in place in the sinus (arrow) for local thrombolytic infusion.

consciousness and intracerebral hemorrhage have been associated with a worse prognosis.[34,70]

Anticoagulation is the basis of treatment of cerebral sinus thrombosis. Heparin intravenously is considered first drug of choice because it provides adequate anticoagulation, halts the thrombotic cascade, prevents pulmonary embolism, allows for quick titration to therapeutic levels, and gives the option of stopping anticoagulation quickly if emergency hematoma evacuation needs to be performed.[71–73] Trials that have not shown a significant benefit of heparin therapy versus placebo in the treatment of sinus thrombosis have been highly criticized for their designs and heterogeneity in the population studies.[24,72,73] However, none of these studies found new or increased size of intracerebral hemorrhages in the setting of heparin. Thus, in the setting of an acutely ill patient with sinus thrombosis and hemorrhage, heparin is still generally considered a first-line agent, even in the presence of hemorrhage.[34] No studies to date have compared fractionated heparin with unfractionated heparin in this patient population.

Warfarin provides a good alternative to heparin for non-hospitalized patients, and is often instituted concomitantly in those who are hospitalized. The optimal length of anticoagulation is unknown, and the risk of thrombosis recurrence is about 2%.[34] It is not unreasonable to base the length of treatment by following the patients with MRI until the thrombus resolves or stabilizes.

There have been no studies investigating the role of aspirin or clopidogrel for the treatment of cerebral sinus thrombosis. In patients who cannot tolerate warfarin, one can theorize that these medications may be an alternative to preventing further platelet aggregation; however, the true benefit is unknown.

Patients with rapidly progressive thrombosis and diffuse brain swelling (with or without multiple hemorrhage) should be considered for endovascular therapy. If, after institution of heparin therapy there is clinical worsening, direct-infusion thrombolytic therapy should be considered. There are several reports demonstrating the feasibility of direct infusion of thrombolytic agents into an occluded dural sinus.[74–78] With improved catheter technology, access to the intracranial cerebral circulation (even the deep venous system) can be achieved via the common femoral vein (Figure 9.15),[79–81] although direct access via a burr hole of the straight sinus has also been found successful when no other access is possible.[82] Alteplase (rT-PA) has pharmacologic advantages over urokinase, including a short half-life[83] and the lowest level of

fibrinogen degradation products,[84] which may reduce the risk of hemorrhagic complications.

Despite the use of thrombolytic therapy in adults, there is conflicting literature in expanding to the application of these results to children. There are several case reports highlighting successful thrombolytic therapy in neonates and children.[75,85–89] One study in a small number of patients compared thrombolytic therapy with the of use of heparin.[90] In this study neurologic function at discharge was found to be better in the thrombolytic group. Major hemorrhagic complications have also been reported.[76] A consecutive cohort of seven children with symptomatic venous thrombosis reported successful lysis in only one child, as well as major complications.[89] Of note, a large population of children with deep venous thrombosis reported a failure of thrombolytic therapy to revascularize the sinuses in a significant percentage of the patients,[87] emphasizing the difference in the coagulation system of children and adults.[87]

Various mechanical revascularization techniques have been used in the dural sinuses: clot disruption using guidewires, rheolytic thrombectomy catheters,[91] balloon thrombectomy with thrombolysis, transluminal balloon angioplasty with or without stenting, and surgical thrombectomy. There are no trials comparing endovascular treatment of CVST with heparin (Figure 9.16).[92]

Dural sinus stenoses and non-thrombotic occlusion

Dural sinus stenosis may occur as a result of high-flow angiopathy, such as that seen with arterial–venous malformations and fistulae. Alternatively, venous stenosis and, ultimately, occlusion can be caused by extravenous compression secondary to primary and metastatic tumors (in the parenchyma, dura, or cranial vault), epidural hematoma, infection, or abscess. The clinical presentation of dural sinus stenosis and occlusion may be asymptomatic and found during diagnostic work-up for another primary disease process. Alternatively, symptomatic stenosis and extravenous occlusion may present with a gradual onset of non-specific symptoms such as headache. However, in

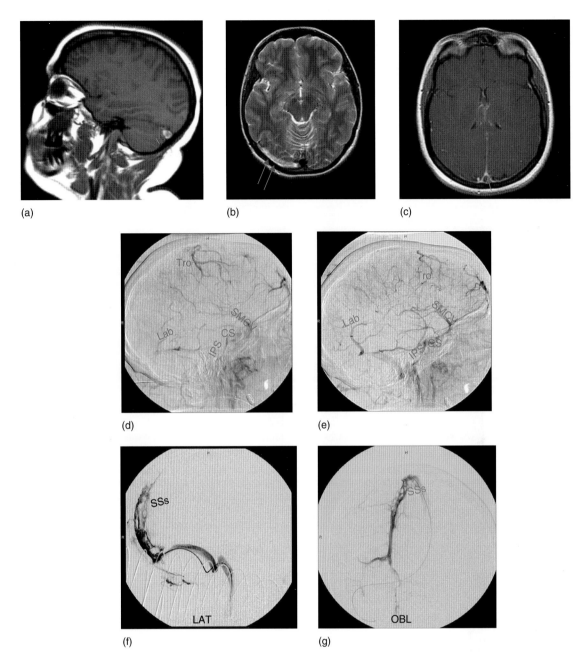

Figure 9.16

a) Parasagittal T1 MR demonstrates thrombus in the transverse sinus. b,c) Axial T2 and T1 post-contrast demonstrating thrombus in the dural sinuses. d,e) Lateral carotid injections, venous phase demonstrates lack of filling of major dural sinuses.

f,g) Catheterization of superior sagittal sinus demonstrates multiple large filling defects consistent with thrombus.

rare instances, patients may present with symptoms similar to the acute thrombotic occlusion as described above. In most instances, venous stenosis and occlusion is diagnosed during the work-up of a related disease, such as pseudotumor cerebri or tumor.

CT venography and MR venography may suggest the presence of a stenosis or occlusion, however, the gold standard in such cases continues to be catheter angiography.[26,54] In cases of stenosis or asymmetry of the transverse sinus, venous pressure monitoring can be performed to determine the presence or absence of increased venous pressure.[93] The intravascular treatment of venous stenosis may include venous angioplasty or stenting;

however, their long term efficacy has not been systematically studied or reported.[94–96]

Conclusion

Cerebral venous sinus thrombosis, although rare, has a varying symptomatic presentation from minor headaches to a moribund state requiring emergency intervention. Stable patients may be treated with anticoagulation and monitored with serial imaging.

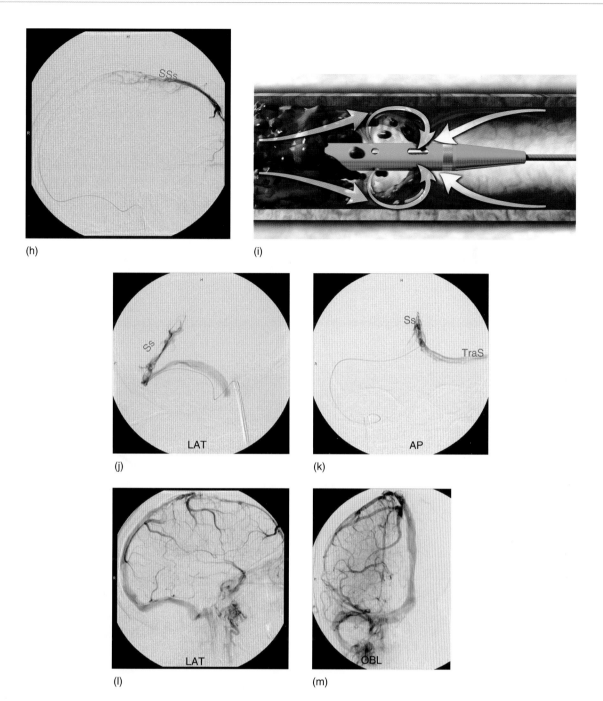

Figure 9.16 (*Continued*)
h,i) Catheter position immediately prior to thrombectomy with Angiojet. j,k) Straight sinus receiving thrombolytics (unable to pass Angiojet to straight sinus). l,m) Lateral and AP venogram demonstrating restoration of flow.

However, patients with a declining neurological status may benefit from endovascular intervention in addition to medical management. In some cases, surgical decompression is warranted because of increased intracranial pressure.

References

1. Lasjaunias P, Berenstein A, ter B, rugge KG et al. Intracranial venous system. In: Lasjaunias P, Berenstein A, ter Brugge KG, and et al (eds). Surgical Neuroangiography, 2nd edition. Berlin, Germany: Springer-Verlag, 2001: 631–95.

2. Ture U, Yasargil MG, Al-Mefty O. The transcallosal–transforaminal approach to the third ventricle with regard to the venous variations in this region. J Neurosurg 1997; 87: 706–15.

3. Cure JK, Van TP, Smith MT. Normal and variant anatomy of the dural venous sinuses. Semin Ultrasound CT MR 1994; 15: 499–519.

4. Mamourian AC, Towfighi J. MR of giant arachnoid granulation, a normal variant presenting as a mass within the dural venous sinus. AJNR Am J Neuroradiol 1995; 16: 901–4.

5. Roche J, Warner D. Arachnoid granulations in the transverse and sigmoid sinuses: CT, MR, and MR angiographic appearance of a normal anatomic variation. AJNR Am J Neuroradiol 1996; 17: 677–83.

6. Leach JL, Jones BV, Tomsick TA et al. Normal appearance of arachnoid granulations on contrast-enhanced CT and MR of the brain: differentiation from dural sinus disease. AJNR Am J Neuroradiol 1996; 17: 1523–32.

7. Liang L, Korogi Y, Sugahara T et al. Normal structures in the intracranial dural sinuses: delineation with 3D contrast-enhanced magnetization prepared rapid acquisition gradient-echo imaging sequence. AJNR Am J Neuroradiol 2002; 23: 1739–46.

8. Alper F, Kantarci M, Dane S, Gumustekin K, Onbas O, Durur I. Importance of anatomical asymmetries of transverse sinuses: an MR venographic study. Cerebrovasc Dis 2004; 18: 236–39.

9. Widjaja E, Griffiths PD. Intracranial MR venography in children: normal anatomy and variations. AJNR Am J Neuroradiol 2004; 25: 1557–62.

10. Konez O, Burrows P, Mulliken J. Sinus pericranii: angiographic assessment and correlation with cross-sectional imaging for intracranial vascular anomalies and endovascular treatment. Radiology 2001; 221: 393.

11. Beers GJ, Carter AP, Ordia JI, Shapiro M. Sinus pericranii with dural venous lakes. AJNR Am J Neuroradiol 1984; 5: 629–31.

12. Bigot JL, Iacona C, Lepreux A et al. Sinus pericranii: advantages of MR imaging. Pediatr Radiol 2000; 30: 710–12.

13. Higuchi M, Fujimoto Y, Ikeda H, Kato A. Sinus pericranii: neuroradiologic findings and clinical management. Pediatr Neurosurg 1997; 27: 325–28.

14. Sadler LR, Tarr RW, Jungreis CA, Sekhar L. Sinus pericranii: CT and MR findings. J Comput Assist Tomogr 1990; 14: 124–27.

15. Robson CD, Mulliken JB, Robertson RL et al. Prominent basal emissary foramina in syndromic craniosynostosis: correlation with phenotypic and molecular diagnoses. AJNR Am J Neuroradiol 2000; 21: 1707–17.

16. Taylor WJ, Hayward RD, Lasjaunias P et al. Enigma of raised intracranial pressure in patients with complex craniosynostosis: the role of abnormal intracranial venous drainage. J Neurosurg 2001; 94: 377–85.

17. Upton ML, Weller RO. The morphology of cerebrospinal fluid drainage pathways in human arachnoid granulations. J Neurosurg 1985; 63: 867–75.

18. Poulishok JT, Levine JE. Cerebrospinal fluid absorption. In: Kapp JP, Schmidek HH, eds. The cerebral venous system and its disorders. Orlando, Florida: Grune and Stratton, 1984.

19. Bogousslavsky J, Pierre P. Ischemic stroke in patients under age 45. Neurol Clin 1992; 10: 113–24.

20. de B, ruijn SF, Stam J, Vandenbroucke JP. Increased risk of cerebral venous sinus thrombosis with third-generation oral contraceptives. Cerebral Venous Sinus Thrombosis Study Group. Lancet 1998; 351: 1404.

21. Martinelli I, Sacchi E, Landi G et al. High risk of cerebral-vein thrombosis in carriers of a prothrombin-gene mutation and in users of oral contraceptives. N Engl J Med 1998; 338: 1793–7.

22. Ameri A, Bousser MG. Cerebral venous thrombosis. Neurol Clin 1992; 10: 87–111.

23. van GJ. Cerebral venous thrombosis: pathogenesis, presentation and prognosis. J R Soc Med 2000; 93: 230–3.

24. Stam J. Thrombosis of the cerebral veins and sinuses. N Engl J Med 2005; 352: 1791–8.

25. Stiefel D, Eich G, Sacher P. Posttraumatic dural sinus thrombosis in children. Eur J Pediatr Surg 2000; 10: 41–4.

26. Bousser MG, Ross R, ussel RW. Cerebral Venous Thrombosis. London: WB Saunders, 1997.

27. deVeber G, Andrew M, Adams C et al. Cerebral sinovenous thrombosis in children. N Engl J Med 2001; 345: 417–23.

28. Ludemann P, Nabavi DG, Junker R et al. Factor V Leiden mutation is a risk factor for cerebral venous thrombosis: a case-control study of 55 patients. Stroke 1998; 29: 2507–10.

29. Hillier CE, Collins PW, Bowen DJ et al. Inherited prothrombotic risk factors and cerebral venous thrombosis. QJM 1998; 91: 677–80.

30. Cantu C, Alonso E, Jara A et al. Hyperhomocysteinemia, low folate and vitamin B12 concentrations, and methylene tetrahydrofolate reductase mutation in cerebral venous thrombosis. Stroke 2004; 35: 1790–4.

31. Cantu C, Barinagarrementeria F. Cerebral venous thrombosis associated with pregnancy and puerperium. Review of 67 cases. Stroke 1993; 24: 1880–4.

32. Lanska DJ, Kryscio RJ. Risk factors for peripartum and postpartum stroke and intracranial venous thrombosis. Stroke 2000; 31: 1274–82.

33. Krayenbuhl HA. Cerebral venous and sinus thrombosis. Clin Neurosurg 1966; 14: 1–24.

34. Ferro JM, Canhao P, Stam J et al. Prognosis of cerebral vein and dural sinus thrombosis: results of the International Study on Cerebral Vein and Dural Sinus Thrombosis (ISCVT). Stroke 2004; 35: 664–70.

35. Vandenbroucke JP, Rosing J, Bloemenkamp KW et al. Oral contraceptives and the risk of venous thrombosis. N Engl J Med 2001; 344: 1527–35.

36. Wilder-Smith E, Kothbauer-Margreiter I, Lammle B et al. Dural puncture and activated protein C resistance: risk factors for cerebral venous sinus thrombosis. J Neurol Neurosurg Psychiatry 1997; 63: 351–6.

37. Ferro JM, Canhao P, Bousser MG et al. Cerebral vein and dural sinus thrombosis in elderly patients. Stroke 2005; 36: 1927–32.

38. Enevoldson TP, Russell RW. Cerebral venous thrombosis: new causes for an old syndrome? Q J Med 1990; 77: 1255–75.

39. Vidailhet M, Piette JC, Wechsler B et al. Cerebral venous thrombosis in systemic lupus erythematosus. Stroke 1990; 21: 1226–31.

40. Daif A, Awada A, al-Rajeh S et al. Cerebral venous thrombosis in adults. A study of 40 cases from Saudi Arabia. Stroke 1995; 26: 1193–5.

41. Farah S, Al-Shubaili A, Montaser A et al. Behcet s syndrome: a report of 41 patients with emphasis on neurological manifestations. J Neurol Neurosurg Psychiatry 1998; 64: 382–4.

42. Carhuapoma JR, Mitsias P, Levine SR. Cerebral venous thrombosis and anticardiolipin antibodies. Stroke 1997; 28: 2363–9.

43. Wermes C, Fleischhack G, Junker R et al. Cerebral venous sinus thrombosis in children with acute lymphoblastic leukemia carrying the MTHFR TT677 genotype and further prothrombotic risk factors. Klin Padiatr 1999; 211: 211–4.

44. Hillmen P, Lewis SM, Bessler M et al. Natural history of paroxysmal nocturnal hemoglobinuria. N Engl J Med 1995; 333: 1253–8.

45. Deschiens MA, Conard J, Horellou MH et al. Coagulation studies, factor V Leiden, and anticardiolipin antibodies in 40 cases of cerebral venous thrombosis. Stroke 1996; 27: 1724–30.

46. Corvol JC, Oppenheim C, Manai R et al. Diffusion-weighted magnetic resonance imaging in a case of cerebral venous thrombosis. Stroke 1998; 29: 2649–52.

47. Yoshikawa T, Abe O, Tsuchiya K et al. Diffusion-weighted magnetic resonance imaging of dural sinus thrombosis. Neuroradiology 2002; 44: 481–8.

48. de B, ruijn SF, Stam J, Kappelle LJ. Thunderclap headache as first symptom of cerebral venous sinus thrombosis. CVST Study Group. Lancet 1996; 348: 1623–5.

49. Kothare SV, Ebb DH, Rosenberger PB et al. Acute confusion and mutism as a presentation of thalamic strokes secondary to deep cerebral venous thrombosis. J Child Neurol 1998; 13: 300–3.

50. Majoie CB, van SM, Venema HW, den H, eeten GJ. Multisection CT venography of the dural sinuses and cerebral veins by using matched mask bone elimination. AJNR Am J Neuroradiol 2004; 25: 787–91.

51. Einhaupl KM, Masuhr F. Cerebral sinus and venous thrombosis. Ther Umsch 1996; 53: 552–8. [in German]

52. Linn J, Ertl-Wagner B, Seelos KC et al. Diagnostic value of multidetector-row CT angiography in the evaluation of thrombosis of the cerebral venous sinuses. AJNR Am J Neuroradiol 2007; 28: 946–52.

53. Jacewicz M, Plum F. Aseptic cerebral venous thrombosis. Einhaupl K. Cerebral Sinus Thrombosis. New York: Plenum Press, 1990: 157–70.

54. Dormont D, Anxionnat R, Evrard S et al. MRI in cerebral venous thrombosis. J Neuroradiol 1994; 21: 81–99.

55. Macchi PJ, Grossman RI, Gomori JM et al. High field MR imaging of cerebral venous thrombosis. J Comput Assist Tomogr 1986; 10: 10–15.

56. Medlock MD, Olivero WC, Hanigan WC et al. Children with cerebral venous thrombosis diagnosed with magnetic resonance

imaging and magnetic resonance angiography. Neurosurgery 1992; 31: 870–6.

57. Zimmerman RA, Bogdan AR, Gusnard DA. Pediatric magnetic resonance angiography: assessment of stroke. Cardiovasc Intervent Radiol 1992; 15: 60–4.

58. Isensee C, Reul J, Thron A. Magnetic resonance imaging of thrombosed dural sinuses. Stroke 1994; 25: 29–34.

59. Forbes KP, Pipe JG, Heiserman JE. Evidence for cytotoxic edema in the pathogenesis of cerebral venous infarction. AJNR Am J Neuroradiol 2001; 22: 450–5.

60. Rother J, Waggie K, van BN et al. Experimental cerebral venous thrombosis: evaluation using magnetic resonance imaging. J Cereb Blood Flow Metab 1996; 16: 1353–61.

61. Ducreux D, Oppenheim C, Vandamme X et al. Diffusion-weighted imaging patterns of brain damage associated with cerebral venous thrombosis. AJNR Am J Neuroradiol 2001; 22: 261–8.

62. Forbes KP, Pipe JG, Heiserman JE. Evidence for cytotoxic edema in the pathogenesis of cerebral venous infarction. AJNR Am J Neuroradiol 2001; 22: 450–5.

63. Kuwahara S, Abe T, Kawada M et al. A case of cerebral venous thrombosis with reversible brain parenchymal lesions: usefulness of diffusion weighted imaging and measurement of apparent diffusion coefficient. No To Shinkei 2001; 53: 79–83. [in Japanese]

64. Ogami R, Ikawa F, Kiura Y et al. Diagnosis of acute phase of venous infarction by diffusion-weighted image: case report and review of the literature. No To Shinkei 2001; 53: 979–83. [in Japanese]

65. Lafitte F, Boukobza M, Guichard JP et al. MRI and MRA for diagnosis and follow-up of cerebral venous thrombosis (CVT). Clin Radiol 1997; 52: 672–9.

66. Lewin JS, Masaryk TJ, Smith AS et al. Time-of-flight intracranial MR venography: evaluation of the sequential oblique section technique. AJNR Am J Neuroradiol 1994; 15: 1657–64.

67. Liang L, Korogi Y, Sugahara T et al. Evaluation of the intracranial dural sinuses with a 3D contrast-enhanced MP-RAGE sequence: prospective comparison with 2D-TOF MR venography and digital subtraction angiography. AJNR Am J Neuroradiol 2001; 22: 481–92.

68. Farb RI, Scott JN, Willinsky RA et al. Intracranial venous system: gadolinium-enhanced three-dimensional MR venography with auto-triggered elliptic centric-ordered sequence—initial experience. Radiology 2003; 226: 203–9.

69. Stefini R, Latronico N, Cornali C et al. Emergent decompressive craniectomy in patients with fixed dilated pupils due to cerebral venous and dural sinus thrombosis: report of three cases. Neurosurgery 1999; 45: 626–9.

70. de B, ruijn SF, de H, aan RJ, Stam J. Clinical features and prognostic factors of cerebral venous sinus thrombosis in a prospective series of 59 patients. For The Cerebral Venous Sinus Thrombosis Study Group. J Neurol Neurosurg Psychiatry 2001; 70: 105–8.

71. Diaz JM, Schiffman JS, Urban ES, Maccario M. Superior sagittal sinus thrombosis and pulmonary embolism: a syndrome rediscovered. Acta Neurol Scand 1992; 86: 390–6.

72. Einhaupl KM, Villringer A, Meister W et al. Heparin treatment in sinus venous thrombosis. Lancet 1991; 338: 597–600.

73. de B, ruijn SF, Stam J. Randomized, placebo-controlled trial of anticoagulant treatment with low-molecular-weight heparin for cerebral sinus thrombosis. Stroke 1999; 30: 484–8.

74. Barnwell SL, Higashida RT, Halbach VV et al. Direct endovascular thrombolytic therapy for dural sinus thrombosis. Neurosurgery 1991; 28: 135–42.

75. Higashida RT, Helmer E, Hallbach VV et al. Direct Thrombolytic therapy for superior sagittal sinus thrombosis. AJNR Am J Neuroradiol 1989; 10: S4–6.

76. Horowitz M, Purdy P, Unwin H et al. Treatment of dural sinus thrombosis using selective catheterization and urokinase. Ann Neurol 1995; 38: 58–67.

77. Tsai FY, Higashida RT, Matovich V, Alfieri K. Acute thrombosis of the intracranial dural sinus: direct thrombolytic treatment. AJNR Am J Neuroradiol 1992; 13: 1137–41.

78. Scott JA, Pascuzzi RM, Hall PV, Becker GJ. Treatment of dural sinus thrombosis with local urokinase infusion. Case report. J Neurosurg 1988; 68: 284–7.

79. Smith TP, Higashida RT, Barnwell SL et al. Treatment of dural sinus thrombosis by urokinase infusion. AJNR Am J Neuroradiol 1994; 15: 801–7.

80. Holder CA, Bell DA, Lundell AL et al. Isolated straight sinus and deep cerebral venous thrombosis: successful treatment with local infusion of urokinase. Case report. J Neurosurg 1997; 86: 704–7.

81. Spearman MP, Jungreis CA, Wehner JJ et al. Endovascular thrombolysis in deep cerebral venous thrombosis. AJNR Am J Neuroradiol 1997; 18: 502–6.

82. Chahlavi A, Steinmetz MP, Masaryk TJ, Rasmussen PA. A transcranial approach for direct mechanical thrombectomy of dural sinus thrombosis. Report of two cases. J Neurosurg 2004; 101: 347–351.

83. Eisenberg PR, Sherman LA, Tiefenbrunn AJ et al. Sustained fibrinolysis after administration of t-PA despite its short half-life in the circulation. Thromb Haemost 1987; 57: 35–40.

84. Sobel BE, Gross RW, Robison AK. Thrombolysis, clot selectivity, and kinetics. Circulation 1984; 70: 160–4.

85. Griesemer DA, Theodorou AA, Berg RA, Spera TD. Local fibrinolysis in cerebral venous thrombosis. Pediatr Neurol 1994; 10: 78–80.

86. Andrew M, Paes B, Johnston M. Development of the hemostatic system in the neonate and young infant. Am J Pediatr Hematol Oncol 1990; 12: 95–104.

87. Andrew M, David M, Adams M et al. Venous thromboembolic complications (VTE) in children: first analyses of the Canadian Registry of VTE. Blood 1994; 83: 1251–7.

88. Andrew M, Vegh P, Johnston M et al. Maturation of the hemostatic system during childhood. Blood 1992; 80: 1998–2005.

89. Monagle P, Phelan E, Downie P, Andrew M. Local thrombolytic therapy in children. Thromb Haemostasis 1977; 77: 504.

90. Wasay M, Bakshi R, Kojan S et al. Nonrandomized comparison of local urokinase thrombolysis versus systemic heparin anticoagulation for superior sagittal sinus thrombosis. Stroke 2001; 32: 2310–7.

91. Chow K, Gobin YP, Saver J et al. Endovascular treatment of dural sinus thrombosis with rheolytic thrombectomy and intra-arterial thrombolysis. Stroke 2000; 31: 1420–5.

92. Canhao P, Falcao F, Ferro JM. Thrombolytics for cerebral sinus thrombosis: a systematic review. Cerebrovasc Dis 2003; 15: 159–66.

93. King JO, Mitchell PJ, Thomson KR, Tress BM. Cerebral venography and manometry in idiopathic intracranial hypertension. Neurology 1995; 45: 2224–8.

94. Higgins JN, Owler BK, Cousins C, Pickard JD. Venous sinus stenting for refractory benign intracranial hypertension. Lancet 2002; 359: 228–30.

95. Malek AM, Higashida RT, Balousek PA et al. Endovascular recanalization with balloon angioplasty and stenting of an occluded occipital sinus for treatment of intracranial venous hypertension: technical case report. Neurosurgery 1999; 44: 896–901.

96. Vilela P, Willinsky R, Terbrugge K. Treatment of intracranial venous occlusive diease with sigmoid sinus angioplasty and stent placement in a case of infantile multifocal dural arteriouvenous shunts. Intervent Neuroradiol 2001; 7: 51–60.

10

The decision-making process: treatment planning for cerebrovascular disease

Peter A Rasmussen

Introduction

The decision-making process for the treatment of patients with cerebrovascular disease can be thought of as an algorithm. As with any complex decision-making process, two approaches can be used. One strategy is to start by determining what the desired end result is for the patient. Then, a clinician may think backwards from the end result through each of the steps that are required to achieve the final goal, eventually arriving at the initial presenting clinical scenario. In the other approach, the physician may start by thinking through the larger and more general issues first and then move through the smaller and more technical issues, finally arriving at a plan. My personal strategy is the latter, where I begin by asking several broad questions that which narrow down the options tremendously in a rapid fashion, allowing me to crystallize my thoughts on the treatment paradigm to be offered to the patient.

A typical example occurs in the outpatient clinic when trainees present their patients with aneurysms to me, and invariably one of their questions is 'should we clip or coil?' Equally invariably, I must always first ask 'should we treat at all?' Indeed, this is the central and most important question that needs to be answered first. The question 'should we treat?' is often the most difficult and the most personal decision a clinician must ask. This statement distills down to an equation that balances benefit of treatment against risk of treatment. If the perceived benefit of treatment is greater than the risk it poses to the patient (i.e. the natural history), generally speaking, treatment with one modality or another should proceed.

When a physician asks that question, he or she needs to have a clear endpoint in mind. For the patient with the asymptomatic aneurysm or arterial–venous information (AVM), I can accept nothing less as an outcome than returning the patient back to his or her previous living arrangement and vocation without a neurological deficit. If the patient has a ruptured aneurysm or AVM, my goal is to create no additional neurological injury with the proposed treatment.

Physicians and patients are truly fortunate in the early part of the 21st century to have more than one treatment technique. Imagine, if you will, practicing neurosurgery in the 1970s, when every hemorrhagic cerebrovascular problem encountered could only be addressed by microsurgery. Although this readily reduces the decision-making to a binary process (surgery or no surgery,) more recent experience has suggested that microsurgery is not always the best option for the patient. Today, we have at our disposal three broad categories of treatment for identified causes of hemorrhagic stroke: surgery, endovascular embolization, and stereotactic radiosurgery. For contemporary treatment of ischemic stroke there is now a broader range of medical therapy as well as surgery and endovascular techniques.

Aneurysms

Long regarded as the gold standard, microsurgery has been challenged by endovascular techniques such that they have become, if not the dominant treatment strategy for the management of cerebral aneurysms, at least a very strong rival. Indeed, in Europe the vast majority of cerebral aneurysms, both ruptured and unruptured, are treated by endovascular coiling. Although the debate over which technique is superior will not end yet, microsurgeons would be remiss if they did not at least think about an endovascular treatment opinion or option.

The most compelling data for the equivalence, if not superiority of, endovascular coiling techniques in the management of cerebral aneurysms come from the International Subarachnoid Aneurysm Trial (ISAT).[1] This large, randomized, multi-center, international trial explored a policy of endovascular treatment compared with microsurgical clipping for the management of ruptured intracranial aneurysms. The conclusion of this study was that patients with ruptured aneurysms whose lesions were amenable to treatment by either technique had a significantly better chance of disability-free survival at 1 year if treated by an endovascular strategy. This study provided, for the first time, nearly overwhelming evidence for the superiority of endovascular techniques. Several points of contention were immediately noted by neurosurgeons worldwide (the overwhelming preponderance of small anterior circulation aneurysms in the trials, the durability of coiling techniques, and the paucity of posterior circulation aneurysms randomized). More candidly, however, the low number of posterior circulation aneurysms is related to the fact that most clinicians recognize that these lesions are generally treated with much greater ease and better outcomes via the endovascular route.[2] Such aneurysms were not randomized and were almost universally treated by coiling. With regard to the large number of small aneurysms randomized, these aneurysms are precisely the lesions amenable to surgical treatment.

Durability issues have been addressed by the Cerebral Aneurysm Rerupture After Treatment (CARAT) study, which was an ambi-directional cohort study of patients with ruptured intracranial aneurysms treated with coil embolization at nine high-volume US centers in the late 1990s.[3] In this study of over 1000 patients, a slightly higher rate of re-rupture was noted in patients treated with endovascular occlusion; however, this difference did not persist after adjustment for potential confounding variables. Mean time to re-rupture was 3 days and almost no patient re-ruptured after 1 year.

This brings me to the first question that I ask myself during my therapeutic decision-making process: Is the aneurysm rup-tured or unruptured? Clearly, based on the above discussion, if the aneurysm has ruptured, strong consideration must be given to treating the aneurysm by endovascular techniques. If the aneurysm is unruptured, ISAT does not give guidance on what technique should be used and other factors in the equation must be factored into the decision.

Location

Location of the aneurysm plays a role in the decision-making process regardless of the treatment technique being contem-plated. From the microsurgical viewpoint, location has different implications from those of the endovascular viewpoint. To a surgeon, location dictates the approach, and some surgical approaches are technically easier and are performed more frequently than others. For example, the surgical exposure to mid-basilar trunk aneurysm is performed infrequently and carries with it high morbidity and technical demands. Conversely, the standard pterional approach to an anterior circulation aneurysm is performed routinely and with very low morbidity. However, that does not mean that all anterior circulation aneurysms are best approached microsurgically. Some common locations of anterior circulation aneurysms are extremely diffi-cult for the neurosurgeon to approach (e.g. a superior hypophy-seal aneurysm arising from the supraclinoid carotid.) Furthermore, a superiorly pointing anterior communicating artery aneurysm can be surgically approached, but its intimate association with the central perforating arteries places the patient at increased risk of neurological morbidity.

From an endovascular standpoint, location does not reflect the approach (since it is nearly always the same – trans femoral); rather, location may have implications in regards to the mor-phology of the aneurysm. Considering location alone, an endovascular strategy for tackling a mid-basilar trunk aneurysm would be preferable over a microsurgical approach. Conversely, middle cerebral artery (MCA) aneurysms are often dysplastic by their nature, and often extending into the MCA bifurcation itself. The dysplastic component often portends a wide neck, and the branching pattern of the MCA can make obtaining an angio-graphic working angle difficult. Thus MCA bifurcation aneu-rysms are generally more suitably treated with microsurgical clipping where open exposure allows direct visualization and reconstruction of the parent vessel.

However, I do not believe that a surgically accessible location, such as the posterior communicating segment of the internal carotid artery (ICA) should cause a surgeon to make a blind recommendation for clipping. Rather, other factors such as the morphology of the aneurysm, the presence of calcification in the dome, the size, and patient co-morbidities should carry more weight.

Age

The age of the patient should play a role in the decision-making process. Treatment morbidity and mortality is clearly higher in patients over the age of 50 years with unruptured aneurysms larger than 12 mm treated by microsurgical techniques than those treated by endovascular techniques. For those patients over the age of 70 years with unruptured aneurysms, a poor outcome is seen 35% of the time regardless of the size of the aneurysm, poor outcome being defined at 1 year as death, a Rankin score of 3–5, or impaired cognitive status.[2] However, a similar impact of age on outcome was not observed in the ISAT trial, leaving unclear the answer to the question of the impact of age on treatment technique for patients harboring ruptured aneurysms.[1] Most likely the influence of the neurological devastation incurred by the patient secondary to the rupture of the aneurysm is at least as powerful as the influence of age and the treatment technique.

Frequently, neurosurgeons are concerned that endovascular coiling may not provide a young patient with durable aneurysm occlusion for the remainder of his or her life. Personally, I have not found this to be a concern with the exception of aneurysms that occur at the ICA terminus. In my opinion, aneurysms at this location have a higher rate of re-canalization than aneurysms at other locations. Therefore, I generally recommend microsurgical clipping for patients under the age of 60 with aneurysms at the ICA terminus. In other locations I have not found this to be of concern, and I would refer the reader to the durability data sup-plied by the CARAT study of ruptured aneurysms.[3] Empirically, the durability of endovascular coiling of unruptured aneurysms is superior to that of the ruptured aneurysms followed in the CARAT study; therefore, durability should not be of concern in unruptured aneurysms.

Morphology

During the infancy of endovascular devices and techniques, a relative contraindication to coil embolization was wide-necked aneurysm morphology. Because retention of the coils in the aneu-rysm sac depends upon a friction fit between the loops of the coil and the wall of the aneurysm, a wide-necked aneurysm posed substantial technical challenges to the endovascular neurosur-geon. Indeed, a dome-to-neck ratio of less than 2 was thought to be the limit of the technique.[4] However, with technological advances in both device and technique, nearly all aneurysm morphologies and dome-to-neck ratios are treatable with coil embolization (Figure 10.1).

Stent-assisted and balloon-assisted techniques have now been developed that allow for embolization of nearly all cerebral aneurysms. These devices have been designed and manufactured to clinician specifications to allow for low-risk treatment of wide-necked side-wall and terminus aneurysms. The first of these technologies and techniques, balloon-assisted coiling (or balloon remodeling technique), was originally designed for the treatment of wide-necked side-wall aneurysms such as in the dorsal carotid

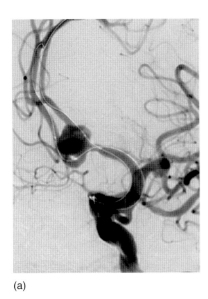

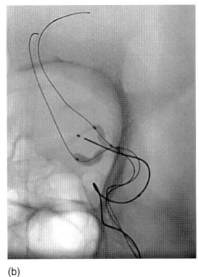

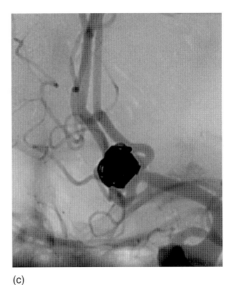

(a)   (b)   (c)

Figure 10.1

(a) Left inferior oblique digital subtraction angiogram showing a wide-necked anterior communicating artery aneurysm in a 74-year-old woman with a strong family history of subarachnoid hemorrhage and death. Given her age, we favored endovascular management of this lesion. This view shows two compliant balloons, one in each A branch, ready to be inflated for parent vessel protection. Prior to the development of compliant balloon technology and the confidence and experience with balloon remodeling technique it is likely this aneurysm would have been deemed 'un-coilable'. (b) Left inferior oblique radiograph showing a micro-catheter in the dome of the aneurysm, poised to begin coiling of the aneurysm, and the two compliant balloons in their inflated configuration offering parent vessel protection. (c) Left inferior oblique unsubtracted angiogram showing the final configuration of the coils and end result of the balloon-assisted coiling procedure.

wall. As interventionalists' confidence and skills with this technique have increased, larger and bifurcation aneurysms are now tackled routinely (see Figure 10.1). In my opinion, the use of a balloon does not add substantially to peri-procedural morbidity or mortality.

It was long thought that the use of a stent intracranially to prevent prolapse of the coils into the parent vessel would be the ultimate solution to the wide-neck aneurysm problem. The main technical challenge in the past was due to the fact that stents of sufficient flexibility were not available to navigate the tortuosity of the cerebral arteries. With the development of the highly flexible nitinol Neuroform (Boston Scientific, Natick, Massachusetts) and Enterprise (Cordis Neurovascular, Miami Lakes, Florida) stents, a larger repertoire of aneurysms have been treatable by endovascular techniques. Although designed for treatment of side-wall aneurysms, these devices can be used for the treatment of bifurcation aneurysms as well.[5]

is of no importance and adds nothing to the technical difficulty of the procedure, in fact this 'armor coating' may reduce the risk of iatrogenic hemorrhage. The presence of thrombus, however, is an entirely different matter.

Prior to the introduction of intracranial stents for the treatment, a partially thrombosed aneurysm dome had been a relative contraindication to endovascular management. Although the initial angiographic result can be perfect, over time there may be substantial aneurysm recanalization due to a migration of coils into the thrombus mass, leading to a major recanalization of the aneurysm. With the addition of stents, aneurysms appear to re-canalize less frequently. Although the presence of thrombus still represents a relatively mild contraindication to coil therapy, large or giant partially thrombosed aneurysms can be managed with coiling provided the treatment is assisted with a stent in the parent vessel. At present, this is the preferred method of handling partially thrombosed giant aneurysms because it carries with it a lower risk of morbidity for the patient.

Thrombus and calcification

From a microsurgical standpoint the presence of thrombus in the dome and of calcium in the aneurysm wall adds to the technical difficulty of the procedure. During aneurysm manipulation and microsurgical clipping, thrombus inside the dome can embolize to the distal circulation, leading to infarction. Similarly, presence of calcium in the aneurysm wall can make clipping difficult and accurate reconstruction of the parent vessel impossible. From an endovascular standpoint, calcification in the aneurysm wall

Co-morbidities

Generally speaking there is minimal debate in the neurological community that patients with significant medical co-morbidities are better served by endovascular management – shorter procedure times, absence of brain retraction, minimal blood loss, and minimal cranial invasion intuitively should be less stressful on a compromised organism. What is debatable is what constitutes significant medical co-morbidity.

Unlike patients with cervical carotid atherosclerotic disease, in whom multiple trials have delineated what constitutes high medical risk for carotid endarterectomy, no such scientific data are available for the operative management of cerebral aneurysms. Co-morbid conditions can roughly be defined as advanced age, recent myocardial infarction (< 6 weeks), chronic obstructive pulmonary disease and other pulmonary disorders, disorders of coagulation, and chronic renal insufficiency. Some authorities feel that subarachnoid hemorrhage itself is a medical co-morbidity and the recommendation should lean toward endovascular therapy in this setting. Clearly those patients suffering acute cardiomyopathy secondary to subarachnoid hemorrhage are better served by endovascular therapy. The presence of one of these conditions may suggest that one technique may be preferred to another for a given patient. Chronic renal insufficiency may lead to a recommendation of microsurgery in order to avoid the renal toxicity of contrast agents. The most rational strategy for approaching the patient with medical co-morbidities may be to seek the opinion of an anesthesiologist familiar with both techniques regarding the relative risk that an individual patient will be exposed to from an anesthetic standpoint.

Adjunctive devices

Adjunctive devices such as highly flexible stents and highly compliant balloons have greatly expanded the spectrum of aneurysms amenable to endovascular techniques. Unfortunately, their use adds an extra dimension to the complexity of the treatment. This is clearly in violation of the KISS principle ('keep it simple, stupid') and consequently the risk of a complication is increased and must be factored into the decision algorithm. Nevertheless both devices enable an interventionalist greater flexibility in treatment strategies for a given patient.

Balloon-assisted embolization techniques require the use of intermittent balloon inflations to protect the parent vessel from coil prolapse and compromise. This can lead to ischemic complications from both thromboembolic and hemodynamic etiologies. Although it is not accurately known how long these balloons can be inflated during aneurysm treatment, some knowledge can be gleaned from the experience of vascular neurosurgeons and their utilization of temporary clipping for proximal control.[6,7] It can be argued that balloon inflations may be tolerated longer in the endovascular laboratory than in the operating room, because collateral vessels in the brain may be partially compromised by the brain retraction.[8] Alternatively, thromboembolic complications can occur, especially if the patient is not heparinized during the procedure.

As opposed to stent-supported coiling, balloon-assisted techniques require an operator to perform two relatively complex tasks simultaneously: accurate inflation of the balloon and coil insertion into the aneurysm. These maneuvers require a high degree of concentration, and given the only minor differences in radio-opacity of the catheters, some confusion can arise as to when the coil has reached the detachment point. This combination of events raises the risk of morbidity ever so slightly during this procedure.

Stent-supported coiling, on the other hand, does not require simultaneous performance of complex tasks. The stent can be introduced initially at the start of the procedure or it can be placed at the end of the procedure after the coils have been placed to protect the parent vessel. Since these tasks are done serially and not in parallel, in my opinion this technique may carry a slightly lower risk of peri-procedural morbidity. However, the use of an intracranial stent is essentially limited to patients harboring unruptured aneurysms and requires the use of antiplatelet agents, which increases the risk of morbidity should the aneurysm or other vessel be perforated. Regardless of which technique is employed, the interventionalist needs to factor in this slightly higher risk of morbidity in the decision-making process.

Family and social history

For those patients who harbor ruptured aneurysms, family and social history have little role in the decision-making process, because these patients require definitive aneurysm treatment. For those patients with unruptured aneurysms, family and social history frequently plays a large role in counseling on whether to proceed with treatment or not.

A family history of a first-degree relative with a ruptured aneurysm will frequently lead me to recommend or offer treatment to those patients whose aneurysm is 4–6 mm in size. Generally, if an aneurysm is 7 mm or greater in size, I recommend that the patient be treated, and if the aneurysm is 3 mm or smaller I would recommend conservative management.[2] If there is a strong family history of several first-degree relatives with subarachnoid hemorrhage or one family member with subarachnoid hemorrhage and death, I would strongly recommend treatment of aneurysms even as small as 3 mm.

Similarly, those patients who are active cigarette smokers or users of cocaine, especially crack cocaine, are at increased risk of subarachnoid hemorrhage as well. I am more likely to recommend active treatment of unruptured aneurysms in these patients, with similar reasoning to that given above for a positive family history.

Arterial–venous malformations

In contrast to cerebral aneurysms, the decision to treat AVMs is more complex, and for the most part falls under the realm of the art of medicine. Even when the AVM has ruptured, the decision to move forward with surgical or endovascular therapy is not always clear. Compared with cerebral aneurysm treatment, morbidity from a surgical standpoint is often substantially higher. In addition, stereotactic radiosurgery is another treatment modality that needs to be considered.

The factors to consider in the decision-making process include age and expectation of the patient, the location of the lesion, the presence or absence of medical co-morbidities, the symptomatic or asymptomatic nature of the lesion, the modality of treatment being considered, and angiographic determinants of hemorrhage risk such as central venous drainage, the presence of nidal aneurysms, or a peri-ventricular location.[9]

Before a decision can be made to recommend active treatment over conservative management and one treatment modality over another, a full evaluation of the patient must take place. This includes an accurate seizure history, a description and a classification of headache, and a history of possible cognitive or neurological decline. Furthermore, the age of the patient, social history, employment history, and patient expectation must be factored into the decision-making process. If the clinician is entertaining the thought of offering the patient treatment, a full imaging evaluation must follow, which includes MRI scanning (I find T2-weighted sequences the most helpful) and high-quality, high-resolution, fast filming (4 frames per second) four vessel cerebral angiography. In my opinion, treatment recommendations cannot be made without both angiography and MRI.

A clear understanding of the natural history of cerebral AVMs is required when counseling patients. Unfortunately, there is a shortage of scientific data available to guide us on the hemorrhage risk of the asymptomatic AVM. Most of the data that are available are based on symptomatic AVMs, and these data are often subjected to institutional referral bias. There also is a strong correlation between the age of the patient and the hemorrhage risk. Most hemorrhages occur in the 20–40-year age group. Consequently, the age of the patient is very important when counseling on their risk of hemorrhage.

In addition, when quoting to patients the microsurgical risks of post-operative neurological deficits, some guidance can gleaned from the literature (Tables 10.1, 10.2).[10-12] Keep in mind, though that *your* surgical morbidity and mortality may not be as good as Spetzler and Martin's. When entertaining the thought of microsurgical treatment of a cerebral AVM, the surgeon must be brutally honest about his or her surgical skill set as to what is the expected neurological havoc that will be brought to the patient during the operation.

To treat or not to treat

AVMs are formidable lesions to tackle both from a microsurgical and an endovascular technical standpoint. Conversely, stereotactic radiosurgery from an operator standpoint is relatively easy. Each of these treatment modalities carries with it different and distinct morbidities. Morbidity associated with microsurgical and endovascular treatment of an AVM may be as high as 30–50% depending on the size and complexity of the lesion. The same lesion may have a morbidity associated with radiosurgery in the low single digits. Therefore, the modality

of treatment to be offered plays a vital role in deciding on whether or not to treat the patient. For instance, a 2.5 cm lesion located in the thalamus may carry an exceptionally high surgical morbidity; however, the risk of radiosurgery is exceedingly low and will probably afford the patient the same likelihood of cure. So, if such a patient had an asymptomatic thalamic AVM and the only modality available was microsurgery, the decision would likely be not to treat; however, if radiosurgery is available the decision would be likely to treat.

Age

As mentioned above, patients who present with hemorrhages tend to be in the 20–40-year age group. Consequently when evaluating patients much younger or older than this, caution must be exercised as to how strongly one recommends treatment. Moreover, patients less than 18 years of age tend to be prone to AVM recurrences or the development of new AVMs after their initial treatment.[11]

Generally speaking, I am reluctant to recommend active treatment of an asymptomatic AVM for a child during his or her high school years for several reasons. First, the risk of hemorrhage in this age group is very low. Second, if treatment is undertaken there's a strong likelihood that the AVM will either recur or re-grow in the same location, necessitating further treatment. Third, if the child develops neurological and cognitive deficits in response to the treatment and this leads to loss of IQ and stigmatization, this will make it very difficult for the child to receive a high school diploma, and his or her social development will be greatly retarded. I much prefer to wait for the child to graduate from high school so that he or she is fully socially developed and has received a high school diploma before exposing the child to the risk of treatment. I feel this is safe as the risk of hemorrhage during adolescence is quite low.

Similarly, if the patient is aged over 45 years, the risks of microsurgery are increased. In my experience, even with the performance of pre-operative embolization, the chance of post-operative hemorrhage secondary to normal perfusion pressure breakthrough is quite high. This needs to be factored into the

Table 10.1 Determination of arterial–venous malformation grade

Graded feature	Points assigned
Size	
< 3 cm	1
3–6 cm	2
> 6 cm	3
Eloquence of adjacent brain	
Non-eloquent	0
Eloquent	1
Venous drainage	
Superficial only	0
Deep	1

Table 10.2 Correlation of grade of arterial–venous malformation with surgical morbidity and mortality

	Deficit	
Grade	Minor	Major
1	0	0
2	5	0
3	12	4
4	20	7
5	19	12

treatment decision-making process. Frequently, patients in this age group are asymptomatic or minimally symptomatic and therefore are at low risk of hemorrhage. I feel that very young patients and older patients need a low-risk treatment alternative given their favorable natural history. Usually this treatment option includes radiosurgery because of its low treatment morbidity.

Role of embolization

Using a groin puncture, floating a microcatheter to an AVM nidus, and injecting an embolic agent resulting in a cure is every interventionalist's dream, and it is the holy grail of endovascular therapy. Although there is some reported success in curing an AVM[12] with embolization alone, by no means can this be guaranteed a priori. Personal experience suggests that even angiographic obliteration following embolization does not necessarily mean that the patient is cured. It is possible that the radio-opacity of the embolic agent cast does not allow for adequate visualization of residual nidus, which can leave the patient susceptible to hemorrhage. Moreover, embolization therapy is not a benign procedure and carries with it morbidity as high as 30% per embolization session.

Because of the low rate of cure following embolization and the risk of leaving unprotected nidus, I view embolization as a pre-surgical adjunct or a palliative treatment for those patients with so-called Spetzler–Martin grade VI ('surgically incurable') AVMs who are having progressive neurological decline secondary to steal phenomenon. In addition, pre-radiosurgical embolization has been associated with a decreased rate of cure. Embolization prior to radiosurgery makes visualization of the nidus during treatment planning difficult. It is often thought that embolization can shrink the size of a large AVM down to one that is more conducive to radiosurgery. In reality, it is difficult to actually reduce the volume of the nidus in a manner that will facilitate radiosurgical planning; therefore, generally speaking, I do not routinely offer patients embolization prior to radiosurgical treatment.

Location

No other factor portends the risk of post-operative (surgical) neurological morbidity than the location of the lesion. Whether the lesion is in so-called eloquent brain or in a deep location, surgical approaches to these regions and potential iatrogenic injury to the surrounding area frequently makes surgical resection hazardous. High surgical risk locations can be defined as eloquent regions as outlined by Spetzler and Martin,[10] who described the sensorimotor, language, and visual cortex, the hypothalamus and thalamus, the internal capsule, the brainstem, the cerebellar peduncles, and the deep cerebellar nuclei as being eloquent regions.

When treating AVMs with radiosurgery in and near these locations, the fact that these territories are thought to be eloquent is less important. Generally speaking, a radiation dose will be chosen that is very unlikely to lead to tissue destruction of the adjacent regions, and therefore the risk is lower. For this reason, lesions in eloquent locations are, in my opinion, are generally best treated by radiosurgery.

Imaging and angiographic determinants

As mentioned above, full evaluation with MRI and catheter angiography is required prior to making definitive treatment recommendations to the patient. These imaging studies should be reviewed to ascertain the location and size of the lesion, its relationship to eloquent structures, the surgical corridors available, the presence of aneurysms both on the feeding pedicles and in the AVM nidus, and the adequacy of venous outflow. The size of the lesion can have direct impact on the utility of radiosurgery. Generally speaking, lesions larger than 3–3.5 cm are not amenable to radiosurgical treatment. Lesions smaller than this are readily treatable by radiosurgery with a cure rate approaching 80%.[13]

Recently we, and other centers, have begun treating AVMs larger that 3–3.5 cm with radiosurgery. This can be accomplished by treating a half or a portion of the AVM at one session, then having the patient return in the future for a second radiosurgical session that treats the balance of the AVM.[14] Chance of cure in what would be an otherwise untreatable lesion has been reported to be as high as 50%. In addition, AVM symptoms such as seizures can often be stabilized with this technique.

Timing of treatment

For patients with asymptomatic or unruptured AVMs, timing of treatment can proceed at the mutual convenience of the physician and the patient. For patients with AVMs who present with recent hemorrhage, timing of treatment and modality can be somewhat more complicated.

Although there has been a trend among some practitioners to move towards early surgical and endovascular treatment of ruptured AVMs, my personal preference is to wait 4–8 weeks after the ictus before proceeding with surgical resection or radiosurgery. During this interval, the hematoma will resorb, reactive cerebral edema can resolve, and the hematoma cavity has a chance to mature. Operating on a ruptured AVM prior to resolution of the hematoma and edema can be technically challenging and may increase operative morbidity through increased brain swelling, errors in differentiating nidus from 'angry' adjacent brain, and difficulty with retraction. Even proceeding with radiosurgery can be problematic because the edema and hematoma may make accurate targeting of the lesion difficult. Since there is often a 1–2-year latent period before resolution of the AVM, a 4–8 week delay in initiating radiosurgical treatment will have no deleterious effects in terms of subsequent hemorrhage risk.

There are some circumstances when urgent therapy is warranted in the acute setting. After presentation with intracerebral hemorrhage, if an AVM is suspected the patient should undergo diagnostic angiography. If this demonstrates an AVM, the images should be searched for the presence of angiographic features that may increase the patient's risk of early re-bleeding. Angiographic determinants of risk of subsequent hemorrhage, such as intranidal aneurysms, peri-ventricular location, and a venous stenosis, put the patient at higher risk of re-bleeding.[9] In this setting, I favor early elective embolization to decrease the shunt and reduce the risk of subsequent re-bleeding. Nidal aneurysms should be assumed to be the source of the hemorrhage and these should be obliterated. In addition, if the patient needs urgent craniotomy for hematoma evacuation to alleviate elevated intracranial pressure and mass effect, pre-operative embolization may add a margin of safety and reduce intra-operative blood loss. Of course, pre-surgical embolization should be sought only if the patient is neurologically stable and can tolerate the procedure prior to craniotomy.

Atherosclerotic stenoses

Surgery of atherosclerotic cerebrovascular disease, particularly at the carotid bifurcations, is one of the commonest surgical procedures performed.[15] The body of medical literature devoted to the subject since the time of Fisher's first account is not only staggering in volume, but also impressive in its evolutionary sophistication. Publication of the North American Symptomatic Endarterectomy Study and the Asymptomatic Carotid Artery Surgery trial extended the concepts of Kaplan–Meier survival curves and odds ratios beyond the realm of public health and biostatistics and into the greater community of surgeons and neurologists. The demonstration of benefit in the reduction of long-term (> 30 days) stroke morbidity and mortality is unique to surgery; this type of data for stenting must await completion of the Carotid Revascularization Endarterectomy versus Stent Trial (CREST).[16] In North America, much credit also goes to the American Heart Association for the inclusion of cerebrovascular disease in its domain, aiding in the recognition and management of risk factors.[17]

Table 10.3 High-risk conditions for carotid endarterectomy

Previous radiation therapy to the neck

Previous carotid endarterectomy with recurrent re-stenosis

High cervical internal carotid or below-the-clavicle common carotid artery stenoses

Severe tandem lesions

Contralateral carotid artery occlusion

Contralateral laryngeal nerve palsy

Age >80 years;

Severe pulmonary disease

Significant cardiac co-morbidity

- Congestive heart failure (New York Heart Association class III or IV) and/or known severe left ventricular dysfunction
- Open heart surgery needed within 6 weeks
- Recent myocardial infarction (>24 hours and <4 weeks)
- Unstable angina (Canadian Cardiovascular Society Class III or IV)

offer brain imaging, and is thus less desirable in symptomatic patients.

Symptomatic versus asymptomatic

Beyond age and co-morbidities that may have an impact on long term survival, there are two key data points in clinical decision making for ischemic disease:

- Is the stenosis symptomatic?
- How severe is the stenosis?

Symptoms in the vascular distribution of a stenosis may be clinically crystalline or obtuse. Certainly, the aid of a neurological expert is invaluable in establishing causation.[18] In the unusual case in which uncertainty persists (especially for cortical symptoms), diffusion-weighting imaging may be a highly sensitive adjunct in establishing parenchymal injury even when symptoms are transient.[19,20] Alternatively, the case for revascularization of asymptomatic lesions rests almost exclusively with the severity of the stenosis in the context of the individual patient's overall health and the risk of intervention.

Severity of Disease

While measured in a specific fashion,[21] severity of stenosis can be established a number of ways: CT, MRI, duplex ultrasound, or conventional angiogaphy. CT and MRI have the added benefit of establishing the integrity of the brain parenchyma and the presence of hemorrhage and of providing a potentially qualitative assessment of cerebral perfusion. Duplex ultrasound, while inexpensive, is an indirect measure of stenosis severity, moreover, it is highly operator-dependent and does not

Timing of treatment

Also important is the relationship of symptom onset and severity to the risk of stroke, and hence the benefit of earlier revascularization. The risk of stroke is greatest in the initial weeks and months after the first symptoms.[22] Patients with contralateral occlusion or poor collateral flow are also at additional risk. The risk of stroke is also noted to be greater in those with hemispheric symptoms than in those presenting with retinal ischemia.[23]

The risk and the reward for carotid endarterectomy are well established, while endovascular treatment of carotid disease is indicated and approved for a relative minority of patients (Table 10.3). Alternatively the EC–IC bypass trial failed to demonstrate benefit of surgery for intracranial occlusive disease,[24] while preliminary experience with specifically designed stent systems has demonstrated early technical success as well as symptomatic relief in selected patients with intracranial stensoes.[25] Demographic and angiographic considerations may play a role in selecting those patients least likely to suffer re-stenosis.[26]

Acute ischemic stroke

Clinical decision-making in cases of acute stroke is often difficult, owing to the urgency presented by time constraints: high stakes 'beat the clock'. Under such circumstances, efficiency of communication is of paramount importance: the time of onset, the age of the patient and his or her baseline functional status, the blood pressure, the heart rate and rhythm, National Institutes of

Health Stroke Scale (NIHSS), medications and anticoagulation status, serum glucose level, imaging results (if available), and contact information for informed consent must be noted immediately (Table 10.4). While obtaining this information, there is a constant mental calibration of the availability of intravenous thrombolytics and their odds of success, the shortest route to an angiography suite, the availability of nurses and technologists, and the time to prepare and access the cerebral circulation via endovascular means. There can be no wasted motion, the corollary of which is that such a high level of coordinated care requires significant pre-planning and education.

In virtually every instance, treatment should be initiated at the earliest possible moment and without delay, (e.g. intravenous thrombolytic therapy if within the 3-hour window from symptom onset). This is the inherent appeal of the so-called 'bridging protocols', in which intravenous lytic therapy is begun at the earliest possible moment, even while mobilizing additional resources for intra-arterial treatment.[27]

Nevertheless, with larger vessel occlusions we know that it is unlikely that intravenous treatment alone will be sufficient.

Table 10.4 Acute stroke checklist

Time of onset

Age of patient

- Able to consent
- Pregnancy status

Right/ left handed

- NIHSS
- Able to consent

Vital signs

- BP
- Heart rate and rhythm
- Anti-coagulation status

Contra-indications to thrombolysis:

- Recent surgery
- Systolic BP > 180 mm Hg
- Coagulopathy
- > 3 hrs post ictus
- Known intra-parenchymal CNS neoplasm

Imaging available:

- Blood?
- Parenchymal changes in over 1/3 vascular territory
- Vascular occlusion*
- Perfusion mismatch*

Contact information:

- Parent/ spouse/ medical power of attorney
   ○ Cell phone
- Living will
- Immediate activation of emergency endovascular technologist, nurse, physician

*Desirable but not essential.

In such cases, particularly those transferred from other facilities, it is always tempting to obtain additional imaging prior to proceeding, potentially at the risk of additional delays. This is particularly true at off-hours when personnel must be summoned from home. Clearly older patients temporally removed from the 3-hour window and with even subtle changes on CT will not do well. Conversely, younger patients seen and treated early with an essentially normal presenting CT scan should be given every benefit of the doubt; the team should be dispatched as soon as possible, with little or no time spent admiring additional imaging studies. It is to be hoped that with the ever-expanding use of faster and safer mechanical thrombectomy devices, the pool of eligible patients for these treatments will expand as well.[28]

Finally, it is easy to succumb to the temptation of treating patients emergently referred for acute stroke when expectations of family and even referring physicians are unrealistically high, even in the presence of significant time delays, contraindication to thrombolysis or anticoagulation, or imaging evidence of early completed infarction. Figure 10.2 is an illustrative case of a 17-year-old with unrecognized vertebral artery dissection and delayed appreciation of basilar ischemia. By the time appropriate diagnostic imaging was obtained 24 hours after the onset of symptoms, the patient was 'locked-in.' Despite diffusion-imaging evidence of an early infarction and the long time delay, there was every expectation that something *must* be done. Remarkably, in consultation with the parents and the interventionalist, the attending neurologist indicated that he had seen patients recover from such severe deficits. Relieved from the responsibility of attempting too much too late, the patient was managed medically. Six months later the young woman stopped to acknowledge the cerebrovascular team at the breakfast table following morning rounds, to thank them for their efforts. Presently she is attending college, studying to be a physical therapist.

Conclusions

Complex cerebrovascular lesions are difficult to manage and require thoughtfulness and a high level of technical skill to effect successful cure. Along the way, there are many pitfalls and opportunities for complications leading to an untoward result. This can take an emotional toll on the physician, and he or she should be constantly on guard for the emotional pain that results from a substantial complication. It is wise in my opinion when facing a challenging lesion to share the decision-making process with a colleague. Enlisting a partner in the care of these patients allows for sharing of the emotional burden if the patient does poorly and prevents second-guessing of a unilateral or solo treatment decision. The corollary to this is that open surgery and endovascular treatments are less competitive than complementary.

It is also important to remember that although these are challenging lesions, their treatment is not about this being a challenge to the physician: it is about their successful treatment for the patient. Each of these is not a test of an individual's skill and surgical or endovascular prowess. Instead, these lesions are a serious problem for the patient, and it is selecting the best treatment with the greatest chance of cure and lowest chance of morbidity that is what matters. Remember, it is not about the surgeon, it is about the patient.

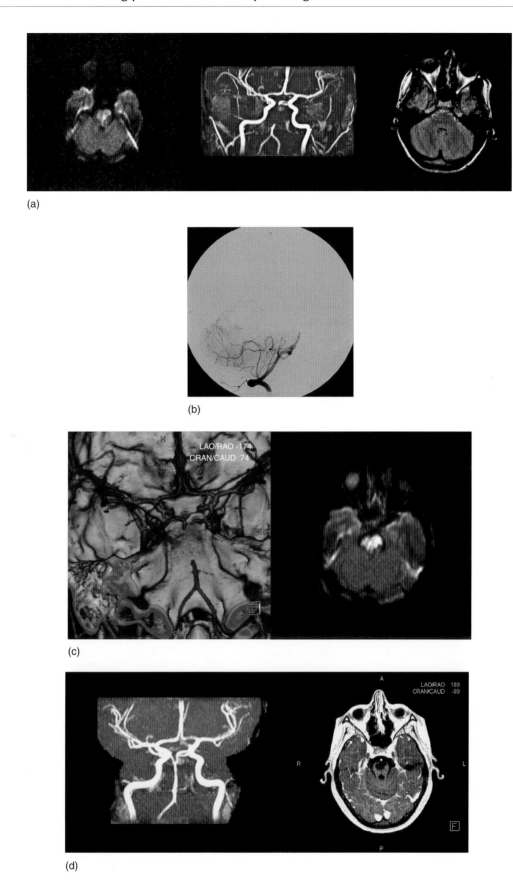

(a)

(b)

(c)

(d)

Figure 10.2

(a) Diffusion-weighted image 24 hours after the onset of symptoms in a 17-year-old female with unrecognized vertebral artery dissection, now 'locked in'. (b) Corresponding fluid-attenuated inversion recovery image. (c) MRA angiography demonstrating embolic occlusion of the basilar artery and confirmatory angiogram demonstrating basilar occlusion and collateral flow via the vermian artery arcade. (d) Follow-up diffusion image demonstrating the full extent of infarction and six-month follow-up T1-weighted scan post-contrast showing chronic infarct. The patient had recovered significant neurological function, with only mild residual dysarthria.

References

1. Molyneux AJ, Kerr RS, Yu LM et al. International subarachnoid aneurysm trial (ISAT) of neurosurgical clipping versus endovascular coiling in 2143 patients with ruptured intracranial aneurysms: a randomised comparison of effects on survival, dependency, seizures, rebleeding, subgroups, and aneurysm occlusion. Lancet 2005; 366: 809–17.

2. Wiebers DO, Whisnant JP, Huston J III et al. Unruptured intracranial aneurysms: natural history, clinical outcome, and risks of surgical and endovascular treatment. Lancet 2003; 362: 103–10.

3. Johnston SC, Dowd CF, Higashida RT et al. Predictors of rehemorrhage after treatment of ruptured intracranial aneurysms: the Cerebral Aneurysm Rerupture After Treatment (CARAT) study. Stroke 2008; 39: 120–5.

4. Debrun GM, Aletich VA, Kehrli P et al. Selection of cerebral aneurysms for treatment using Guglielmi detachable coils: the preliminary University of Illinois at Chicago experience. Neurosurgery 1998; 43: 1281–95.

5. Chow MM, Woo HH, Masaryk TJ, Rasmussen PA. A novel endovascular treatment of a wide-necked basilar apex aneurysm by using a Y-configuration, double-stent technique. AJNR Am J Neuroradiol 2004; 25: 509–12.

6. Ogilvy CS, Carter BS, Kaplan S, Rich C, Crowell RM. Temporary vessel occlusion for aneurysm surgery: risk factors for stroke in patients protected by induced hypothermia and hypertension and intravenous mannitol administration. J Neurosurg 1996; 84: 785–91.

7. Samson D, Batjer HH, Bowman G et al. A clinical study of the parameters and effects of temporary arterial occlusion in the management of intracranial aneurysms. Neurosurgery 1994; 34: 22–8.

8. Moret J, Cognard C, Weill A, Castaings L, Rey A. [Reconstruction technic in the treatment of wide-neck intracranial aneurysms. Long-term angiographic and clinical results. Apropos of 56 cases]. J Neuroradiol 1997; 24: 30–44.

9. Marks MP, Lane B, Steinberg GK, Chang PJ. Hemorrhage in intracerebral arteriovenous malformations: angiographic determinants. Radiology 1990; 176: 807–13.

10. Spetzler RF, Martin NA. A proposed grading system for arteriovenous malformations. J Neurosurg 1986; 65: 476–83.

11. Lindqvist M, Karlsson B, Guo WY et al. Angiographic long-term follow-up data for arteriovenous malformations previously proven to be obliterated after gamma knife radiosurgery. Neurosurgery 2000; 46: 803–8.

12. van Rooij WJ, Sluzewski M, Beute GN. Brain AVM embolization with Onyx. AJNR Am J Neuroradiol 2007; 28: 172–7.

13. Karlsson B, Lax I, Soderman M. Can the probability for obliteration after radiosurgery for arteriovenous malformations be accurately predicted? Int J Radiat Oncol Biol Phys 1999; 43: 313–9.

14. Sirin S, Kondziolka D, Niranjan A et al. Prospective staged volume radiosurgery for large arteriovenous malformations: indications and outcomes in otherwise untreatable patients. Neurosurgery 2006; 58: 17–27.

15. Rosamond W, Flegal K, Friday G et al. Heart disease and stroke statistics—2007 update: a report from the American Heart Association Statistics Committee and Stroke Statistics Subcommittee. Circulation 2007; 115: e69–171.

16. Hobson RW. CREST (Carotid Revascularization Endarterectomy versus Stent Trial): background, design, and current status. Semin Vasc Surg 2000; 13: 139–43.

17. Adams HP Jr, del Zoppo G, Alberts MJ et al. Guidelines for the early management of adults with ischemic stroke: a guideline from the American Heart Association/American Stroke Association Stroke Council, Clinical Cardiology Council, Cardiovascular Radiology and Intervention Council, and the Atherosclerotic Peripheral Vascular Disease and Quality of Care Outcomes in Research Interdisciplinary Working Groups: The American Academy of Neurology affirms the value of this guideline as an educational tool for neurologists. Circulation 2007; 115: e478–534.

18. Rothwell PM, Slattery J, Warlow CP. A systematic review of the risks of stroke and death due to endarterectomy for symptomatic carotid stenosis. Stroke 1996; 27: 260–5.

19. Molloy J, Markus HS. Asymptomatic embolization predicts stroke and TIA risk in patients with carotid artery stenosis. Stroke 1999; 30: 1440–3.

20. Barth A, Remonda L, Lovblad KO, Schroth G, Seiler RW. Silent cerebral ischemia detected by diffusion-weighted MRI after carotid endarterectomy. Stroke 2000; 31: 1824–8.

21. Fox AJ. How to measure carotid stenosis. Radiology 1993; 186: 316–8.

22. Johnston SC, Gress DR, Browner WS, Sidney S. Short-term prognosis after emergency department diagnosis of TIA. JAMA 2000; 284: 2901–6.

23. Mayberg MR, Wilson SE, Yatsu F et al. Carotid endarterectomy and prevention of cerebral ischemia in symptomatic carotid stenosis. Veterans Affairs Cooperative Studies Program 309 Trialist Group. JAMA 1991; 266: 3289–94.

24. Failure of extracranial-intracranial arterial bypass to reduce the risk of ischemic stroke. Results of an international randomized trial. The EC/IC Bypass Study Group. N Engl J Med 1985; 313: 1191–200.

25. Fiorella D, Levy EI, Turk AS et al. US multicenter experience with the Wingspan stent system for the treatment of intracranial atheromatous disease: periprocedural results. Stroke 2007; 38: 881–7.

26. Turk AS, Levy EI, Albuquerque FC et al. Influence of patient age and stenosis location on Wingspan in-stent restenosis. AJNR Am J Neuroradiol 2008; 29: 23–7.

27. The Interventional Management of Stroke (IMS) II Study. Stroke 2007; 38: 2127–35.

28. Kelly ME, Furlan AJ, Fiorella D. Recanalization of acute middle cerebral artery occlusion using a self-expanding, reconstrainable intracranial microstent as a temporary endovascular bypass. Stroke 2008 (NYP).

Index